A(

Solving the Mys

Get ready for a fascinating journey into the realm of scientific discovery in that most complex and storied human organ; The Heart. The Voyage is led by a truly remarkable tour guide; an icon of modern scientific investigation, a scientist versed in art, architecture, dance, and literature with an almost magical command of story-telling.

Herbert I. Machleder, M.D.
Emeritus Professor of Surgery, UCLA
Past Chief of Staff, The UCLA Hospital and Medical Center

"Thinking outside the box" barely skims the surface of his brilliant mind.... Dr. Buckberg's theories have changed the way we practice cardiac surgery.

Marc R. Moon, M.D.
Chief, Cardiac Surgery
Director, Center for Diseases of the Thoracic Aorta
Washington University School of Medicine

...a real "page turner" ...a fascinating cross between a high-end spy novel and a scientific treatise on the causes of heart disease. Buckberg leaves nothing on the table... and we feel his pain as he explains why some of his most transformative ideas have not yet become mainstream.

Dr. Alan Russell
Highmark Distinguished Career Professor
Director, Disruptive Health Technology Institute
Carnegie Mellon University

At some point, nearly every person or someone they love is touched by heart disease. It occurred with me when my father needed a quadruple bypass and mitral valve repair. As it happens, I married one of my father's heart surgeons, Brad Allen, who I discovered was also a medical researcher and has collaborated with Dr. Buckberg for over 35 years. He would often tell me of these amazing discoveries coming from this research, but I never truly understood until I read this book. Written in understandable language, it shows how many beliefs we have (and even our doctors have) about different heart diseases may actually not be true, and explains how these remarkable discoveries could literally save thousands of lives.

Jaclyn Smith
American Actress and Businesswoman

Solving the Mysteries of Heart Disease is a memoir, a detective story, and a love affair with the heart. These adventures of Dr. Buckberg are entertaining, but also carry an important message about modern medicine.

Paul Micevych, Ph.D.
Chair, Dept of Neurobiology
Director, Lab of Neuroendocrinology of the Brain Research Institute
David Geffen School of Medicine at UCLA

...a fascinating journey.... Getting a wide acceptance of new concepts and innovative treatments is probably as difficult as climbing the Everest Mountain. Courage and tenacity are, among others, the key characteristics of Gerald Buckberg.

Daniel Loisance, M.D.
Professor Emeritus
Former Head of the Cardiac Surgery Department at Henri Mondor Hospital Paris XII
Member of the Académie Nationale de Médecine

This remarkable work chronicles the scholarly and yet deeply personal account of the research achievements of one of our most respected cardiac surgeons. Although written for the general public, practicing physicians would gain a great deal by reading it.

Ralph B. Dilley, M.D.
Surgeon-in-Chief, Scripps Green Hospital, Retired
Clinical Professor of Surgery
UCSD School of Medicine

SOLVING THE MYSTERIES

of

HEART DISEASE

Life-Saving Answers *Ignored* By The Medical Establishment

GERALD D. BUCKBERG, M.D., D.Sc.

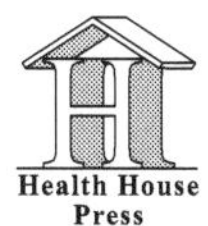

A special thanks to Jim Novack, a wonderful wordsmith
whose contributions helped make this book possible.
www.jamesnovack.com

Solving the Mysteries of Heart Disease

For information about this title, contact the publisher:
Health House Press
info@healthhousepress.com

ISBNs: 978-0-9998472-0-6 (hardcover)
978-0-9998472-3-7 (softcover)
978-0-9998472-2-0 (eBook)

Printed in the United States of America

NOTE TO READERS

This memoir defines my career as a cardiovascular surgeon and researcher, and uses this background to explain my conviction that answers to major cardiac illnesses exist now, but are not currently used.

The basis of this belief is widely documented by reports of my work published in major cardiovascular journals with worldwide distribution. The stepwise progress from experimental to clinical application has been validated by national and international studies in patients. Each conclusion is carefully reported with clear-cut references. This information is attainable by all physicians, but not appreciated or used due to the rigidity of conventional thinking.

I bring this information to the non-medical public. My stimulus for this action came from the mother of a surgical colleague who watched television news to become aware of an innovative, but little-known treatment. She asked her son (who had never heard of this approach), "Why don't you consider this?" He was not confined by convention... and pursued learning about it.

I hope that readers will ask their doctors to look at this book's solutions, whose supportive evidence is furnished by included references. The book does not provide answers for the reader's individual treatments, but rather encourages them to bring these concepts to their physicians, whose medical knowledge and professional judgment will guide their response.

This book is independently authored, without being affiliated with or endorsed by the David Geffen School of Medicine at UCLA, where I am a faculty member and cardiac surgeon. Its opinions are mine, and do not necessarily reflect the views of my mentors, teachers, or colleagues that conduct research and cardiac surgery.

Patients' stories are authentic, though such individuals have been given fictional names to avoid identifying any real person, living or dead.

FOREWORD

BY JAMES L. COX

Note: *James Cox is a distinguished scientist who found a treatment that offsets atrial fibrillation in most patients. He is internationally heralded, since this disease affects over 3 million patients in the United States alone, and is a major cause of strokes worldwide. Dr. Cox is unique in his creativity, and his innovative work has had an astounding impact.*
In 2015, Dr. Cox was the recipient of the Scientific Achievement Award from the American Association for Thoracic Surgery. Similar to a Nobel Prize for the profession, this is the association's highest award, and has honored the legends of cardiac surgery, such as Drs. Kirklin, Shumway, DeBakey, Cooley, and Carpentier. Dr. Buckberg was the sixth person to receive this award, in 2007.

Gerry Buckberg is a "Level One." Let me explain. Many years ago when my cardiology colleagues at Washington University in St. Louis had successfully created the world's first and only computerized system capable of digitally mapping the complex cardiac rhythm abnormality called Atrial Fibrillation, our initial data output consisted of a hodge-podge of numbers that made no sense to anybody. During that time, I happened to meet the Emeritus Professor and Chairman of the Department of Pure Mathematics at Cambridge University. During the course of our conversation, he asked me to describe my current research interests and I made the seemingly innocuous statement that I was studying a "chaotic" rhythm of the heart. With the mere mention of the word "chaotic," the old man's ears perked up and his eyes suddenly began to sparkle. He said, "Well, you know, my people at Cambridge are the world's experts on the Chaos Theory!" He began to quiz me relentlessly about what I meant by a "chaotic rhythm" because his group had proven that there is nothing in all of nature that is truly chaotic ... everything in nature has a pattern to it and anything that appears to be chaotic is simply the result of our own ignorance and inability to discern its underlying pattern.

After several hours of discussion, my new friend proposed that I come to Cambridge with a stack of our raw data so that his "people" could examine it for nature's underlying organized activity, which he was certain was there. So... I had the unexpected privilege of giving an hour lecture to the members of the Department of Pure Mathematics at Cambridge University! While I was there, I met the new Departmental Chairman of Pure Mathematics, who informed me that all members of his profession know and accept the fact that there are three levels of mathematicians in the world and that the intellectual level of each mathematician is based solely on pure brain power. Apparently, mathematicians are less "politically correct" than cardiac surgeons!

The vast majority of accomplished mathematicians are "Level Threes" and they address the solution of "Level Three Problems" because, while brilliant, they are intellectually incapable of solving more complex mathematical problems. There are usually 20–40 "Level Two" mathematicians in the world at any given time and they spend their time trying to solve "Level Two Problems." However, they don't bother with the simpler "Level Three Problems" and they accept the fact that they are intellectually incapable of solving "Level One Problems." Throughout history, there has usually been only one "Level One" mathematician alive in the world at any given time. The only exception that the Cambridge Professor could recall was in the early 20th century when two "Level One" mathematicians were alive at the same time ... Albert Einstein and Niels Bohr.

I'm sure that there have been a few "Level One" scientists in the history of cardiac surgery but there is only one that I know of for sure ... Gerry Buckberg. His ability to tackle problems that the rest of us see but cannot solve has been nothing short of astounding. Because of his scientific contributions in the field of myocardial preservation alone, he has probably saved more lives than any cardiac surgeon of our generation. He converted cardiac surgery from being the most dangerous of all surgeries into routine and safe procedures for the rest of us to perform. I have repeatedly referred to him as "The only true genius of our generation of heart surgeons," and I stand by that statement.

This is a particularly interesting statement to come from me because when we were young, Gerry Buckberg and I were serious antagonists ... I thought he was wrong in practically everything he said and I don't think he even bothered to think about me at all. When I was only 29 years old, we locked horns for the first time at the Surgical Forum of the American College of Surgeons meeting in San Francisco. The next year, we got serious about our differences. I presented a 10-minute talk "disproving" his paper from the previous year in San Francisco and we were supposed to have a 5-minute discussion period following my presentation. The session was chaired by Dr. Gerald Austin of Harvard, one of the most powerful surgeons in the world. Nevertheless, Dr. Austin allowed our post-presentation "discussion" to go on for a full 25 minutes in front of a standing-room-only crowd. It was a defining moment for my relationship with Gerry Buckberg because it cemented my disdain for him. Again, I don't think he even knew my name.

An interesting thing happened over the ensuing 30 years or so. I slowly developed first, a kind of neutrality regarding his ideas, then an acceptance of them, then an ardent respect and admiration for them that resulted in my ultimately becoming an avowed "Buckberg Groupie." I became convinced that he was the most brilliant man I'd ever met and I remain certain that is true. Over the years, we have become collaborators on multiple projects, co-authors on multiple publications, and the dearest of friends. When I was President of the American Association for Thoracic Surgery in 2001, I asked Gerry Buckberg to be my "Guest Scientific Lecturer" at our annual meeting in San Diego. As expected, his lecture was groundbreaking and breathtaking, weaving together all of nature, from the spiral DNA helix to the spiral helix of the galaxies, into a mind-blowing elucidation of how the ventricles of the heart perform their vital function.

Late in our lives, I learned that Gerry Buckberg is the epitome of the Renaissance Man. Not only is he one of the most important cardiac surgeons of our generation, but he is also an accomplished and talented painter and creator of a ballet in which he integrates classical music with modern dance into a visual spectrum of the normal and abnormal rhythms and heart motions. His mind's capacity and his inherent talent are apparently limitless, the *sine qua non* of a "Level One." This book is his story, told in layman's prose. It is a story that everyone who is interested in how revolutionary ideas evolve should read, for there are few people in life who have something of general importance to teach all other people, regardless of their chosen profession. Gerry Buckberg is that person for our time.

James L. Cox, MD
Department of Cardiac Surgery
Northwestern University
Chicago, Illinois
April 2018

INTRODUCTION

Exploring Uncharted Territories

Before you is the lifelong adventure of a heart surgeon and cardiac researcher whose mission has been the solving of mysteries. Discovering solutions that will evolve into new treatments that improve and save lives — possibly including yours or those of your loved ones. This journey will introduce you to a range of seemingly *impenetrable riddles*... of your heart. Many of these puzzles — the solutions to which have the potential to impact millions of people all over the world — were long thought unsolvable. For while our country directs immense attention toward cancer, the reality is that diseases of the heart claim more lives every year, at enormous personal and financial costs.

This story reveals how the solutions to many of these major cardiac issues have been uncovered by our efforts at UCLA's David Geffen School of Medicine and around the globe, and explains how this new knowledge can bring about a surprising "revolution" in health care.

Yet today, the progress made possible by this knowledge has not happened.

While the general public reasonably expects the medical profession to welcome changes that can transform healthcare... that is frequently not the case. A fundamental, powerful, and ageless barrier prevents the embracing of new techniques and technologies. This obstacle is *a rigidity of thinking.*

I did not anticipate this when I first became a cardiac surgeon / researcher. My commitment was to care for my patients and set off upon the challenging investigations needed to find long-sought answers. I would make rounds to visit patients at five in the morning and often not complete my surgical procedures and research until ten at night. This lifestyle made others ask, "Why was I so steadfast in my dedication?"

The answer springs from my childhood.

I grew up as "a kid in the Bronx." My family didn't have much money or socio-economic status. Yet my mother and grandmother were absolutely regal in this environment. Their presence elicited from others a deep respect, gratitude, and devotion for a simple reason. Their lives were built upon giving and helping others. Their smiles, grace, and positive attitudes were palpable to me as a child, as I observed their lack of interest in taking anything back (short of knowing that what they did was useful). Their joy came from giving. My hope was to someday experience this splendor that characterized my mom and grandmother.

As it turned out, the opportunity arrived fairly early on.

A heart attack claimed my grandfather when I was 14 years old. This sudden end to my grandparents' 54 years together created a great loneliness for my grandmother. Suddenly, she lived alone. Though she would never complain, a glance at her eyes and the absence of her customary smile told the true story.

Their house was only a block away from ours. I decided to stay with my grandmother, sleeping in the room next to hers. She spoke only Yiddish, but this lack of communication did not prevent me from being there with her every night for a year and a half. I still recall Grandma coming into my room and singing lovely Russian lullabies and folk songs to me as I drifted off to sleep.

It was my first profound experience of giving without expecting anything in return. Yet I received much: the lovely smile returned to her face, and I felt my being there helped bring the light back to her eyes. While I didn't recognize it then, that experience would set the stage for building a life of devoting my energies to helping others.

As I entered the field of medicine, I soon realized that the mentors and role models I most admired were just like my mother and grandmother. They mirrored their generous qualities by dedicating themselves to improving the health of their patients.

I became a cardiac surgeon / researcher because of my need to better understand my grandfather's sudden illness, coupled with my desire to heal ailments centered around the organ most central to our being — our heart. I was excited to learn the latest techniques in open-heart surgery, since we could solve many underlying problems. But I was deeply troubled to see that many hearts were damaged during the operations, even when each of the surgeons performed the procedure with perfect technique. Was this simply, as many believed, the best that could be expected when operating on such a fragile organ? That attitude was unacceptable to me and I was driven to find an answer — one that could be shared with others in medicine, and used to improve outcomes for our patients and their families.

I had astounding success at my start, as I uncovered why an area inside the heart would die after a perfect operation, and I then developed a method to protect the heart from this damage during the procedure. My introduction of "blood cardioplegia" (a way to safely stop the heart's beating movement, so that surgeons can precisely correct the heart problem) is now used by 85% of cardiac surgeons in the United States and nearly that many worldwide, and has benefited over 25 million people.

But this was only the beginning.

The life of a researcher is much like that of an explorer. Yet most successful researchers achieve one significant finding, and it predominantly defines their career. This holds true even for Nobel Laureates, who (with the exception of just four) have all been honored with a single award for their extraordinary work.

I ended up pursuing ten different major research goals. I appreciate that this approach may seem scattered. Yet it more aptly represents the difference between an explorer who searches out one island... vs. someone whose broad vision sees that there are many islands before them, each needing exploration. For me, the yardstick is always the research's quality, not its quantity. Therefore, my team and I focused on a single project over a three to six year period. There were no detours into other research until we completed each full endeavor.

In addition to losing my dear grandfather to a heart attack, I later watched my father suffer the devastation of congestive heart failure. I wanted to help people, but I also wanted answers. Thus, I entered this world of cardiovascular research to solve unresolved problems. The number of patients that this could affect would vastly exceed those I could help by individual treatment in my operating room. I embarked on *a voyage of discovery that has raised new questions — and resulted in my finding answers that contradict many commonly accepted medical beliefs.*

The breadth of our research covered questions such as:

- Must congestive heart failure incapacitate and ultimately kill the patient, or can the heart's health be restored?
- Must "sudden death syndrome" (cardiac arrest — when the heart stops and CPR is applied) end up killing 90% of its victims, and leave its rare survivor with brain damage, or can this be avoided?
- Must part of a patient's heart muscle die after an acute heart attack and create a weakened heart in many who survive?
- Must a successful replacement of a diseased heart valve sometimes turn into a fatal event because the heart's inner lining dies?
- Must some babies (called "blue babies" due to deficient oxygen in their blood from a heart defect) suffer permanent heart and brain damage after an otherwise successful surgical correction of their congenital problem?
- Must the large muscle in the middle of the heart (the septum) become almost routinely damaged during many successful heart surgeries?
- Must modern pacemakers continue to create the same abnormal heartbeat contractions that were first reported as long ago as 1925?
- How does the *true* structure of the heart (largely unacknowledged in medicine) determine its function and lead to new findings that will save countless lives?

The pages that follow describe the exciting chase that led to solutions to every one of these compelling questions — plus others.

In each case, the starting point for our research was a problem we saw in the patients. A game plan evolved where we'd begin by seeking a deeper understanding *of why* something happened... then correcting it experimentally... and then finally using this new knowledge for the successful treatment of patients. Once this was done, I could establish guidelines for others to reproduce these treatments. Only then did we move onto the next challenging investigation.

This path into uncharted territory meant we could not to be put off by failure. Rather, each defeat brought with it fresh questions that would lead us onto the next step. Also essential was my willingness to advocate solutions that would *contradict conventional thinking* — an approach that must be coupled with an unbending drive to continue forward, even if our answers are not initially accepted. The ultimate reward is to come to a complete understanding of a problem's underlying cause, and its successful medical solution. Solutions that can be used by others.

Each story of discovery will be told in just one or two chapters. But each task represented a daunting puzzle at the time. Addressing them needed inventive approaches. My hero, Albert Einstein, famously stated, "Imagination is more important than knowledge."

Creativity always played a vital role in my life, starting when I was young and interested in art. This interest in the crossover between science and art remains strong, and five chapters toward the end of this book talk about how I merged the two to develop new outlets to communicate my work. Importantly, those chapters also discuss how a creative mindset enables one to find answers to difficult problems.

Despite these exhilarating breakthroughs in treating cardiac problems... unexpected difficulties have tempered the joy of our successes. The welcoming reception our blood cardioplegia work received was never repeated. Instead, each new life-saving discovery was met with rigorous resistance.

We found solutions to major heart disorders afflicting millions of people... but *no one is listening.*

I had unknowingly encountered a parallel for this dilemma early on, while applying for medical school. When asked to name my favorite book, my answer was *The Cry and the Covenant,* about Ignaz Philipp Semmelweis, a Hungarian physician in the 1800s who realized the frequent occurrence of childbed fever in the maternity ward was due to infections caused by the delivering doctors. This was before the emergence of the germ theory. The titans of medicine shunned Semmelweis because he asked them to wash their hands.

As I would learn firsthand, resistance to dramatic new ideas that can reverse awful illnesses has not lessened. Though the positive results of our studies were confirmed in patients, first by myself and then by other leading physicians around the globe, they were disregarded by those who determine the "medical standard of leading care." Yes, ours reflected "radical changes" from how treatments are currently done, but they were even "more radical" in another pivotal way: their success rates were remarkably higher than the outcomes with traditional methods.

While this has certainly been frustrating, it has never deterred me from searching for the next answer. I know that *the truth will win*. These innovative approaches will eventually be adopted *because they work.*

The question is, how long must that take?

I am pleased to share our quest, which spans over 50 years of research and heart surgery practice. It's a story of formidable twists and turns, met by a readiness to think outside the box, and energized by an unrelenting thirst for discovery. This memoir is written to breach the medical barricades I have encountered. I'm writing directly to the general public to let you know that *answers to major cardiac illnesses exist now, but are not currently used.*

It is your turn to discover what has been learned. Please read on and join me on my voyage.

Gerald D. Buckberg M.D., D. Sc.
Distinguished Professor of Surgery
David Geffen School of Medicine at UCLA
Department of Cardiothoracic Surgery

TABLE OF CONTENTS

There will be a number of opportunities for readers to view videos that illustrate some of the research findings discussed throughout the book. To view any video, type the address link shown below each video into the search bar of your web browser.

eBook readers can click directly on the link beneath each video.

CHAPTER 1

Truth Will Win... But When?

"I think you need to take this call."

Twenty years ago, my administrative assistant stood in my office doorway. Normally, she wouldn't be so insistent unless it was one of my patients or one of my interns with a pressing question. It wasn't either of those.

"So who is it and what's it about?" I asked.

"Some doctor in Birmingham, Alabama. He didn't take time to explain, other than to say it was urgent. You need to take the call."

I picked up the phone. "This is Dr. Buckberg. Who is...."

He didn't let me finish. "It's Connie Athanasulcas. We met at the Duke conference. I drove you to the airport."

I remembered him. Well-respected cardiac surgeon, bright, articulate, assured. His tone now, however, seemed to make clear he wasn't looking for a thank you or merely to renew acquaintances.

"Tell me what's going on."

Connie explained that he had just completed a coronary artery bypass graft to improve blood flow to the heart of a 65-year-old woman. It was a routine operation. Since the 1980s, the survival rate has been around 98%. Of course, for a patient, nothing is routine about open-heart surgery, and complications can still occur.

"Everything went as expected," he confirmed. "But then I was in the visitor's room and speaking with the patient's family when my pager went off. I rushed back to the ICU."

His patient was having ventricular fibrillation — where the heart's electrical activity becomes disordered and the main pumping chambers contract in a rapid, unsynchronized way. This causes the heart to quiver, rendering it incapable of pumping blood. It is a lethal event, requiring cardiopulmonary resuscitation (CPR), which provides external compression that can squeeze the heart, allowing it to keep a patient alive by circulating blood to the body.

By the time Connie arrived, his ICU staff was administering CPR and applying a defibrillator to try shocking the heart back into a normal rhythm. All to no avail. His patient was dying. She was becoming part of the 2% death rate.

The standard belief at the time was that after 15 minutes of unsuccessful resuscitation, the heart and brain sustain irreparable damage and any attempts to revive the patient should stop. Even before those 15 minutes are up, there is only a 10% survival rate, and half of those few survivors will suffer severe brain damage. For Connie and his patient, time was running out.

That's when he called me.

Just two weeks earlier, I'd met Connie for the first time at Duke University, where I was giving a series of talks on coronary artery surgery. One of my talks described a new approach to treating sudden death (cardiac arrest, where the heart suddenly stops) that my team at UCLA had recently developed and used successfully on patients in our hospital.

My lecture revealed our early findings for 14 patients with whom we had administered CPR for *an average of 55 minutes* before they were put on a heart-lung machine (which takes over circulation and oxygenation of blood throughout the body) — which then allowed us to surgically repair the underlying problem causing sudden death. We even had one patient to whom we successfully administered CPR for 150 minutes!

This was unheard of at the time.

Our approach, employing groundbreaking treatments following a greatly extended use of CPR, had never been done before. As I mentioned, conventional wisdom was that CPR lasting longer than 15 minutes *always resulted in 100% mortality.* Yet we found 11 of our 14 patients had complete heart and brain recovery — nearly an 80% survival rate.

While my presentation at Duke was well-received, you never really know what will come from these talks. Oftentimes ideas are exchanged, but then are quickly forgotten as everyone returns home to their comforting practice of "business as usual."

Connie hadn't forgotten.

Calling from his ICU, Connie quickly filled me in on his patient's status. The situation was uncannily similar to what I had discussed during my Duke lecture. I wasted no time and went over the exact procedure he'd need to follow. It was important we act fast.

"First, you need to ensure that whoever is performing CPR is told to press hard enough on the chest to maintain adequate blood pressure — greater than 60 mm Hg — to make sure sufficient blood is reaching the brain." (Most CPR only provides about one-third the amount of blood needed by organs.)

"Next, proceed immediately to the operating room. Put the patient back on the heart-lung machine, as you will need to operate on her again. You need to decompress the heart with a vent tube to ensure it is empty. Then make certain each bypass artery you put in is open, since a blocked or closed artery could cause the unexpected fibrillation."

Connie was in new territory now, as we had already passed the supposedly always-lethal 15-minute limit of CPR.

"Connie, proceed immediately with this. Now, let me talk to your perfusionist."

Mike Rose, the perfusionist (who runs the heart-lung machine), got on the phone. Fortunately, Mike had visited me a year earlier at UCLA to learn about our methods for protecting the heart during cardiac surgery, so I knew he was up to speed on our methods. I told him to administer a "cardioplegic solution" to the patient for 20 minutes. This solution is a mixture of the patient's blood that is modified by adding specific substances (using an ingredient composition I designed) that protected the heart.

"After Connie decompresses the heart and checks the newly implanted arteries, you deliver this solution. Then supply regular blood to the heart for 30 more minutes."

I hung up as the clock was ticking. It was in their hands now.

Less than an hour later, Connie called with an update.

It was great news.

He confirmed the implanted coronary vessels were indeed open. As soon as they had completed delivering the special cardioplegic solution and begun normal blood flow, the heart's activity returned so vigorously that his patient was easily taken off the heart-lung machine. In fact, no supportive drugs were needed to improve the heart's ability to properly contract. He said the entire surgical team was amazed. So was Connie. He was grateful, too.

Four days later, Connie called back to report that the patient had been discharged and had suffered no brain damage. Connie said it was like a miracle.

Of course, it wasn't a miracle. It was just good science.

This was validation for me on several levels. First, we had saved a life, which is why we do this. Second, Connie was the first person outside of my team to perform this new technique for treating sudden death, and he learned about it at a seminar.

Finally, and this is the case with all of my research after being proven true, I could envision the immense impact this groundbreaking approach would have as word spread and more and more doctors like Connie adopted this new technique.

Think about it.

We had changed the belief that more than 15 minutes of CPR meant certain heart and brain death, 100% of the time. Now it had been proven that the heart and brain could last through as much as 150 minutes of CPR, with nearly 80% survival!

This would change the way CPR is taught in the classroom and how emergency responders would treat sudden death when picking up and transporting the patient to the hospital. Emergency rooms would soon be equipped with heart-lung machines and more technicians would be trained for their relatively easy hook-up. Surgeons would have more time to treat and correct the underlying conditions that caused the sudden death in the first place.

Hundreds of thousands of lives would be saved every year around the world! Victims of heart attack, drowning, suffocation, seizure, drug overdose, electrocution — all the things that cause the heart to suddenly stop — these people could have a second chance to live.

This was not a small advance, but a revolutionary shift in the way we think about and treat sudden death. Our study, conducted at one of the world's leading institutions in cardiac research, led by recognized investigators in the field, with its techniques successfully proven in patients — had yielded an entirely new approach to treating a condition that strikes without warning and causes devastating results in half a million people yearly. It was nothing less than stunning.

For me and everyone involved, it was cause for rejoicing. And it was the first step in another of a series of significant steps to transforming cardiac care.

20 Years Later: Where are We Now?

Today's *standard protocol* for dealing with sudden death states: after 15 minutes of unsuccessful resuscitation, the brain and heart sustain irreparable damage and all attempts to revive should cease.

Essentially, nothing has changed in 20 years!

Only a few minor enhancements have occurred in the treatment of sudden death patients. The protocol is nearly identical to what it was two decades ago. This lack of growth and progress has been nothing less than stunning.

I have not let this rejection stop me. I and others have continued to publish papers. We have conducted additional clinical studies with nearly identical results in 34 patients, with patients undergoing an average of 72 minutes of CPR before our treatment successfully brought them back to life.

We have applied for grants for further research based upon our outcomes. They have not been forthcoming. In fact, we were told by the National Institutes of Health reviewers that our findings were "not significant" — even though no one, either nationally or internationally, had ever achieved such a consistent reversal of an injury that was considered lethal.

Only my travels around the world, training surgeons and perfusionists one at a time, has advanced this new approach to sudden death. Why? It turns out that leaders in the medical community in positions to influence change... don't always like to consider new methods. This rigidity also results from an unwillingness to consider an uncomfortable premise: that presently accepted conventional approaches — fail many patients.

This chronic obstruction to progress is not limited to my work on sudden death. It happens with most of my clinical discoveries. Throughout my long career, we have introduced what should be remarkable and historic shifts in thinking about major cardiovascular issues — in managing heart attacks, sudden death (and possibly stroke), congestive heart failure, pacemakers, the relationship between a heart's structure and its ability to function correctly, and others.

While some of our breakthrough discoveries have become widely implemented, many others still have not.

Truth remains truth, yet I have learned firsthand over these five decades of research and practice, that willingness within the general medical community to adopt *truly innovative* avenues of treatment... is startlingly rare.

Different Perception

There is no demand for change when one perceives what they are doing as successful. If we can now save 15% of people from sudden death, that's a considerable improvement from when it was 10%, and many feel that this "50% increase" in survival reflects a fine contribution. I don't disagree, but my point of view is a bit different: how do we address the 85% of sudden death patients that die because of our present approaches?

People like Connie are the exception: someone who is willing to listen and leave the comfort zone of repeating yesterday. Yet instead of being hungry to explore new ideas and methods, too many of our colleagues follow entrenched patterns that lead to well-known, yet unacceptable (to me) outcomes. Such rigidity leaves our patients at risk of suffering the limitations of conventional treatments.

It comes down to a choice: embracing scientific inquiry, or maintaining a steadfast adherence to traditional ways. Perhaps not a momentous problem if this was simply an academic debate. But lives hang in the balance. From my point of view, when people can be helped, you do whatever you can to save them. Especially if there have been proven results.

Phenomenal Quest

Despite all this, I remain optimistic. Our profession has the marvelous opportunity for each practitioner to gain pride in helping others by facing the imperfections in our current methods. Understanding flaws in the process now leads us to ask the next questions and steers us toward finding their solutions. This is the nature of growth.

We must recognize that the attitude of remaining content with past successes can quickly turn into a barrier to future growth. A balance must exist between welcoming the positive achievements of standard treatments — even when they may help 95% of the population — while simultaneously asking why the other 5% are not benefited. Acknowledging that we fail in those 5% creates a stimulus for future progress.

The nature of life is motion. We can witness this by looking out at the world... or peering deep inside ourselves to understand why our heart might fail to perform its assigned tasks. Any form of stagnation — even when fueled by self-satisfaction — opposes natural evolution. Our medical education must always continue to progress.

How lucky I am to have been taught by some of the greatest minds in medicine; to be given the opportunity to conduct leading-edge research on some of the most debilitating and prevalent medical conditions known to man; to travel the world and share ideas and solutions with other professionals... and now with the general public.

This is the story of a kid from the Bronx who just wanted to be the local dentist, but through a series of fortunate events, encounters, and lessons, became a passionate contributor to cardiovascular research and surgery, touching the lives of many. While not all of my discoveries have been utilized to their full potential, that has never slowed me down. There is always so much more to learn and do.

As you read this book, you will realize that we have found practical and effective answers to many of the most pervasive and serious heart ailments that I described in my introduction. The upcoming chapters will reveal that *solutions exist, but they have not been used — despite their initial and successful applications with patients from around the world.*

I am confident that these ideas will succeed because the truth will win... but when?

CHAPTER 2

A Series of Fortunate Events, Encounters, and Lessons

I have been curious for as long as I can remember. But my early observations and pursuits aimed more toward art than science. I loved to draw.

I had no problems in school, so I was surprised when summoned to meet the principal of my public junior high school. Having no clue about what I had done, I was completely caught off-guard when he grinned and said:

"You're doing very well here. We'd like you to go to Science High School or Stuyvesant High School."

These were the two premier high schools in New York and to be encouraged in that direction was quite an honor. So what was my answer?

I wasn't interested in either, since I did not care for science. I just wanted to play basketball.

In truth, I did have other ambitions. I'd grown up in a lower middle-class environment in New York's Bronx. Life wasn't easy for most families and I saw you had to work for everything you got. So I would take jobs at different neighborhood businesses: the tailor shop, grocery, vegetable store. I delivered packages from the meat store. As I got older, I'd work summers as a busboy and waiter at lodges in the Catskill Mountains in upstate New York to make money for college (while playing basketball in my free time). I paid for all of my education myself.

I believed I would earn my future, rather than expect it to be given to me. I didn't want to rely on anyone else. In fact, I always wanted to be *independent* of other people. I wouldn't learn until years later that this was the wrong goal. My life would never be independent, but rather *interdependent*.

During my youth, I looked and found only two in my world that seemed truly self-reliant: my doctor and my dentist. Respected. Professional. Comfortable. Autonomous. That was what I wanted most. So when it came time to make a decision about my future, I consulted with both men. Unexpectedly, it was my doctor who advised dentistry, suggesting that path would allow me to achieve my aims with less work.

So as a teenager considering college, my decision to pursue a profession in the health sciences was hardly altruistic, but came simply from my desire to be self-sufficient. I became a pre-dental student at Alfred University, and then, during my sophomore year, transferred to Ohio State University to continue my studies.

Alas, my time in dentistry was short-lived.

In fact, all it took was one visit to the dental lab with my cousin Herb Urell, who was already in Ohio State's dental program. As I watched him grinding and drilling on a set of model teeth, I quickly realized this was not how I wanted to spend my next eight years in school, let alone an entire career. Suddenly, I didn't know what I would do.

Fortunately, I found my answer the next day during my first class — in zoology. The teacher presented a lesson on the organization of the cardiovascular system. A red dye was injected into the blood vessel system of a frog and the sight was unbelievable! I still remember sitting in the lab, looking at the inside of the frog and thinking, "My God, this is beautiful. It's so organized. Artistry in nature."

At that instant, I realized, "I'm going to be a doctor."

This lovely visualization of the arrangement of the blood supply, its graceful balance from side to side, the blood nourishing all the organs in an elegant way stoked a flame of curiosity that burns even brighter today.

I fell in love with the heart.

So my goals changed by my sophomore year in college. Self-sufficiency was not going to cut it as my primary ambition. I also needed to be thoroughly interested, highly engaged, and willing to be challenged. I was going to be a cardiologist.

The Investigator

Applying to medical school was an education in itself. Each applicant visited different institutions in the hope that this personal appearance would help them in the selection process. Interviewers frequently would ask what we were reading. I always cited *The Cry and the Covenant,* written by Morton Thompson.

It described Phillip Semmelweis, an Austro-Hungarian physician who worked in a maternity ward in Budapest in the 1800s, and focused upon his discovering why women were mysteriously dying of "childbed fever" after giving birth. He observed this almost always happened in women whose babies were delivered by the doctors in the hospital. In sharp contrast, almost no deaths occurred in women whose babies were delivered by midwives at their homes. Naturally, he wondered "Why?" He reasoned that better results should be expected in women whose babies were delivered at hospitals.

He realized that after the doctors delivered the baby, they would go across the street to the autopsy suite to examine bodies of the women that had died the day before. The doctors then returned to the hospital to deliver more babies.

Germs were not a consideration in health care yet. But Semmelweis wondered if the doctors could be transmitting the infection from the dead women to the live mothers.

To test this, Semmelweis had the medical students and interns in the maternity ward wash their hands between patients. Miraculously, the women whose babies they delivered immediately stopped dying.

The answer was simple. He told the doctors to just "wash your hands."

Imagine the reaction of these *leaders of medicine, who consider themselves to be titans,* after being told *they* were responsible for this spread of childbed fever because *they* transmitted a lethal infection due to their dirty hands. Their reaction was immediate and fierce. They became infuriated and castigated Semmelweis.

He had the truth, but no one was listening. Sadly, he spent the rest of his life trying to make others aware of this correctible cause of a major disease, but to no avail. He ended up dying without ever knowing he was right.

Truth eventually won out. Germ theory and general cleanliness guides physicians' actions today as they move from one patient to another.

His story impacted me. I was stirred by the beauty and majesty of the creative discovery, and was saddened by the opposition to such truth, and stunned by the reaction that created barriers to believing such a simple and straightforward solution.

I thought, "How could this be?"

Little did I realize that this classic issue confronts any new idea that may change conventional thinking. The innovative path toward discovery is often challenged by initial rejection, *yet my pursuit of such truths would become the motivation for the journey* I would take during my next five decades of my medical career.

A formidable journey that was first set in motion when I entered medical school.

First Failure, First Lesson

The challenges started as I took my initial anatomy test at the University of Cincinnati College of Medicine, which I entered in 1957.

I had learned the material backward and forward. I was confident. So when our papers were handed back, I was aghast to see the big "D" on my test.

It was the first-ever D of my scholastic career. In my chosen field of study! I was shocked. Destroyed. I thought my medical career was over. I walked out of that class in a daze. Everything I dreamt about was not going to happen.

I went back to my fraternity and didn't tell anyone what had occurred. I just sat alone on the back porch staring out. Other fraternity members were going about whatever they were doing, talking with each another, laughing, shouting. None of it mattered. They could've been a million miles away. I heard nothing they said. I was in my own world, and not a very pleasant one.

How could this happen to me?

I tried to calm myself and look at the problem. How could I fail when I always worked so hard? How did I get a D in the very subject I wanted to study? I was an A student.

I didn't screw up because I was stupid. That much I knew. What I came to realize is I didn't truly understand what I had studied, and I did not recognize what was really being asked on this test.

That's when I had a realization.

As I looked out from the porch, a new understanding began to form. I had memorized specifics about each and every artery, vein, muscle, joint, and nerve in the body. What I had *failed* to understand was their *inter-relationships.* The body is a whole, and my trying to separate its components by aiming to become an expert in each piece would never replace the importance of understanding *the interactions* of one part upon another — the hallmark of their relationships.

It became an epiphany that would change my life.

It was here that I first began to realize that the real objective was *interdependence.* This process existed within the body — and between those with whom I would study, work, and explore the riddles of medicine.

Yearning for Learning

The irony is the distress caused by my early failure on this exam simultaneously introduced another critical lesson, one that has served as a fundamental guidepost during my entire professional career. As I would learn from many of the great minds that I'd come to admire, failure is not the end, but rather, only stimulates the next beginning. You cannot be afraid of it. It is one of your greatest motivators.

I compare this process to ascending a mountain that represents education. Every mountain has a series of peaks and valleys, and what educators and practitioners must decide when one peak is reached, is whether to remain self-satisfied, relish the success of overcoming this peak, and look down at other climbers... or to take advantage of this privileged vista and look upward to see the next peak that is not apparent to those still in the valley. Pursuing the latter means creating a plan to descend into a new valley, and a willingness to do the hard work needed to reach the subsequent peak.

That lowly D surely placed me deep in the valley, but I now understood what it took to reach the mountaintop: never giving up, *while welcoming* the next unanswered question. I was going to climb to the peak, and eagerly look for the one that would follow.

I was developing the mind of a researcher.

This newfound appreciation and dedication to learning served me well, as both my grades and my understanding of the interconnections of the human body greatly improved. I was a hard worker, nearly always studying till midnight or one in the morning. My drive was never for the grades, but to solve whatever problem presented itself. By the end of my second year in medical school, I could easily see myself as the cardiologist I first envisioned when I dissected the frog.

Yet another revelation would be coming my way.

New Direction

As a result of my new outlook, I was particularly excited to be taking a summer fellowship in cardiology (a fellowship is a period of specialty training).

During one of our rotations, my fellow student cardiologists, faculty, and I were faced with a patient who was believed to have narrowing of the aortic valve (called aortic stenosis). He was being evaluated for chest pain and early signs of heart failure. The role of our cardiology team was to confirm this diagnosis.

We were to do that by first placing a blood pressure measuring tube into the main artery (aorta) that distributes the blood throughout the body, and then through the aortic valve into the left ventricle (one of the two ventricle chambers in the heart, which fills with blood and then contracts to pump it into the body). From these two measurements, we would be able to establish the difference in pressure between the aorta and ventricle chambers — and determine if the patient had narrowing of the aortic valve.

A catheter (a small flexible tube through which we can give or withdraw fluid, or slip in an instrument) was to be inserted through an artery. It would be aimed toward the heart and then pushed past the heart valve into the ventricle. We spent two hours trying to traverse that bulky valve and it was simply not possible. So we called in the cardiac surgeon.

This was all foreign to me. Up until this point, I didn't know anything about heart surgery at all.

The surgeon came in, thoroughly proficient, full of assurance. We told him what we needed to know. He simply nodded and confidently began.

"Give me the alcohol sponge. Now give me a syringe with a needle on it."

He anesthetized a small spot on the chest and easily inserted the needle directly into the left ventricle, connected it to tubing to measure and record the pressure, and confirmed the diagnosis — all within a minute!

It was so simple that it was unbelievable. He knew what the job required and went about it immediately and efficiently.

Yet the most impressive event occurred the next day, when he joined our discussion of this case in the cardiology / surgery conference. To my astonishment, the cardiologist and cardiac surgeon seemed to have an equal understanding of the disease process and its management. Soon after, I attended the operation on this patient, my job being to watch the blood pressure on the recording machine while I observed the surgeon performing all the steps needed to correct the narrowed valve.

I was astounded by the orchestration of movement between the surgeon and the assistant, the anesthesiologist, and the scrub nurse. It had a great flow to it, like music. It was fully a demonstration of the inter-relationships of working with a team — that interdependence I spoke of before. The camaraderie was something I relished and hoped to embrace throughout my career. Their enthusiasm was palpable. It seemed to me that they were having all the fun.

All of this was an eye-opener for me. My goal suddenly changed.

I wanted in on the action.

I wanted to be a cardiovascular surgeon.

CHAPTER 3

A Compelling New Path

Dreams sometime do transform into reality. Imagine the excitement when this kid from the Bronx gets selected to serve his internship at the renowned Johns Hopkins Hospital in Baltimore, Maryland, where I would have daily face-to-face contact with the legends of surgery in America. What a place to launch a surgical career!

And as it would turn out, what an auspicious time to be there.

The era of open-heart surgery had just begun in 1953 with the invention of the heart-lung machine by John Gibbon. During surgery, this apparatus takes over for the heart and lungs by utilizing a pump that circulates the blood through the body... while an oxygenator simultaneously adds the right levels of oxygen to the blood as it removes carbon dioxide. This allows the surgeon to stop the heart — and perform the needed delicate procedures in a motionless environment. Unfortunately, the initial mortality rate using these new machines was disturbingly high, at over 50%. Working with The Mayo Clinic, Gibbon was able to improve his device and by 1956, the mortality rate dropped to 20%, and then 10% by 1957.

I would arrive at Hopkins just four years later, in 1961.

In the early days, when the mortality rate was 50%, only the pioneers would perform open-heart surgery with a heart-lung machine. But when the success rate went up to 90%, a new generation of surgeons embraced the technology and began creating all types of new procedures. Many of these treatments are now commonplace. They define the practice of heart surgery and include replacing damaged heart valves, bypassing obstructed arteries to create new pathways to bring blood flow to the heart, treating traumatic heart wounds, and repairing congenital defects in the heart muscles of children.

Role Models

Leaving the classroom behind, my interning at Hopkins offered a steady infusion of wisdom from the masters, beginning with Alfred Blalock, Professor of Surgery and Director of the Department of Surgery. Dr. Blalock was world-renowned for developing an innovative procedure before the heart-lung machine was invented. It helped children with cyanosis (known as "blue baby syndrome," where insufficient blood travels to the lungs for oxygenation due to heart defects) — and gave life to these fragile infants where no possibility had existed before.

I saw in him the kind of surgeon I wanted to be: smart, dedicated, caring, highly skilled, and willing to try new things — even after experiencing heartbreak when he realized his innovative operation didn't fix these children forever. Yes, it offered them life since it would flow more blood to the lungs to receive oxygen, but he also knew there would be problems later as they grew, since his procedure couldn't correct the hole in the ventricle that was the source of the problem.

Yet he was the quintessential leader. Dr. Blalock had never used the newly developed heart-lung machine or the novel surgical procedures emerging from its capability. But he could foresee that this apparatus would someday allow for the development of a more complete solution to fixing heart defects like those in blue babies, and so made his goal to provide support and encouragement to his students to begin evolving new ways to care for damaged hearts.

It was here that I witnessed that the magic of true excellence starts by appreciating work done by others. One must then become an educator and pass your baton to those who can execute the next steps of this endless path of growth.

As many of his residents subsequently became famous all over the globe, this beautiful lineage of contribution continued to flourish as they similarly trained their own residents. Watching Dr. Blalock's selfless actions gave me new goals with regards to how I would conduct my future research, and encourage and support my own students.

Earliest Mentor

Johns Hopkins brimmed with faculty members that had a powerful impact on my career. After all, the climb up the mountain path is made upon the shoulders of those who have pursued the journey before you, and I was at a place that provided a lovely trail.

My first rotation at Hopkins was on the heart surgery team, and its chief was Dr. Henry Bahnson, an early adopter of the heart-lung machine and who became my first "hands-on" mentor. He was a phenomenal surgeon who had a commanding presence: tall, self-possessed, humble, and someone who knew exactly what he was doing.

He was a man's man, a gentleman, and everybody's hero. (**Figure 1**)

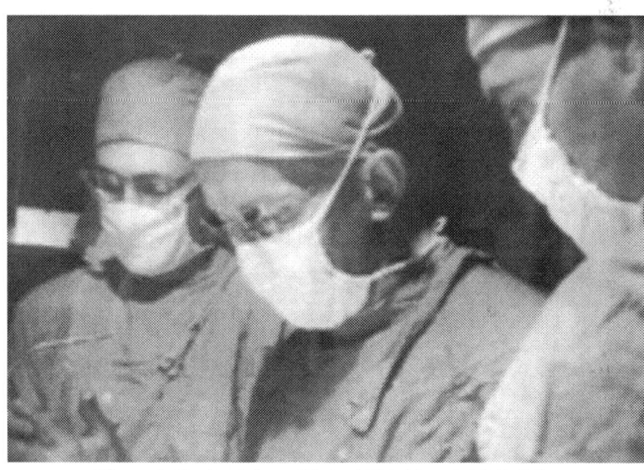

Figure 1: During internship in 1961, I (on right) helping Henry T. Bahnson at Hopkins, where open-heart surgery was just starting.

You'd climb the hill with him without question. Sometimes literally. We used to make rounds with him to see all the patients. Sometimes he would bypass the elevator and run up eight flights of stairs, jumping two at a time. We'd barely keep up and when we'd get to the top, he'd turn to us and say, "All right, tell me about our patients."

Only problem was the other intern and I couldn't breathe!

He was a true leader, in part because he had fallibility. He wasn't full of braggadocio like so many others. You see those types all the time that care only for themselves and not about anybody who works with them. They'll sacrifice anyone to reach their ends, blaming problems on others and never taking the fall. Dr. Bahnson wasn't that way. To him, winning meant *we* won, not he won.

He wasn't always perfect in diagnosis or treatment (no one is), but was always willing to listen and learn, and led by doing the right thing.

I met him for the first time in an intensive care unit where we were examining a patient that was having some trouble. I said, "Dr. Bahnson, I think the problem is his calcium levels are too high." I followed up by naming a particular drug we could use to bring the calcium down.

He just smiled at me a moment and asked, "So tell me about his drug."

It wasn't so much that Dr. Bahnson didn't know what the drug was, but rather, he marveled that an intern could stand there and try to figure out what to do and make suggestions. Here I am, a new intern telling the guy who's the head of heart surgery what I think was going on and remarkably, he wanted to listen. This too had a pivotal impact on me — because I realized that great people had open ears. You not only hear, but *you listen*. We tried the drug and it worked.

Dr. Bahnson's attention went far beyond just surgical technique. He always engrossed himself in any problems that arose even after the technical surgery procedure was done. Again, with an open mind, he would seek all input, determine a strategy, and then lead others toward a solution. This was particularly important at the time, since this new era of open-heart surgery introduced fresh problems that had to be overcome. These problems became the "seeds" for the growth of future breakthroughs.

Hidden Dilemma

One such problem was that while the heart-lung machine allowed intricate surgical procedures to take place, we still needed to understand why the heart's performance was often impaired afterward, despite our having performed a perfect technical correction of the underlying defect.

While we didn't know precisely why this happened, we suspected the heart might have been damaged when it was made quiet (stopped beating), which was done since operating upon a moving heart was difficult. But this speculation only suggested the problem's source without solving it, so the mystery persisted. Our dilemma was that *the repaired heart often appeared more hurt than helped.*

While the patient survived the operation, new issues arose because the impaired performance of the damaged heart reduced blood flow to other organs, so that kidney, liver, and brain failure developed. These complications created terrible problems for the patient, and intense frustrations among their physicians who had to try to overcome these new ailments. Moreover, we didn't know the long-term impact of this heart injury at the time, though now recognize it subsequently leads to an increased death rate.

The steps of the researcher's eternal learning process became evident through this quandary as Dr. Bahnson brought us to the peak of one mountain (showing us how to fix the heart's obvious problem) — and simultaneously taught us to look toward the more challenging peak ahead (avoidance of this lethal injury). I remained haunted by this enduring puzzle of damage resulting from an otherwise flawless heart procedure. This riddle continued long after I left Hopkins, and my initial research efforts were galvanized into finding its solution.

Never Give Up

Such challenging situations can really test a person, and reveal traits that foretell how they conduct their future professional life.

Among the many outstanding individuals at Hopkins was Warfield Firor, the prior surgeon-in-chief, President of the American Surgical Association (our premier society), and chairman of the Joint Conference Committee on Graduate Training in Surgery in the United States. Dr. Firor was a general surgeon that did not do cardiac operations, but he remained clinically active and had a patient named Libby B. who experienced persistent intestinal obstructions. He had operated on her many times, but the obstruction recurred again and again. Finally, he concluded it was a terminal situation and ordered an ongoing morphine injection so she could pass away comfortably.

I was intrigued by Libby's expressive features and the glint in her eyes. I thought Dr. Firor was being hasty. He knew I disagreed with his prognosis, as my ceaseless telephone calls kept bringing him back to surgically try to relieve the intestinal blockage.

I'd phone him, "Dr. Firor...."

"Buckberg. Again? When are you going to let go of this?"

"I have another idea, sir. You have to operate on her another time."

He did, and one of these procedures was completely successful. Libby survived the illness and went home, her sparkling eyes seeming ever more beautiful.

While I knew Dr. Firor was very pleased that she recovered, I also knew I'd really been bugging him. Still, he kept teaching me, leading me to become a better surgeon at every step. He was committed to the work he did.

For that reason, when I was to leave Hopkins in December of 1963 for the rest of my training in Los Angeles, I phoned Dr. Firor at his home to thank him for his instruction. He hadn't known I was going and appreciated the call, adding, "Don't leave yet. Please go to the operating room desk and await my arrival."

While surprised that he wanted to say goodbye in person, I was delighted and waited for him. In he came, in the middle of winter, wearing an old brown coat, dark brown muffler, shabby hat, and carrying a paper bag under his arm. He thanked me for helping him with Libby and presented me a gift. Inside this brown paper bag was an old book about Harvey Cushing, the world's most famous brain surgeon who started neurosurgery at Hopkins and with whom Dr. Firor had studied when his own training began.

I was puzzled why he would give a cardiac surgeon a book about a neurosurgeon. Then Dr. Firor asked me to open the book.

Today, treasured mementos line the edge of my tall cherry wood bookcase, where four books live upon the top shelf. One, wrapped in a shaggy cover, is this book about Harvey Cushing. Inside, the personal inscription that Dr. Firor had written to me that night when I was about to leave Hopkins:

> To Gerald Buckberg, who has been
> irrepressible but not irrestrainable
> determined but not obstinate
> energetic but not aggressive
> tough but not rough
> kind but not soft
> irreverent but not uncouth, etc
> From Warfield M Firor, in appreciation of the fun we've had working together at the Johns Hopkins Hospital, December 14, 1963.

This was unexpected. I knew how much he meant to me, but truly did not know what he thought of me, especially after our experience with Libby.

Even today, I remain touched by what he wrote back then to a very young, fairly green intern. Dr. Firor recognized he was working with someone truly concerned with caring for sick people, someone who was not overly concerned with what his professor or others might think of him, but dedicated to doing everything he could to help patients get better. Dr. Firor was a bedrock in my formation. He recognized and encouraged my positive traits, and kindled our shared outlook: that passionately pursuing solutions to help people is fun.

UCLA

I exchanged the cold winters of the east with the sunnier climate of Southern California as I traveled next to UCLA, where I was to spend six months in cardiac surgery during the final year of my residency. My good fortune traveled with me and I continued to be surrounded by eminent leaders in the field.

One of those I was privileged to work with was Dr. William Longmire, the founding chief of surgery of the UCLA School of Medicine and internationally respected surgeon. Not only that, he had a history at Johns Hopkins

Hospital. He'd been on the surgical team with Dr. Blalock that successfully conducted the first "blue baby" procedure.

Dr. Longmire was an inspiring individual who had mastered many phases of surgery, and was the ideal person to demonstrate the qualities of a dedicated physician by taking care of both patients *and* their families. From him, I could see the primary attribute of a cardiac surgeon was to be a complete physician, combining knowledge, precision, and teaching with the full understanding that all of these qualities should be directed toward the ultimate goal of quality patient care.

Despite a demanding travel and lecture schedule, Dr. Longmire continually demonstrated these caring traits by visiting his post-operative patients immediately after his trips. The knowledge that he would return from a trip at 2:00 a.m. and immediately go to the hospital before heading home had an impact on all of his resident surgeons. Dr. Longmire made us understand that you could be the greatest surgeon in the world, but if you did not put your patients and their families first, you were still a lousy physician. The doctor-patient relationship became the central theme of his clinical practice.

It was a lesson I learned under the most uncomfortable of circumstances.

One morning at 5:00 a.m., a resident called to inform me of a brief convulsion in one of Dr. Longmire's patients. From what the resident said, I determined the cause was low calcium, which I had him cure by calcium restoration. I did not call Professor Longmire, knowing I would be meeting him at 7:00 a.m. for an operation.

As we both arrived and prepared for the surgery at the scrub sink, Dr. Longmire spoke to me first, saying only one thing:

"How would you feel if you came to see one of your patients and the family asked you if their mom would convulse again... and you had no idea what happened earlier?"

He had visited the patient and their family early that morning before coming to surgery. Before I could reply or apologize, he walked off into the operating room. I had no choice but to follow.

A ten-hour liver resection ensued under the technical mastery of this surgical genius — without a word exchanged between us. In his silence, he taught me a profound lesson about the completeness of surgical care.

The Search Continues: We Begin to See the Enemy

The dilemmas of heart surgery are universal.

My time on the cardiac rotation at Johns Hopkins Hospital had lasted only two months, but I repeatedly witnessed an outcome of a heart becoming seriously damaged, despite the performance of a faultless technical operation. This injury caused deaths from impaired heart function. Yet the problem was not isolated, as the same thing was also occurring at UCLA.

Even when the outcome was not fatal, temporary impaired heart performance was *expected* whenever the patient was on the heart-lung machine more than 60 minutes. Yet, we could only deal with the symptoms of this damage, since answers to the overriding question, "Why does the heart function diminish after an excellent technical repair?" were unknown.

The frustration was overwhelming to me. My visit to the pathology department to look upon the now-still body that had previously pulsed with life, stirred a mixture of deep sadness and intense curiosity. The common denominator of these deaths was always extensive damage to *the inner shell* of the left ventricle (inner muscle closest to that chamber), as shown in **Figure 2**.

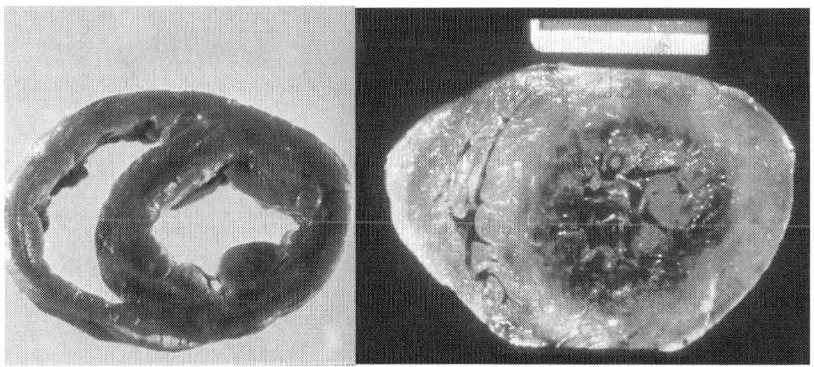

Normal Heart　　Thick Heart with Dead Inner Shell

Figure 2: These are cross sections of the heart.
In the healthy heart (left image), the left ventricle is on the left side,
the midline structure shows the septum, and the thin wall on right side is the right ventricle.
The thickened heart of a patient (right image) shows a massive amount of blood
in the inner shell of heart wall due to bleeding (hemorrhaging) into dead tissue, caused by
extensive damage developed despite a technically perfect operation.

We knew the blood vessels supplying this region were unobstructed, so the problem had to be elsewhere. Like others, I desperately wanted to reverse this cause of death, and my search for an answer would drive me toward a deeper exploration of its cause and prevention.

But before that could occur, I had a two-year military obligation that began once I completed my residency at UCLA.

Military Man

I entered military service in 1967 and served in the Air Force at Wright-Patterson Air Force Base in Dayton, Ohio. I would treat people stationed on-base as well as soldiers flown back to the states for surgery. It was here that the first glimmer of insight unexpectedly arose toward how to address the heart muscle damage that commonly occurred during cardiac surgery.

During the Vietnam War, a strategy of rapid retrieval of injured soldiers was developed so that medics could enter the battlefield to treat them. In the past, medics would have to wait for the battle to finish before they would retrieve the soldiers to bring back to the hospital. But these brave paramedics were now trained to go out in the field during the fighting just after the soldiers were wounded. Typically, the injured soldiers had lost a lot of blood and the medic would transfuse the victim, providing them fluids through an intravenous needle. They could not give them blood since they couldn't know their blood types, so they administered large quantities of saline solution directly into the veins to replace the massive blood loss.

While this certainly saved many who would have otherwise perished, there was a problem. It was causing a massive amount of lung congestion, a condition that was called *Vietnam Wet Lung*. As a result, they were losing these young healthy soldiers.

Upon learning of this, my natural response was, "Why did this happen? We have to figure this out." I got involved.

I attended a meeting organized by the military in Washington, DC, with representatives invited from major academic institutions to consider this problem. A surgeon from New Orleans suggested that the lung swelling happened because the major lung veins went into spasm for some reason and narrowed, and thus prevented good drainage of blood through those veins, resulting in congestion. Sounded interesting.

To determine if this diagnosis was accurate, I went back to Dayton to see if I could reproduce this in animals. I caused the animals to go into shock by removing a lot of blood, and then measured their lung vein pressures. To perform the measurement, I developed a curved cannula (a tube with a handle) (**Figure 3**) through which we passed a catheter into a tiny hole in the heart's left atrium, and then passed it into the lung (pulmonary) vein.

Yet the pressures we measured in the veins remained normal. With this, we determined there was no such problem with the major lung veins, so the theory proposed by the surgeon from New Orleans was wrong.

(The cause of Vietnam Wet Lung was later found to be the use of water or saline transfusions. This differs from what occurs when *blood* transfusions

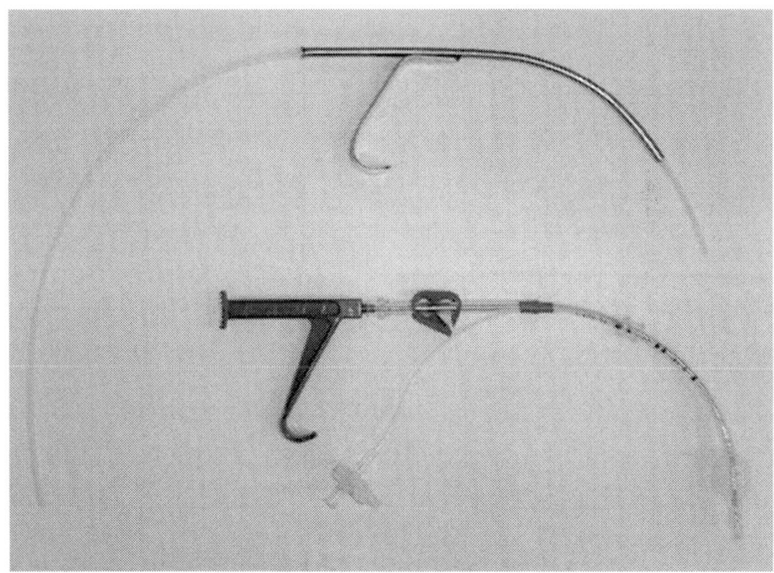

Figure 3: Upper example is tubing device (cannula) for entering lung veins from left atrium. Lower example shows similar device for entering the coronary veins from right atrium.

are used to replace what had been lost, since the infused blood remains in the arteries and veins. By contrast, the *water or saline solutions* will leave the tiny capillary blood vessels and enter the tissues, and this leakage is most evident in the lungs. The medics were giving massive saline infusions that saved lives, but inadvertently caused the lung congestion that followed.)

While I was able to evaluate the validity of this surgeon's theory, I also realized something else: the device I'd created that was used on the left side of the heart — might also prove to be a valuable tool on the right side of the heart — and permit us to study ways to better protect the heart during cardiac surgery. After all, if the catheter could be easily placed into heart's left atrium and into a vein within the lung — why couldn't it be passed into the right atrium (via a tiny incision) and just as easily be passed into the coronary veins — to take blood samples and help us study heart metabolism?" (**Figure 4**)

We tried this... and it worked!

This major forward step would later permit advances in understanding the heart's metabolism during both health and disease. What I couldn't yet foresee was this cannula technology would also allow another important

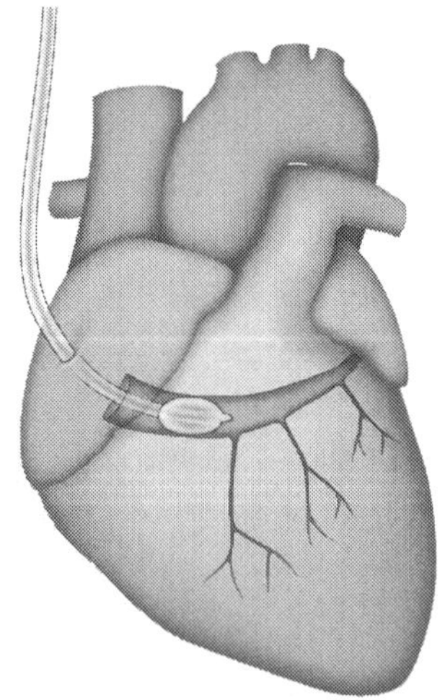

Figure 4: Tubing device shown passing from right atrium to coronary veins (called coronary sinus)

discovery to emerge while I was at UCLA ten years later — one that would help finally unfold the mystery of why damage to the inner shell of the heart caused death after open-heart surgery. This would play a vital role in allowing surgeons to safeguard the heart during cardiac operations. This will be described in the next chapter.

One of the most valuable things I learned during my medical training is that you never know where that next inspiration will come from. After all, sometimes it can be as simple as an apple falling off a tree (as when Newton discovered gravity). You just need curiosity and an open mind. This cannula — initially used to show that the prior theory about the lungs was wrong — would later be used on the other side of the heart and contribute to the success of cardiac operations.

Setting New Course

By the end of my military service, I had charted a clear path for my professional career.

I would be a clinical surgeon *and* a researcher. This pathway differs from that of the typical researcher, who never sees the problem firsthand in patients. Yet this vital combination allows the laboratory to act as the launchpad toward finding initial answers, and simultaneously sets the stage for subsequent development of treatments that I and others could use to resolve these issues.

I entered the world of *translational surgical research* as I adopted a "bedside to bench to bedside" approach with key steps. First, I had to recognize a persistent problem occurring with patients (bedside), then perform research in the lab (the bench) to develop a solution, followed by testing it in my patients (bedside again), then asking colleagues to test it with their patients. Finally, if successful, I had to teach everybody about it. This has been the game plan of my experimental / clinical explorations for over 50 years. It combines my passions for investigation, discovery, and practice.

Accordingly, after fulfilling my military obligation in 1969, I entered the Cardiovascular Research Institute (CVRI) in San Francisco to become skilled at the rigorous process of defining a medical problem, developing a hypothesis, designing an experiment, and measuring the results... and recognizing that any failures simply point to the next step in the progression toward uncovering the answer.

In short, CVRI would teach me how to be a researcher.

CHAPTER 4

Becoming an Investigator

Recognized contributors to our profession have always had heroes — accomplished individuals that are giants who show us how to build a solid foundation for growth. We never start alone. We do not win some lottery for success. Rather, our internal spirit evolves while relying upon the guidance of these prior leaders.

These mentors provide total commitment to their new students. Julius Comroe, the head of the Cardiovascular Research Institute, was one of these. He was an outstanding scholar and teacher who essentially gave up his career in pulmonary research to create an institution that furnished the educational "seeds" for the development of our future leaders. His unyielding commitment was to infuse us with the fundamentals of knowledge: how to use it, and how to create it. The research fellow always had complete access to his attention. On the other hand, such access was not possible even for recognized international scientists coming to San Francisco; they could not see Dr. Comroe without a prior appointment. (**Figure 1**)

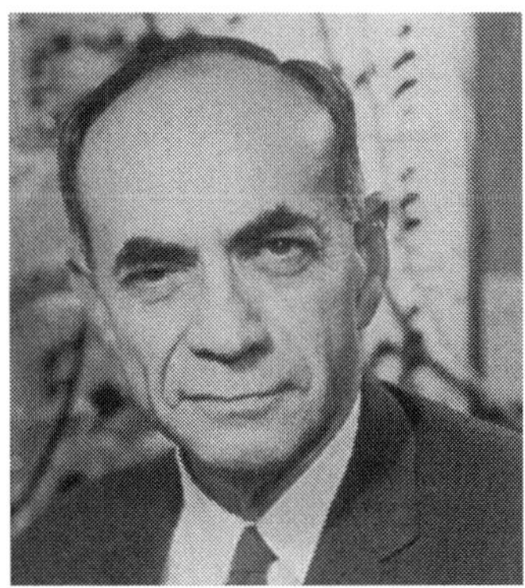

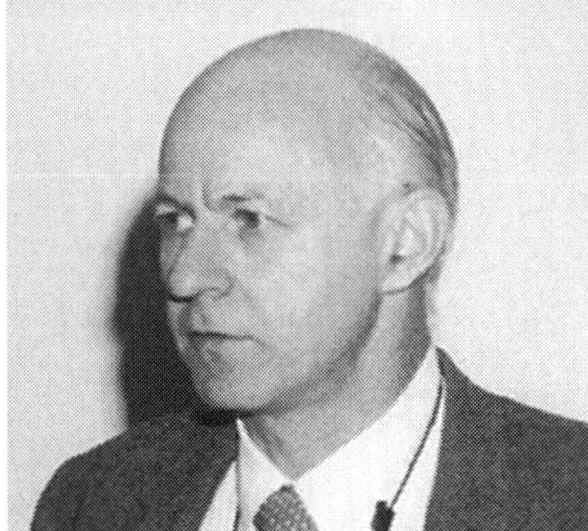

Figure 1: My CVRI mentors, Julius Comroe and Julien Hoffman. Their teaching set the tone for how I taught my students.

I'll never forget his class on teaching us how to review medical literature — information published in journals and texts dedicated to the field of medicine. He asked me to comment on an article published in 1935 about blood pressure responses and the carotid artery. I was given 45 minutes to read this two-page paper, which reached its conclusions from studying only two experimental subjects. Dr. Comroe demanded to know what my editorial decision would be on this brief manuscript that offered only limited investigative data and unsupported concepts.

Of course, I rejected this paper due to its deficient research, essentially no statistics, and imprecise questioning of what was known. Dr. Comroe gracefully accepted my surgical point of view... then informed me that my decision was not shared by the Nobel Committee, who had bestowed their prize onto Corneille Heymans for this unique and scholarly description of the carotid sinus reflex... a fundamental contribution toward understanding normal physiology.

It was an important lesson for me: listen, learn, but do not be so eager to evaluate and dismiss. Rather, consider and grow from what you are shown and go forward from there.

This, as did many lessons gleaned from those who came before me, influenced my professional evolution and helped further set the stage for how I would conduct my future research.

My principal guide at CVRI was Dr. Julien I.E. Hoffman, a cardiologist, physiologist (specialist in functions of all parts of the body), and thoughtful mentor. He taught me how to respond to data I collected through research: how to look at it, find the new questions stimulated by the data, and answer those questions in a way that provided reasons for everything I was asserting.

"You don't simply report your observations — you must understand the biological mechanism underlying the study, and also appreciate the study's limitations."

A methodologist in his research, Julien wanted us to make sure our investigative techniques were done properly. He insisted on absolute certainty about our findings before any report was finalized.

Though demanding, he was patient with surgeons without exception. He welcomed your ability to ask the questions he had not thought of, rather than you simply providing a solution that he already knew was true. He urged different views and evaluated each idea carefully... then would sometimes tell you with incisive, dry wit that your excellent conclusion might not actually be correct. But only after examining all the factors, would he either reject you on a solid basis, or more importantly, encourage your next step.

Removing the "Blinders"

While I was at CVRI, we wanted to create an experiment to finally solve the mystery that had been plaguing me and others: why were so many open-heart surgery patients not surviving, even though their operations had been done in a technically perfect way?

Most of those patients didn't die on the operating table, but sometime *after* the surgery was completed. What I consistently witnessed in the autopsy suites was that the inner shell muscle — the muscle closest to the ventricle chamber responsible for pumping blood into the body — had either died or was severely damaged. Something must have happened to it either during or after the operation, and we wanted to know what it was.

Actually, we *had* to know.

A normal assumption would be that too little blood flow had gone to the area. Typically, that would be from an inadequate blood supply to the heart due to narrowing or obstruction of the coronary arteries. But those vessels were open (not blocked) in these patients. That was not the problem.

Adding to the puzzle was that we *weren't* seeing any damage to the outer muscle of the heart. It appeared to be fine.

So why was there inadequate blood flow — just to this inner shell muscle?

Using Microspheres

We began to measure the blood flow to this inner shell muscle (also called the endocardium). While we were already capable of measuring the amount of blood going to the whole heart through the arteries, never before had anyone been able to repeatedly measure the amount reaching specific regions *inside* the heart through the capillaries.

Until now.

Julien Hoffman developed a breakthrough concept of measuring blood flow with small *microspheres.* The microspheres were tiny man-made polymers — each *just slightly larger* than a red blood cell. They were to be injected into the left atrium of a laboratory animal's heart. Because they were a shade larger than red blood cells, they would become entrapped in the heart's capillaries — vessels so small that only a single red blood cell can barely squeeze through.

Because these microspheres were also radioactive, we would be able to track their locations during the experimental study. We hoped to accurately measure the blood flow to this inner shell of the ventricle by counting how many microspheres had become trapped.

This would be a huge advance — if it worked. Sorting this out became a challenging experiment. The study was carried out by me and three other surgical residents, and Julien Hoffman guided our efforts.

The first step was to determine the distribution of flow *when the heart was normal.* This was equally critical to learning what happens when something goes wrong. If you don't know what normal is — the way the heart *should be* — then you cannot know what has changed and cannot fix the problem.

The experiment began.

We injected the microspheres under ordinary conditions to establish that critical starting point. Their movement was tracked by a spectrometer, and as we had predicted, they became entrapped in the capillaries, revealing to us their flow distribution in the heart's muscles when everything was normal. This established, for the first time, that we could measure blood flow in the inner shell (endocardium) during an experimental study.

It was a great beginning.

These initial results confirmed what would be our baseline: that under normal circumstances, the blood flow to both the inner shell muscle and the outer muscle were the same. But that still left us with the riddle: *what changed to cause damage only to the inner shell muscle.* That's what we would look at next.

Astounding Results

Here's what we knew about the heart before we started: each time it beats, the heart's muscles contract in order to pump the blood from inside the cavity of the heart to move it out into the body. But in doing so, that compression *also* squeezes the arterial blood vessels within the heart's walls — those that carry nourishment to the contracting heart muscle itself. Each squeeze *restricts the amount of blood flowing* through them.

In fact, the blood only flows freely to these heart muscles when the heart relaxes between beats.

While this was true for *both* the inner and outer muscles in the heart, we also knew from previous studies — that this compression on the blood vessels was *greater within the inner muscle* than the outer muscle.

Could that be the clue?

No one knew, because until now, no one had ever been able to measure any of these changes in flow within the inner muscle before.

Yet as we continued our experiment, we learned that during heart contraction — nearly *all blood flow stopped* to the inner shell muscle — while the outer muscle had only minor blood flow reduction.

This was a powerful observation, as it meant that the inner shell muscle could *only* receive nourishment when the heart was at rest between heartbeats — never while the heart contracted (which meant it could not be nourished one-third of the time during a heartbeat).

No wonder this inner shell was the most vulnerable part of the heart and at risk of becoming damaged!

We now tested further, by reducing the blood pressure to match what it would be in patients with a leaky valve in the aorta (main artery connecting to the heart) — a disease condition that open-heart surgery commonly treats. We found the blood supply to the inner shell *was down dramatically* in patients with this condition. This increased the vulnerability, since it got nothing while the heart was contracting.

I reported our findings at an American College of Surgeons Forum for young investigators in San Francisco. It was a meeting where the "next generation" of leaders in research would share what they were working on in their labs. It was an electrifying place to be and I was eager to give my presentation.

Ours was a totally new finding. Though a small study, it was the first time anyone had ever used microspheres to prove a damaged area had too little flow, despite having open arteries.[1]

The audience was intrigued. Someone even posed the question, "Could these microspheres be used to measure blood flow in other organs in the body as well as the heart?"

"Absolutely. The brain, kidney, lungs, intestines — there are all kinds of possibilities. In fact, someone is now doing this in another study at CVRI."

Our results were very well received. It was a wonderful experience to be the happy recipient of much positive acknowledgment and congratulations.

But we weren't done yet.

I knew we only had part of the answer.

Missing Piece

Our findings had told us why there could be damage during an open-heart procedure. But it didn't answer why this happened to some patients and not others. Not every patient had heart damage after surgery.

Under what circumstances would this happen? And could we predict it?

So I began inducing different variations on the experiment: we tried having less blood pressure pushing into the area and saw how that would reduce the blood flow. We made the heart rate too rapid — since faster beats per minute meant less time for the heart to relax and be nourished between each beat. And we increased the opposing pressure in the blood vessels leading out of the heart — since if that opposing force was too high, new blood flow cannot enter.

We hoped we could accurately predict what the flow rate would be to the inner shell in response to these changes we made. And we did find in each of these cases that the blood flow did reduce to the inner shell. But it wasn't consistent. Under certain conditions, the measurement of nourishment would be adequate, while in other yet similar circumstances, it would not. We couldn't directly relate it to the changes we made in the blood pressures or heart rate, and we didn't know why.

Perplexed, I showed our results to my maestro, Julien Hoffman. He looked over everything very carefully, and then asked us this question: "Have you considered factoring in *for demand*?"

What a remarkable insight.

The "demand" is *how much oxygen the heart needs* from the blood. Whether an area is being adequately nourished or is being damaged — will be based on how much blood supply it is receiving — compared *to what it needs* for the tasks it is doing. If an area had a very high requirement for nourishment, you would have a problem even with what normally would be a higher flow level because it still may not be enough.

This would be the missing piece of the puzzle!

It came back again to the issue of independence versus interdependence.

We had been looking at one part: the supply. But we couldn't tell if that blood supply was truly adequate or not, because we weren't looking at the demand. Once we began to factor in the demand that the heart muscle would have for oxygen, we suddenly could bring everything together — and were able to predict when there would be inadequate blood flow to the inner shell muscle.

With this, we finally solved the baffling mystery of why a piece of the heart could die or be injured even though the coronary arteries were open and the surgery was impeccably performed. We now knew it wasn't a matter of obstructions. It was about the balance between the blood supply going to that area and the oxygen demands.

This led to developing what became our "supply / demand ratio" — a mathematical formula that measured this relationship between blood supply and the inner shell muscle's requirements for oxygen from the blood. We called this the DPTI/SPTI ratio (Diastolic Pressure Time Index / Systolic Pressure Time Index). (**Figure 2**)

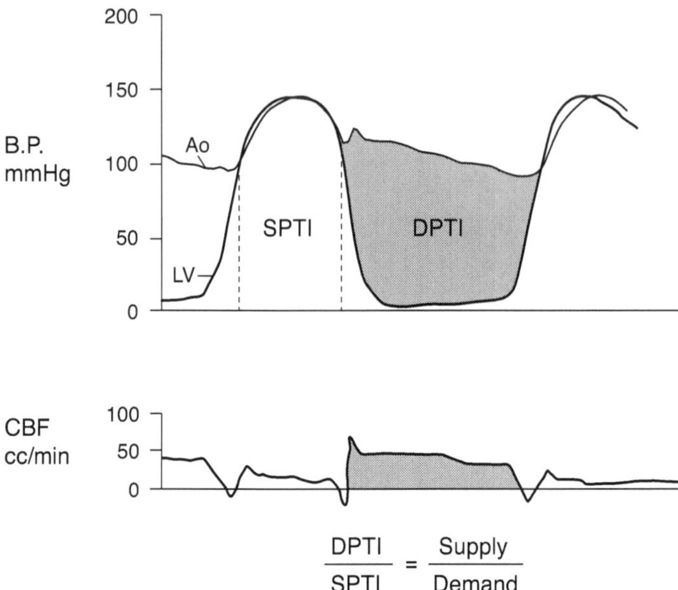

Figure 2: Upper part shows how blood pressures (B.P.) were used to calculate the diastolic and systolic time indexes (that measures supply and demand). Lower tracing shows coronary artery blood flow (CBF) that predominantly happens when the heart relaxes during diastole.

This would become the biggest breakthrough of our study. We took a process (blood flow to the inner shell) that was previously so complex that no one could even measure it... and translated this unique information into a formula that merely used the patient's blood pressure and heart rate. Plugging those numbers into a formula would accurately predict if sufficient blood supply was getting into the inner shell muscle of the ventricle. An exciting and thrilling end result.

Valuable Tool to Improve Care

Our discovery opened the door for much better care during that critical period after open-heart surgery during which we had been losing so many patients. This was vital because it provided guidelines to treat damage that may follow the operation — one that impaired the heart's ability to contract, resulting in worsening of the patient's condition.

Now for the first time ever, any doctor, nurse, or other clinician could take a simple measurement of the patient's blood pressure and heart rate, and put those numbers into our simple formula to determine if damage had occurred and if the blood supply to the inner shell was now adequate. If it wasn't, they could administer the appropriate drugs to support the heart, helping it get past the injury. Simplicity replaced the sophisticated technology of measuring flow into the heart muscle.

By understanding how to deal with an imbalance between the heart's blood supply and its need for oxygen to give it energy, we finally addressed the question I began asking at Johns Hopkins when I first observed hearts being "more hurt than healed" after surgery.

I should also note that even with our terrific and very gratifying results, Dr. Hoffman nearly drove me and the other three research fellows crazy as he came up with additional methods that he wanted us to use to confirm our findings before we published. His message was "You never say anything publicly until you're sure of it, *but* once sure you are correct, don't be afraid to say it." It made me understand that if you are right, nobody can attack you to overturn the truth.

That was another great lesson I've adopted in my own work. When I know I'm right, it doesn't matter what others say. You keep going forward, despite being faced with opposition. Truth will win.

Next Mountain Peak

Our research and hard work were well received. In fact, of the over 450 papers I've published, the paper describing our findings about how to use microspheres to measure flow in remote and inaccessible regions of the heart has been the most quoted article of my entire career.[1]

Yet as great as this advancement was, I still recognized that we were dealing with the *consequences* of something that must have occurred during surgery. Somehow, despite having a technically perfect operation performed, the inner shell muscle was still getting damaged in many patients. Finding the answer to this riddle became the next mountain to climb. My time at CVRI was coming to an end, so I would return to UCLA to address this challenge. My first project.

My schooling wasn't over. I now understood that the surgical skills and scientific methods I had learned before CVRI only reflected the beginning of my education. This boy from the Bronx was now a cardiovascular researcher and surgeon, armed with the tools, passion, and ambition to try to set a worldwide course for fixing broken hearts.

Needless to say, I was excited to use everything I'd learned in trying to understand and solve this devastating complication.

CHAPTER 5

Great Expectations

After completing my fellowship at CVRI, it was my great fortune to return to UCLA and work on the faculty as an assistant professor under James Maloney, the Chief of Cardiothoracic Surgery.

I vividly remember my first day on the job. I had an immediate need to speak with Dr. Maloney, who I knew pretty well by this point. I was aware of the emphasis in academic medicine on publication. Dr. Longmire had informed me some time before of the need to publish many papers on your research, since productivity was viewed as the road to success.

But Dr. Longmire (**Figure 1**) was wise and advised me that, "Sometimes they count them and sometimes they weigh them. ...*But they never read them.*"

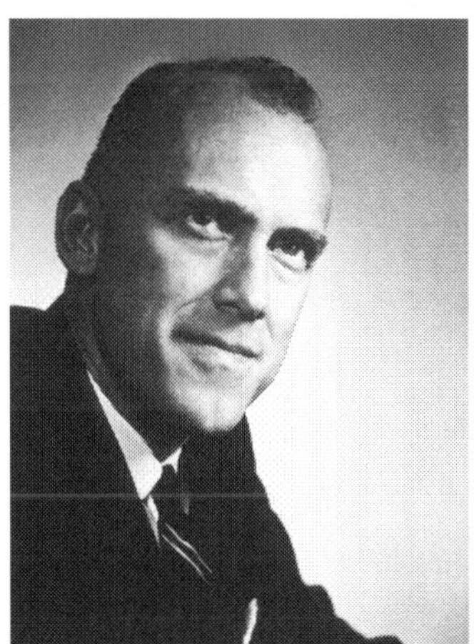

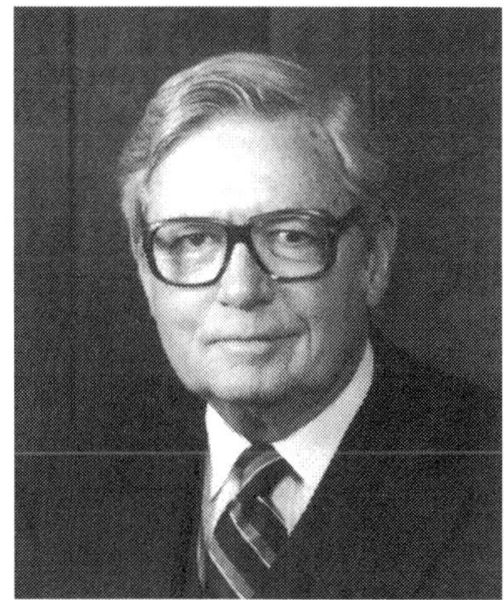

Figure 1: My surgical teachers, James Maloney and William Longmire, who taught me how to use the operating room to ask new questions that needed innovative answers.

In other words, the focus was to publish *something*, but this task was rarely geared toward providing information that would improve the status of medical science. The researcher's mandate of "Publish or Perish" made no sense to me, as I could waste a lot of time trying to play a "paper game" without meaning.

I was not willing to squander my time. There was too much valuable work that needed to be accomplished.

So on day one, I approached Dr. Maloney and said, "Jim, I know the criteria for academic success is to publish numerous abstracts and subsequent papers. But here's something else I also know that is true: I can't work under an obligation of needing to do something just for the sake of doing it. I need to perform research in a way that can make a real difference. I don't want to be in a position where the measure of my success is marked by how many pages I can generate."

It was a pretty bold statement, especially by a brand-new faculty member. But I even went a step further by adding, "If there are such requirements for publication and presentation in this department, I would have no choice but to begin looking for another position immediately."

Dr. Maloney looked at me a long moment. "Let's take a walk."

He escorted me into his lab, through its range of facilities, past various staff working there.

"I hear your concerns," he ultimately replied, "so this is how it will be." He faced me straight on. "Here, you can work on whatever you want. I will provide the equipment and the people. I will offer my thoughts as you show me whatever you are developing. If in two years we need to have this conversation, we'll have it then."

That was unexpected… but music to my ears.

Of course, that conversation would never happen, then or in the future. During the next two years, I would be free to create innovative experimental research that would become translated into new methods and technologies to help patients after heart surgery.

Jim Maloney showed his faith in me that first day and put me in position to succeed at what I wanted to do.

He had a very good reason to do so.

Things were not going particularly well. As with most medical institutions, UCLA was experiencing too many injured hearts after cardiac operations. The survival of our cardiovascular program depended upon the development of new approaches to be used for protecting the heart during open-heart surgery.

This dilemma wasn't helped by the department's response to this problem: focusing only *on the speed* at which a procedure could be performed. This approach was based upon the belief that the longer the surgery, the more damage would occur in the ventricle's inner shell. Besides being a shortsighted concept, outcomes were not helped by the fact that UCLA is a teaching hospital, meaning residents would operate while being overseen by the more veteran surgeons. They performed excellent procedures, but their inexperience meant they required more time to do the operation.

More experienced surgeons at other (non-teaching) hospitals were faster. These prolonged operations at UCLA led to fewer referrals for open-heart surgery from cardiologists.

So the belief at UCLA was that "time was the enemy." But I had explained to Jim Maloney that while this might be true with ordinary or conventional surgical techniques, the true problem wasn't speed. Instead, the basic issue was how well you protected the heart during each procedure, and I was dedicated to discovering new and safer techniques that would allow for longer operations that could be done safely, and would not subject the heart to progressive damage.

This is why he provided me free reign in my research.

As already noted, I first recognized this problem of a heart "more hurt than healed" during my residency at Johns Hopkins, and this complication became a well-recognized dilemma *throughout* the cardiovascular community. The extensive damage to the heart's inner shell that I observed after attending postmortem studies at UCLA was happening everywhere. But *its cause* baffled everyone.

Yet I was lucky, because I had a technique that might uncover the reason.

As the previous chapter described, I learned at CVRI how to measure blood flow in remote regions of the heart (including the vulnerable inner shell) and calculate the relationship between blood supply and blood demand — determining that the heart becomes damaged when demand isn't met. Essentially, I knew what to look for, and had the tools to measure what was happening. I was eager now to embark on a detective's path that might uncover the cause for a major worldwide problem.

Jim Maloney agreed that battling the clock was not a winning solution. He was hoping I would find one.

I was now on a mission.

Forging a New Trail

It was time to begin the work. This study would be my first opportunity to fully apply the "bedside to bench to bedside" approach that I had chosen to adopt when I entered CVRI. It includes three steps:

The first starts with observing and defining a problematic clinical event: the functional damage happening in patients' hearts (the bedside portion) after a technically successful procedure. To gain a more complete picture, I would always consult with the other attending physicians and surgeons to learn what they were observing. Dr. Comroe at CVRI taught me that while others' viewpoints may not always concur with mine, my understanding of a problem grows by listening to differing opinions. For example, I might see *four* things occurring; they might see *a fifth*. I needed to grasp the whole issue.

The second step is to recreate in the lab (the bench) the same disease event, and design research studies that will lead to the development of techniques that will solve the problem. Now, I did not do this alone, but am grateful for the assistance of research fellows from UCLA, as well as other universities both nationally and abroad. We are a team, and they conduct much of the study under my direction, yet they are encouraged to ask probing questions that may take us in different directions. Julien Hoffman had demonstrated the incredible value of remaining open to new ideas. Throughout my career, I was never invested in wanting to *be* right, but rather to find out what *was* right. The power of listening must triumph... and it does.

The third step involves translating a successful laboratory experience into a clinical solution to be used in patients (the bedside), and ultimately used by more and more surgeons as acceptance grows. Admittedly, this last part can be easier said than done, for even with their expressed enthusiasm for new discoveries, many physicians may still not want to use them. In medicine (and in many other endeavors), people have a tendency to do what they did yesterday. This roadblock must continually be overcome, as I would learn throughout my career.

Mission Launches

So I began my first experimental study at UCLA as a new faculty member. I had access to world-class equipment, with staff and research fellows to assist me. There was freedom to order what I needed to duplicate the microsphere measurements that I had performed at CVRI. A perfect launchpad.

Yet these tools were common to all experimental laboratories. The piece typically missing is the ingenuity to develop new ideas, then do experimental studies to test their truth, and finally to use these concepts in sick patients. Again, I was reminded of Einstein's adage, "Imagination is more important than knowledge." Hopefully ours would meet the challenge that we needed to face.

Our experimental subjects would be large pigs, given the similarities of their circulatory systems to our own (in fact, you may know that pig heart valves are sometimes used to replace human valves today). Fortunately, another positive attribute of UCLA was that it had the highest level of animal protection requirements. Its policies for making sure test animals were properly protected were very specific, in their being properly anesthetized and well taken care of before, during, and after experiments.

Ventricular Fibrillation

My work would start on ventricular fibrillation (VF), since purposely inducing VF in a patient was commonly used to quiet the heart so cardiac surgeons could operate more easily. It is very difficult to perform procedures on a beating heart. So a patient would typically be connected to a heart-lung machine that took over pumping oxygenated blood throughout the body — as a *momentary electrical stimulus* is applied to cause the heart to *spontaneously fibrillate.* Instead of a normal pumping motion, the heart would quiver minutely, so that it essentially does not move and cannot perform any useful cardiac action. Once begun, the heart would continue to fibrillate on its own until the procedure was complete, at which time an electrical counter shock (called defibrillation) would be applied to restart the heart's normal rhythm.

The question I posed was: might using ventricular fibrillation during operations be connected to the heart damage we were seeing far too often?

The vast majority of cardiac surgeons didn't believe so, because ventricular fibrillation was used routinely in many centers worldwide. But I wanted to find out for sure.

Our study began with normal hearts. We would induce spontaneous fibrillation with a momentary electrical stimulus in a heart, just as it is done during a surgical procedure. We would then let the heart fibrillate on its own for an extended period (one hour), and then restart the test subject's heart with another electrical impulse to return it to normal function.

Our results showed excellent performance. There was no evidence of any damage to the heart, and no need for drugs to help support its capacity to contract normally.

However, one particularly interesting fact did emerge.

We already knew that blood flow distribution in a healthy beating (not fibrillating) heart is equally distributed to its inner and outer muscles — the flow ratio is 1:1.

Yet when measuring its distribution *during fibrillation* (by using the microsphere protocol we had developed at CVRI) — we discovered the inner muscle *received 40% more blood flow* than the outer muscle.

That was a significant finding since the blood flow to an area will match its oxygen demand requirements (amount of oxygen needed) when it functions normally. Our unanticipated finding revealed that when the inner muscle is fibrillating — it has a 40% higher flow need in order to have its oxygen requirements met.

This observation was especially notable because "normality" in any given circumstance is not necessarily what we *anticipate* (equal blood flow distribution to the inner and outer shells). Instead, our testing of fibrillating hearts demonstrated the *reality*, whereby more flow is needed to the inner shell in order for the heart to maintain normal performance.

This baseline information sets the standard for our analyzing for potential damage (impaired function) after open-heart procedures, where the inner muscle failed to receive the required 40% increase in blood flow.

Consistent Current = Persistent Problem

It was time to create our first experimental effort to mimic what happens during a clinical procedure (meaning one that would occur with a patient).

For this, we changed from inducing fibrillation with a momentary electrical stimulus — *to applying a continuous* alternating current. This continuous approach was used by many cardiac surgeons — who were worried that the spontaneously fibrillating heart (from a momentary stimulus) might suddenly resume beating in the middle of a procedure. The continuous low level current ensured that this did not happen.

Our new results differed dramatically from those using a momentary electrical stimulus to cause fibrillation.

These hearts became swollen and did not beat well! Our chemical tests documented that cell enzymes had leaked, certifying there had been cellular damage. This experimental finding confirmed other recent reports that heart performance was impaired following continuous ventricular fibrillation (VF) using an ongoing electrical current.

Yet our study was unique, because until then, nobody knew *why* this damage happened. *Now we did:* it was inadequate blood flow to the inner muscle.

The expected 40% greater blood flow to the inner shell did not occur *when a constant current was used — and this undernourishment caused severe damage.* The likely cause was further compression of the blood vessels inside its quivering muscle. The continuous current made the ventricle squeeze more vigorously.

The light of understanding was now beaming upon us, and how delighted we were! These studies had finally uncovered and documented why the heart sustained damage when ventricular fibrillation was used during cardiac operations!

But there was one more study that we needed to do... and it yielded remarkable findings on its own.

Unhealthy Hearts Hurt More than Helped

I understood our studies had impact, but I also recognized that our findings were incomplete — because sometimes using only a momentary electrical stimulus in operations did not always work either. Some patients sustained heart damage, and we did not understand how that could be.

It dawned on us that we rarely operated on the normal, healthy hearts that we studied.

Instead, we operate on sick and damaged hearts.

To explore *this* reality, we would mimic another operation, this time inducing fibrillation with the single momentary electrical stimulus — but in a hypertrophied heart — whose thickened muscle walls mirror those of patients with hypertension, aortic stenosis, heart muscle injury, or heart failure — common illnesses that may need surgical corrective procedures.

Our first task was to create a heart containing a sick, thickened ventricle. Toward this end, it was our good fortune to have Christof Hottenrott, a research fellow from Germany, working in our lab. During his two years with us, he created hypertrophy in animal test subjects by narrowing their aorta.

After waiting six to eight weeks for hypertrophy to develop, we then studied ventricular fibrillation after a single momentary stimulus. The ventricle fibrillated on its own for 60 minutes, and heart performance was measured 30 minutes later. This exactly matched how we conducted our studies in normal healthy hearts.

These results were both disturbing and revealing.

Our findings *mirrored those we found when using continuous fibrillation* (continuous current) on the normal heart — as blood flow rate to the inner muscle was *the same* as to the outer muscle (1:1). But the general medical belief that such "equal flow distribution is fine" is simply incorrect during ventricular fibrillation. We knew a 40% higher flow is needed to the inner muscle to match its greater oxygen demands. That meant an equal flow *could not furnish enough oxygen to meet the hypertrophied inner muscles'* need for oxygen (perhaps because thickened muscles were compressing its feeding blood vessels).

A wide range of damage became evident, as these thick-walled hearts experienced acidosis (excessive acidity), leakage of enzymes, bleeding into its inner wall (hemorrhage), and markedly impaired performance. Studies at postmortem examination showed that these test animals developed the same damage that occurred in patients that succumbed to this injury. (Its elaborate name, hemorrhagic sub-endocardial necrosis, means dead inner wall tissue with bleeding into its cells.) (**Figure 2**)

It was now clear to us that the cause of this too-common injury was the dramatic *reduction* in blood flow to the inner wall of the thickened heart. Yet

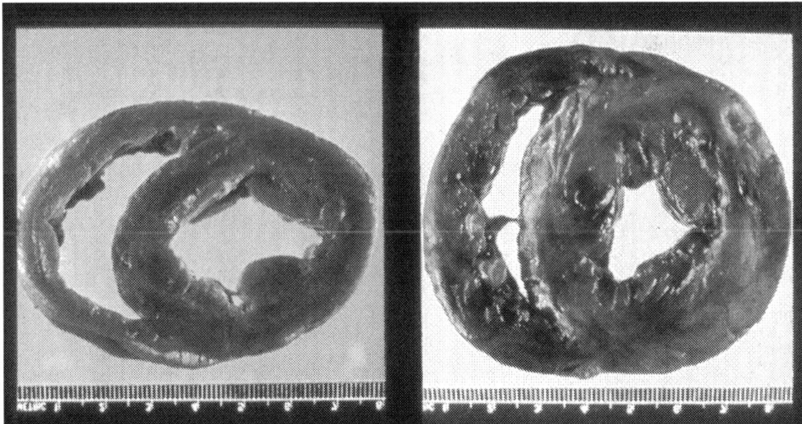

Figure 2: Experimental examples of how the heart appears as you look at it in cross section. The normal heart is shown on the left, and on the right is a thick walled (hypertrophied) heart that underwent ventricular fibrillation. Note development of hemorrhaging (bleeding) and cell death (marked by darkened area) on the inner circumference of the thickened heart — findings that precisely mirror what happens in humans, as described in the last chapter.

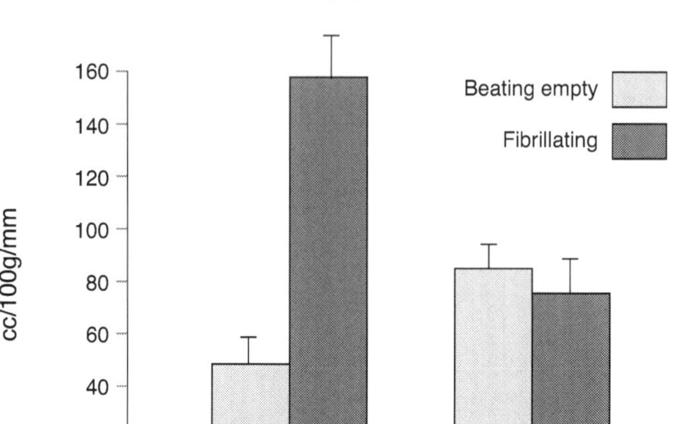

Figure 3: Blood flow to inner shell when the whole heart develops ventricular fibrillation (shown in darker columns) and in a beating empty heart (lighter columns). Flow increases markedly (to meet high demands) in normal heart (on left), but this expected increase falls to occur in hypertrophied quivering heart (on right).

the need for blood flow to this inner wall is substantially higher (40% more than the outer wall) in a normal heart. (**Figure 3**)

Cracking the Riddle = Wide-Reaching Change

Our discoveries about ventricular fibrillation became a turning point. The mystery behind why hearts were being "more hurt than helped" was unraveling. My attitude toward the adverse effect of ventricular fibrillation led me to then state that "fibrillation was the F-word." That belief has never changed.

Finding these answers established the vital link between the lab and the patient, and the cardiac surgical community responded promptly to our discovery! Our seminal studies resulted in the abandonment of using ventricular fibrillation to stop the heart from beating during aortic valve replacement operations in thickened hearts. They also introduced a wariness about its use in other cardiac procedures (such as coronary artery surgery, and correcting congenital problems).

Yet despite these two breakthrough studies, I knew there was something else to be found — and it was even more important. While I was pleased that our findings halted a major cause of heart damage, one that I first witnessed starting at Johns Hopkins, a central question remained:

What should take its place?

Searching for the Alternative

With VF no longer an option, we needed to find another way to quiet the heart. Having a "motionless operative field" is important for our technical repairs during cardiac surgery. The only other alternative was to stop the heart from beating by shutting off its blood supply. This is done by placing a clamp on the aorta (while the heart-lung machine takes over to pump oxygenated blood through the rest of the body). An effective method, as the heart muscle stops contracting almost immediately (and rather miraculously, spontaneously begins beating again when the blood supply is returned).

But a critical issue remained.

Despite this technique's ability to achieve a perfectly quiet operative field, hearts become damaged after about 15 minutes of no blood supply.

Aware of this, many surgeons worked around this 15-minutes ballpark figure by doing a part of the procedure on a stilled heart, then re-nourishing it by restoring blood supply for ten minutes, then shutting it off again to continue their surgery.

The problem was that while this repeated pattern sounded good in theory, the hearts of our patients were still being damaged.

From our research, I felt this all pointed toward one thing. Somehow, these hearts were *still* not being sufficiently nourished during those ten-minute intervals of blood flow. The concept of supply and demand for oxygen re-emerged, just as it did when we developed the DPTI/SPTI ratio (while working with Julien Hoffman at CVRI).

To make operations safer, we now had two goals: first, to minimize the oxygen needs of the ventricle when the heart is stopped, and second, to optimize nourishment to the inner shell when blood flow is restored.

An imposing task… *but there would be no giving up.*

Minimizing Demand

We had learned about the oxygen demands of the ventricle in earlier studies, in which "decompressing the ventricle" (done by inserting a tube to drain out or "vent" its blood) would cause a three-fold lowering of its oxygen requirements. Basically, the heart is still pumping, but with no blood in it.

Cardiac surgeons knew about venting the heart, but often would not do it, as this added an extra step to the procedure. This reluctance was also due to a widespread lack of awareness of how venting reduced the heart's need for oxygen. However, we knew that it worked by lowering the heart's energy requirements and thus would enhance the heart's protection. So we added decompression (venting) to our protocol during clinical surgery.

Maximizing Nourishment

As said, I suspected the heart was not being adequately nourished during those intermittent ten-minute periods of restoring blood flow. We wanted to identify the reasons why, and then put in steps to make sure the heart got the best nourishment possible.

I believed we first needed to keep a sufficient blood pressure so that the heart and all its capillaries were being well fed. This had not previously been a consideration, as maintaining an adequate flow of blood to the body by the heart-lung machine was our top priority.

So we first established minimums for blood pressure.

The second objective was that the blood supply from the heart must deliver adequate oxygen. The red blood cell is the vehicle for nourishment, yet many operations were done by adding extra water to the fluid in the heart-lung machine. This was done to avoid adding donor blood into the circuit. But this approach caused anemia (lowering the amount of red cells in the blood), which impaired nourishment by oxygenated blood.

To accomplish our dual goals (sufficient blood pressure and sufficient oxygen), we created a series of interconnected procedures that safeguarded the heart. These strategies were then combined into protocols that were used in a variety of cardiac operations, that included mitral valve procedures, aortic valve operations, and coronary artery bypass grafting.

These new surgical tactics were used in about 300 patients at UCLA, resulting in a dramatic improvement in patient survival — and an impressive reduction in the number of patients that required drugs to support their hearts when the heart-lung machine was disconnected after the operation was complete! (**Figure 4**)[2]

There was great enthusiasm in the department, and as our successes increased — cardiologists realized that we had hit the target and increasingly referred their patients for cardiac surgery to UCLA. Our cardiology and cardiac surgery teams were pleased.

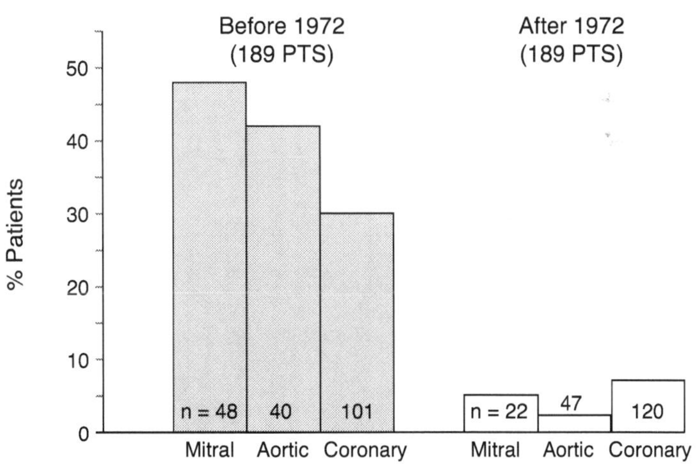

Figure 4: Our new methods of heart protection in 1972 dramatically reduced the need to support the heart with drugs, compared with findings before 1972. (from 1975 AATS presentation)

Big Presentation... Big Surprise

The worldwide problem of cardiac protection was enormous. Its ongoing issues caused the leaders in cardiac surgery to set up a special session at the meeting of the American Association of Thoracic Surgery (AATS) to allow selected members to present different methods of avoiding damage during cardiac repair. This was the first time in the long history of this meeting that people would be pooled from all over the world to address a single topic: myocardial protection. They wanted to get the best people to report what they were doing.

The leaders of the organization knew we had been conducting numerous studies regarding this at UCLA, and so asked Jim Maloney to chair the conference as he was the head of our division.

I was thrilled and looked forward to presenting the paper on applying our newly developed methods that essentially eliminated the need to use supportive drugs after a range of cardiac procedures. I felt that our studies had conquered the world's greatest problem during heart surgery, and wanted to share our findings!

The meeting took place in New York City in 1975. At this time, my normal dress outfit was a suede coat and open-collar shirt. I also had long hair and a big, broad mustache. I looked like a cross between a hippie and Pancho Villa. (**Figure 5a**)

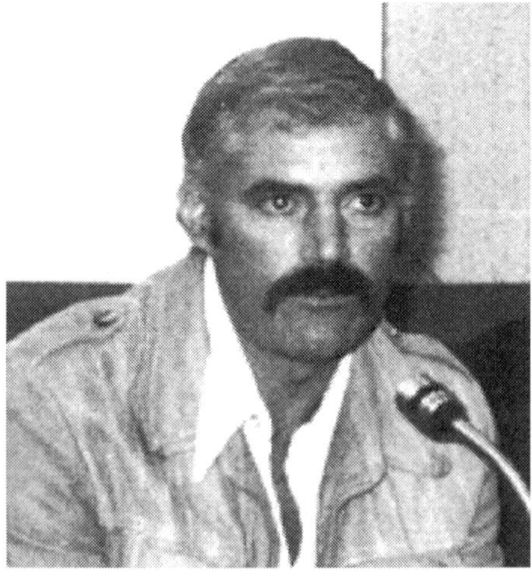

Figure 5a: Dr. Buckberg in his typical dress with suede coat in 1975, before AATS meeting.

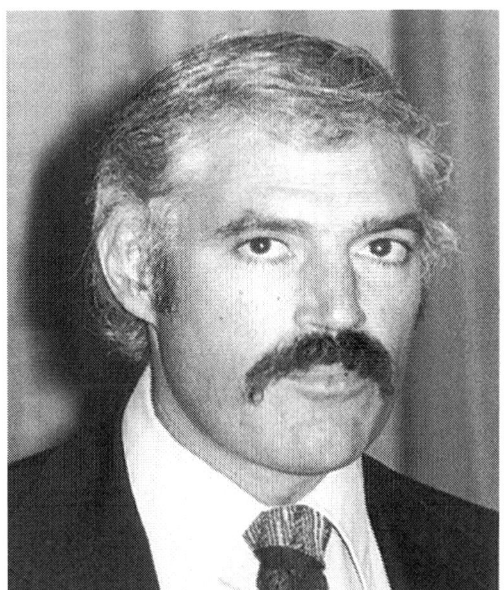

Figure 5b: Dr. Buckberg's "new" outfit at 1975 AATS.
The renegade now dresses "as expected" to let the data do the talking.

Concerned this might prevent others from taking my message seriously, I got a haircut and trimmed the mustache, and attended the meeting in the same three-piece suit I'd worn to my wedding. (**Figure 5b**)

Seeing my new look, several friends asked if I was attending someone else's wedding.

"No," was my answer. "I'm going to a funeral."

From my point of view, I *was* attending a funeral — to bury these ineffective methods of heart surgery and their accompanying damage. All of that would soon come to an end as our new approaches were adopted.

In preparing his remarks as moderator for the meeting, Jim Maloney asked my advice on what he should say as way of introduction to set the tone for the presentations, since this was my field of interest.

I pondered this and had a mischievous idea. I created a fictitious but plausible story of Jim Maloney seeking advice from Ernest Starling, a London professor during the early 20th century who was a legend in circulatory physiology. Jim Maloney was supposedly asking for advice on how to remedy the all-too-frequent situation in which patients did poorly after otherwise typical heart surgery procedures.

Jim Maloney was delighted by the idea, and opened the day's session by telling my fabricated tale of him speaking with Ernest Starling:

"Dr. Starling, I'm so glad to consult with you. Today, we see patients whose hearts are not performing normally and we can do all kinds of wonderful operations to correct them. They perhaps have arteries that aren't getting blood supply — which we fix. They have valves that are leaking or have become narrowed — which we change. There are blue babies with holes in their hearts — and we make them pink again. We do all of these things and the hearts are now technically better — but they look awful. Somehow they're getting damaged during these procedures and patients have been dying."

Dr. Starling was intrigued. "That indeed sounds unusual. How is it you can do all those procedures?"

"We use something called the heart-lung machine. It takes the blood out of the body and oxygenates it and pumps it back in. So we can exclude the heart from the circulation while we perform surgery on it."

"Fascinating. What pressure do you use?"

"Oh, we don't look at pressure. We just use the heart-lung machine to maintain a high blood flow."

"Really, so what pressure is maintained?"

"Probably around 30 or 40."

"Just 30 or 40? That is called shock, is it not?

Dr. Starling further asked, "What are the hematocrit numbers?"

"You mean how many red cells are in the circulating blood? Oh, we don't worry about that, Dr. Starling. We're concerned mostly about flow and volume, so we just mix in water to add to the blood."

"But that creates anemia, does it not?"

"I suppose if you want to get technical about it."

"Right. And what else happens in these procedures?"

"Sometimes if we need to quiet the heart while we operate on it, we give the heart a little electric shock to make it fibrillate or slightly quiver so it essentially doesn't move."

"You mean... electrocution as happens with criminals? Dare I inquire what else you do?"

"Sometimes we go another direction and shut off the blood supply. Completely."

"That sounds awful."

"Oh, it's not a problem — because we also expose the heart and then douse it with ice water in order to lower its needs."

Starling clarified, "You mean... by freezing it."

Jim Maloney then asks Starling, "So that's pretty much it. What do you think?"

Dr. Starling considers all this only a moment before he replies:

"I don't quite understand. You're *surprised* there is a problem?"

I created this hypothetical story for Jim Maloney to focus upon the outrageous things surgeons were doing to the heart — things everyone thought were so terrific. It was a humorous way to start off this conference's historical conversation about protecting the heart. Jim Maloney delivered it flawlessly and the audience thought it was hilarious.

This was followed by numerous presentations of studies addressing the universal problem of heart damage during surgeries. Finally came time for the last paper — mine — on our method of cardiac protection that was producing such great results at UCLA.[2] I walked up to the podium and began extolling our noteworthy findings in cardiac surgery to the most well-attended meeting of thoracic surgeons in the world. Over 4,000 people focused on every word I said during my presentation.

Once finished, I was met with an ovation from the room. This was truly the proudest day of my career to date. I had just made, in my mind, a gargantuan contribution to the future of cardiac surgery.

I relished this experience as I returned to my seat.

That feeling lasted all of 15 minutes.

After my presentation, Georg Rodewald, a surgeon from Hamburg, Germany, approached the stage as he would be the primary discusser of my presentation. He was shaking his head as he passed me in my seat.

"Why is he doing that?" I wondered.

Rodewald went on stage to the same podium and began by saying he didn't understand the need for all the multiple-step solutions I was offering. He simply applied a *cardioplegic solution* to the heart while shutting off the blood supply to quiet it and saw excellent recovery — despite periods of aortic clamping far beyond 60 minutes.

I was stunned. Though he hadn't yet made his research widely public, Rodewald was in effect producing similar results to ours in a much simpler manner while providing a much longer window for a surgeon to perform their procedures.

I sincerely doubt Dr. Rodewald noticed my jaw drop. But after all the time and hard work put in to reach our grand solution, his comments were massively deflating.

Soon after, the conference was over. I could have reacted to this experience in one of two ways. I could have dismissed what he was saying — as do many people in the medical field who reject what's new and continue doing what they've always been doing. But that's not me. I'm not after what is familiar and comfortable even if it makes me feel good about myself.

I'm after what works.

I regarded his new piece of information as a glimpse toward the next peak ahead. On my flight home, Dr. Rodewald's comments reverberated through me. I knew right then where my research would take me next. I was going to study cardioplegia. I wanted to explore these other ways of stopping the heart. Dr. Rodewald had described a chemical method that he was using in Germany. I also learned that others were exploring this approach in different ways. I wanted to discover what would work best.

In our research, I had looked at ways to intermittently still the heart between periods of nourishing it with blood. I never looked at ways to simply and safely stop the heart in a prolonged way during a cardiac operation. Now I would investigate how to do this.

It was a whole new direction.

I had ascended my first peak, and brought my fellow surgeons up with me, to the benefit of many patients. But now was the time to scale the next mountaintop. Rather than feel threatened by Dr. Rodewald's findings, I enthusiastically embraced them.

I couldn't wait to get home and back into the lab — my *bench* where new research needed to be done — where we might develop findings that may be converted into a *bedside* approach that can help patients undergoing cardiac operations.

CHAPTER 6

Discovery: Myocardial Protection and Blood Cardioplegia

The path of scientific discovery is unpredictable, to say the least. Who'd have thought that one man's comments at a conference would change the trajectory of my entire career? It focused my spotlight upon not protecting the laurels of yesterday, but toward exploring tomorrow.

Yet for this fresh round of research, our goal was the same: to uncover a better way to protect the heart during surgery.

At UCLA, we were enjoying success with the intermittent aortic clamping as described in the last chapter, and outside institutions experienced similar achievements. But the methods were admittedly cumbersome, involving extra steps that many surgeons did not want to do. I recognized that our procedures could be greatly improved if we found a safe method that allowed us to extend the clamping period while still avoiding heart damage, as Rodewald had suggested was possible by using cardioplegic solutions.

The possibility of using cardioplegia in this procedure was not new to me, but I had my doubts about its safety. Cardioplegia is the administering of a chemical solution to arrest (stop) the heart's beating during surgery, as well as a way to protect the heart when its natural blood supply is stopped. This approach was introduced in 1955 by Denis Melrose in England.[3] But significant clinical problems had accompanied its use. Sometimes it worked and sometimes it did not, and people died due to ventricle damage. This technique was largely abandoned in the early 1960s.

At AATS, Rodewald presented better cardioplegia results than I'd heard previously. He was among the first to report that you *can* do cardioplegia safely.[4]

Progress had been made elsewhere as well. Recent studies showed that the cardiac damage following use of the Melrose solution[3] was caused by its exceedingly high concentrations of chemicals (including potassium and citrate and other concentrated particles) in the cardioplegia solution that was mixed with blood.[5,6] In the United States, Gay and Ebert used a crystalloid (water-based) solution[6] and showed that using more reasonable concentrations of potassium offset problems with cardioplegia solutions. Finding a safe way to use potassium would be valuable: potassium causes the heart to stop in a flaccid state — non-contracting and limp — making it easier for us to operate. Gay and Ebert also avoided citrate, which could lower the heart's calcium levels dangerously and cause cell injury, and they excluded chemical components that drew fluid from cells, causing them to shrink.

These new studies overturned the devastating problems in the Melrose solution — *and the interest in cardioplegia was suddenly reborn.*

First Bench to Bedside Test: Unexpected Outcome

My experience at the AATS meeting sent my team in a new direction, with a new goal: to learn how to safely stop the heart with a cardioplegia solution. There would be many steps along the way, as the pathways for each of our discoveries would build upon the one that came before it. It would be a three-year quest filled with exhilarating successes — and terrifying failures.

Though the Rodewald and the Gay and Ebert crystalloid (water-based) solutions were much safer than the Melrose approach, they were not perfect, as both still had issues with impaired post-operative heart performance. But we followed their lead and designed our own crystalloid cardioplegic solution. Our experimental studies showed it to be successful following one hour of aortic clamping to stop the heart, yielding results that matched the clinical effectiveness reported by Dr. Rodewald at the AATS meeting. Despite this, we still didn't use this cardioplegic approach in patients because we observed some heart cell membrane damage. Further studies were needed.

My team and I continued trying new mixtures to solve this dilemma. Eventually, we found a way to better protect cardiac membranes by adding lidocaine (a local anesthetic) to the solution. This development gave us the confidence to go to the operating room and begin to use our newly developed cardioplegia solution in patients.

That's when the unexpected happened.

Nobody had ever given this solution that we created to cardiac surgical patients. My first case involved doing a coronary artery bypass procedure on a man who had traveled to UCLA from Santa Barbara, since we were recognized as performing operations more safely than in other centers.

Everything was prepared. I arrived, scrubbed in, and began the procedure with the rest of the operating team. I inserted a needle into the aorta, and after it was clamped, the cardioplegic solution was delivered by my perfusionist, Chuck Dyson. Chucky (as I called him) reported that all was well.

The heart immediately stopped — as it was supposed to. Then we placed grafts beyond the obstructions in the coronary arteries, and the procedure went flawlessly. We finished, and took off the aortic clamp to wait for the heart to spontaneously start beating again.

But the heart did not restart.

We waited. And waited.

"Something's wrong."

The heart was sitting there, limp and still, as if we'd been doing an autopsy.

It retained the flaccidity it had had while we were working on it. Unmoving. Meanwhile, my heart was racing.

"How long has it been?" I asked.

Chucky consulted the clock. "Five minutes."

Everyone was trading looks. Finally, they all turned to me. But I didn't understand this any better than they did. What had happened??

Again I turned to Chucky. "How long now?"

"Ten minutes."

My apprehension was growing exponentially! I went from bedside to bench to bedside, and the second bedside wasn't working. I was confronted with somebody who may never recover. That's all that was going through my mind.

"Fifteen minutes."

I stood there, powerless, in front of that limp heart. I pled with God to come down and help me. Aloud, I pled, "Please, Chucky, make it beat."

But Chucky had no answers either. I was filled with anguish. I'd just caused the most serious kind of cardiac damage possible.

Did my experimental solution cause a fatality in my patient?

Mercifully, thankfully, 23 minutes later, the heart simply started beating. Those were the longest 23 minutes of my life. The patient made an uneventful and full recovery.

It was me, the surgeon, who was damaged.

Eventually, we recognized that the prolonged arrest was due to our initial use of lidocaine having been delivered in concentrations that were too high, but we didn't know this at the time. Currently, new studies use lidocaine at lower doses, more successfully.[7]

I was discouraged, but still believed we could do better. Though we'd had successes in the lab, it was definitely not time to present this protocol to our staff surgeons or publish it. As mentioned, our surgeons and many others in the U.S. and around the world were quite satisfied utilizing the periodic clamping protocols that we had developed and described at AATS.

We returned to the lab.

Though we had successfully shown that our cardioplegic solution could extend aortic clamping for over an hour, our studies still revealed damage to the heart's membrane. We could measure leaking enzymes from the heart to reveal the degree of this tissue damage, and we reviewed other surgeons' experiences and found they too were finding enzyme leaks during the first 24 to 48 hours.[8]

Surgeons carefully watch their patients for six to ten weeks after surgery. But you really need a lengthier follow-up to know if there are any late consequences. It was eventually recognized that there is a *progressive* mortality after the heart is injured during the operation: the ten-year death rate following damage that causes a substantial enzyme leak is four times higher than when no injury occurred.[9]

This striking statistic means that just because someone with significant enzyme leaks gets out of the hospital, it doesn't mean they are out of the woods. Not at all.

The Road to New Thinking

Medical advancements do not start in the laboratory. They come about by observing, then asking the right questions... and most importantly, by listening.

The best part of going to conferences is not presenting my own findings, but listening to the observations of others. Such attention is essential to the investigative mind. Do not be confined to the small tribe of researchers at your institution. Reach out to others around the country and the world. Observe the problems they encounter, and their solutions. This principle of *travel and listen* is a mantra that I teach my students. The "seeds" for growth is to have humility, for retaining this quality will permit your open mind to continually search for new knowledge.

I presented our periodic or intermittent aortic clamping (every 15 minutes) approach at the AATS conference. The technique became a formidable arrow in the quiver of tools available to cardiac surgeons and many began to use it. That led to my first career invitation to be a guest speaker, extended by Dr. John Kirklin (**Figure 1**) at the University of Alabama, to talk about

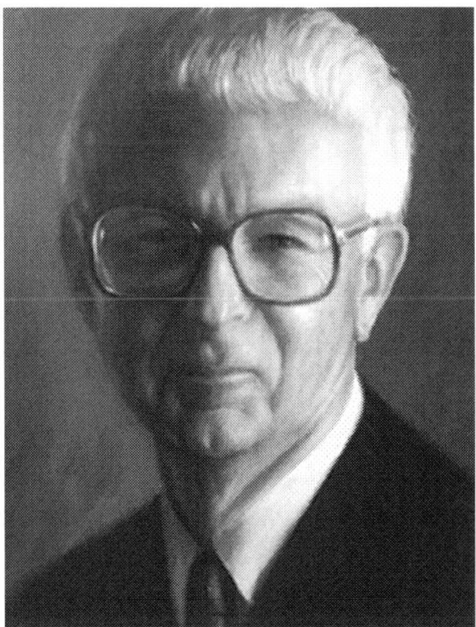

Figure 1: Dr. John Kirklin

the work we had been doing. I was honored. Dr. Kirklin was one of the most prominent and influential cardiac surgeons in the world.

I was escorted to a large classroom holding between 50 and 100 students and colleagues. Dr. Kirklin walked in with his clipboard, taking notes as I spoke about all the various things we'd been doing at UCLA. Then, as is typical in these kinds of presentations, he would challenge whether something I presented would work, and I would use my data to explain my logic.

Dr. Kirklin possessed incredible curiosity. He would hold tenaciously onto the past until a new idea came to light. Once he trusted that the new development was well-founded, he would abandon tradition and move on.

Dr. Kirklin asked probing questions, and in turn, explained that he had used our short intervals of periodic clamping during coronary bypass procedures, though not during aortic and mitral valve replacement. In the aortic and mitral valve surgeries, his team instead used deep hypothermia (placing ice around the heart) to markedly cool the ventricle and lower its energy demands, which allowed for longer periods of aortic clamping. Though I was answering his inquiries about my research, it was actually I who was gaining powerful insights as I listened to his observations.

This heightened when Dr. Kirklin invited me to join him afterward on his rounds in the intensive care unit. It was here that he reported an observation to me that would inspire my experimental and clinical studies for the next 25 years.

We stopped by one patient who just had a coronary artery bypass graft to improve blood flow to the heart using the mammary artery (from behind the chest wall) as the bypass graft. Kirklin explained, "This surgery went very well. It was an excellent graft and I was quite satisfied. Except I noticed something very odd during the operation."

"What was that?" I asked, my curiosity piqued.

"I had my hand on the heart as I completed the graft and took the clip off the artery to return blood flow to the heart. Suddenly the heart went rigid. I literally could feel this. It was soft before and abruptly stiffened."

"Really," I wondered aloud in surprise.

"There's even more to it than that. The heart's initial rigid condition then softened over time, back to normal."

Very odd indeed! His observation indicated that the muscle developed this firm condition immediately after its blood supply was restored. This reflow process is known as *reperfusion*. This rigidity was temporary because the stiff muscle progressively softened.

"What do you think happened?" he asked.

I considered his intriguing question. My response was shaped by my previous studies on the use of cardioplegic solutions to protect the heart. A theory was forming....

"I wonder, could this phenomenon relate to how the heart deals with the calcium in the blood flow being restored to it? It is possible, after a period of being without a blood supply — that it cannot handle the return of normal calcium in the blood for some reason and reacts. Almost like a charley horse."

Dr. Kirklin nodded at this new consideration. Of course, he wouldn't be convinced until it was proven. All he said was, "That is interesting. Very interesting."

I thought so as well. Metabolizing calcium is critically important for both contraction and how the heart uses energy. Could some change occur in a muscle while it is without blood... that compromises the muscle's natural ability to self-correct, such that a hazard is created by simply returning ordinary blood after ischemia (when the heart receives no blood flow)? If so, it would pose a serious challenge to *any* cardioplegia solution that might be used. This needed to be studied.

And I knew just the team to do it.

Changing Winds

As is the nature of research, a new observation created a new question. My course shifted again.

I had gone to Alabama to share my research and returned with new insights. Dr. Kirklin's astute clinical observation led me to the world of *reperfusion* — where blood is returned (called reflow) to the heart after a period during which it received none. My previous fascination with blood flow had now become my passageway into this new realm.

So I returned to UCLA with the stage now set for a series of challenging and paired investigations: step one was learn how to safely stop the heart for prolonged periods of time. Step two was to safely bring it back afterward.

The Stone Heart

Up until this time, the accepted wisdom was simply to restore the normal blood supply. No one had ever researched controlling the conditions and composition of reperfusion blood. *It was uncharted territory.*

I realized that these detrimental effects may not be limited only to those portions of the heart supplied by the bypass graft artery — but that such damage may also develop *throughout* the heart. Proof came from a report by Denton Cooley, a superb cardiac surgeon from Houston, who observed that his patients' entire inner ventricular wall became irreversibly rigid, following 30 minutes of aortic clamping during valve replacement.[10]

"Irreversible" meant the patients had died. He termed this lethal outcome "the stone heart."

Cooley's experience added an intriguing piece to the puzzle: while the damage observed by Kirklin was temporary, Cooley's was permanent. Presumably, this was due to longer periods of lack of blood and insufficient heart protection. While Kirklin had used 15-minute periods of ischemia (no blood to the heart), Cooley had used 30 minutes of ischemia. Those additional minutes somehow shifted a temporary injury that recovers… into lethal damage.

You can imagine the frustration and powerlessness of a surgeon, who after successfully repairing malfunctioning valves or remedying defects that have existed since birth, is confronted with a drastically flawed heart upon restoring blood flow. The family can only join him in lamenting that the damaged heart was injured more than helped, despite his technical success.

The age-old riddle of cardiac surgery.

Calcium Connection

Driven to understand these observations, I initially explored my hypothesis that calcium was one of the culprits: that managing "normal" levels of calcium in the blood returning to the heart was somehow too much for the ischemic heart to handle.

This much I knew: an injured heart does not efficiently move the calcium back and forth between the inside and outside of the cell. Calcium sometimes gets into the cell and does not come out. If there's too much calcium within the cell, the heart has a sluggish contraction, doesn't relax well, and can't use oxygen properly.

But how do we lower the level of calcium when the heart can't do it?

I turned to a protocol used by blood banks. To avoid blood clotting during storage, calcium concentrations are lowered by adding acid citrate dextrose (ACD), which binds the calcium.

We would use ACD to lower the calcium concentration.

But there was a problem. We would want to use only enough ACD to lower the calcium the right amount... but we also knew the blood will clot if it doesn't contain *enough* ACD. Our two parameters might be working against one another. We solved this by adding an additional ingredient — heparin, an anticoagulant. This substituted for the need for ACD to prevent clotting — and freed us to lower calcium by just varying ACD concentrations.

So then the question was: how much ACD is needed?

A significant issue, since we couldn't make calcium measurements in the lab. So we chose to use a practical test of sequentially adding ACD, 1 cc at a time. We'd know the right amount after we observed how the heart's performance recovered.

We added 1 cc of ACD, then 2 cc, and 3 cc, and so on to the reflow blood until we found that 9 cc of ACD was the effective amount.

The results were terrific!

My hypothesis was based on our research that the heart underwent metabolic and chemical changes during ischemia (when no blood was going to the heart). We believed these changes could be remedied by the way in which blood supply was restored. Our results proved this to be true and led us to devise what we called *controlled reperfusion*. Rather than reintroduce a normal blood supply after the heart had been ischemic (stopped without blood), we added citrate phosphorus dextrose (CPD) — a variant of ACD — to control the calcium concentration of the returning blood. It successfully avoided the injured, rigid hearts that were previously observed by both Kirklin and Cooley!

Looking Deeper

We now had a way to *safely reintroduce blood flow to the heart after surgery*. Each of us on the team felt a real sense of pride.

Yet there was more to do.

I now wanted to re-look at how standard methods of heart protection may not prevent damage from occurring during the operation, and uncover ways to bring such an injured heart back to normal.

Topical cooling (hypothermia) is commonly used, and was the first method we studied. This technique, first introduced by Norman Shumway at Stanford University, showed that cooling the heart limits damage when the heart's blood supply is stopped, by slowing metabolism and reducing its need for oxygen.[11] Though it was broadly accepted, we wanted to find out if this topical cooling method avoided problems from occurring in heart function.

Topical ice was placed around the heart in our animal test subject after we stopped its blood supply by clamping the aorta for 60 minutes. But recovery of the heart was impaired after taking the clamp off: ventricular performance returned to only 60% of normal.

Certainly hypothermia was helpful, but its protection was incomplete, since the 60% functional recovery confirmed that an injury was still happening.

Our next step — was to add one variation as we repeated this experiment.

Instead of simply removing the clamp at 60 minutes, we *delivered blood containing CPD* for the first five minutes of reperfusion before returning normal blood flow. We then measured heart performance 30 minutes later.

The result was startling — as there was *85% recovery* of function! So on top of demonstrating a safer way to reintroduce the blood supply — this study of reperfusion also showed an improved performance of a heart *that we knew had sustained an injury* while its blood supply had been stopped.

Suffice it to say, we were all extremely pleased!

Yet we also knew we had only opened the door. We weren't finished.

I believed the problem couldn't just be calcium — it had to relate to other changes as well. Nature is seldom disruptive in only one way. So our next steps were to search out and understand other reasons for the heart injury that occurs when there is normal reflow after a period of no blood supply.

Second Problem — Lactic Acid

We also knew that tissues without a blood supply, including the heart, always produce lactic acid that causes acidosis. This was not a new finding, as high concentrations of lactic acid were known to develop in muscles of marathon runners as they "hit the wall." So we decided to test a new reperfusion solution that *only* contained a buffer to raise pH and counteract this acidosis that harms the heart cells. The buffer called THAM was selected because it had the unique ability to enter the cell, and treat the inside and the outside of the injured heart cells.

As with the calcium study, this buffered reperfusion was delivered for five minutes and then the aortic clamp was removed. The recovery of function was 80%, revealing yet another new alternative reperfusion strategy.

Logic Doesn't Always Work

We were thrilled. I looked at the other researchers and stated, "Well, if we got 85% with reducing calcium and 80% with raising pH — we have it nailed. We put them together and we will have discovered the triumphant answer!"

The next logical step was to blend the two strategies. I fully anticipated that such a mixture would return heart function to 100%. So my cardiac surgery research fellow, David Follette, did exactly that. He used them both together and what did he find?

Only 40% recovery.

These results were even worse than when normal blood was given for reperfusion.

Extremely disappointed, I declared to David, "You must have done something wrong. This has to work. Go do it again."

Wanting my theory to be right, I blamed the investigator for not doing the studies properly. My mistake became immediately apparent.

David tested it 5 more times and got 40% every time.

There was no escaping the truth. I had violated a central principle to good leadership: *give credit, take blame*. I was trying to pass fault onto another, when this limitation rested with me. As I have long said, when a study doesn't work, there are only two possible reasons — either it is not done right, or the idea is wrong.

"Clearly, I don't understand this," I was forced to admit. I thought for a second. "There is someone we need to see."

Convinced the issue still had to do with abnormal calcium, I felt this someone to see was Glenn Langer — a preeminent cardiac physiologist at UCLA and known worldwide as "Mr. Calcium," due to his extensive research in the dynamics of how it functions in the heart. Nobody in the world knew more about calcium.

Our team visited Glenn Langer at his office, where he listened to everything we reported. Acutely aware of the role that calcium played in causing reperfusion damage, Glenn took particular note of our describing the rigid heart that occurred immediately after reperfusing it with normal blood. He concluded this reflected a temporary contracture (a hardening of muscles that can lead to rigidity) — due to the heart's inability to remove excessive calcium from within the muscle cells.

Yet curiously, he could not explain why our results *worsened* when we combined our two successful strategies of reducing calcium and raising pH in the blood we reflowed into the heart.

I pondered that paradox as we returned to our labs. There had to be an answer! I asked David, "Tell me exactly what you observed when you started the reperfusion with our combined solution."

"It was really quite something. As soon as I began reflowing the blood, the heart fibrillated (developing a completely inefficient rhythm) very vigorously."

I sat down and considered this. "I know the problem. The real issue is this fibrillation. It's strangulating the blood supply."

Remembering that Gay and Ebert used potassium in their studies of cardioplegia, I told David, "We have to stop the fibrillation. Let's try adding only potassium to the reflow."

David was enthused by the idea. He added potassium alone to the blood — and got 70% recovery. Definitely a step in the right direction!

Encouraged, I suggested, "Now let's add that to the other components of our blood cardioplegia reperfusion solution."

David tried the delivery of a combination of low calcium, higher pH, and potassium solution — after 60 minutes of having the heart stopped (receiving no blood flow), using only hypothermia for protection. *Would this new solution work better*?

It did. There was 100% recovery.

This remarkable result was tested again many times, and each duplicated the 100% recovery. We were ecstatic! We'd solved the reperfusion problem. We helped an injured heart recover through our goal of creating a new approach — *controlled reperfusion*!

Right for the Wrong Reasons

Everyone on the team was thrilled. Jim Maloney was delighted. This was a huge achievement. While I could have simply been celebrating this success along with the rest of them, one question remained completely unresolved:

How was it possible, before we added the potassium, that we observed powerful ventricular fibrillation — at a time when blood calcium was low?

So why should this question be haunting me? Because logically, we shouldn't have had powerfully fibrillating hearts when there is low calcium, as this prevents the muscle from squeezing strongly. Heart contraction should have been reduced, *not increased.*

This dilemma shines a light upon the beauty of research. There is never a single answer, but rather, each finding leads to the excitement to ask the new questions, whose answers will unfold along the learning pathway.

I continued searching for this seemingly unattainable answer, and eventually found a German physiologist named Piper[12] who discovered that calcium lurches into the injured cell and the muscle as blood is restored to an ischemic heart — causing *hyper*-contracture (overly contracted beyond the normal range) — much like what Cooley reported seeing with the stone heart after he removed the aortic clamp.

Suddenly I realized the "vigorous fibrillation" problem within the heart that David described — was in reality an example of cardiac hyper-contracture. The fibrillation might actually have been fairly low, but the heart muscle cells were being injured as calcium entered them — and the rapid twitching movement was camouflaging the underlying heart's rigidity. The charley horse observed by Kirklin now became lethal to the whole heart.

Interestingly, despite misjudging what the powerful fibrillation was telling us... *we* had added potassium. This was the correct decision, as its use left the heart flaccid, and prevented calcium from entering the heart cells.

It's one of those peculiar aspects of science: *sometimes you arrive at the right conclusion for the wrong reasons.*

But that wasn't important now. We had a blood composition that took a damaged heart showing only a 60% recovery with standard methods (topical hypothermia) and could now give it 100% recovery!

No doubt about it. What we had found was inspiring.

Two Types of People

This successful discovery illustrates my belief, and my approach to research, which I learned from my "bible" of investigation, *An Introduction to the Study of Experimental Medicine,* written in 1865 by Claude Bernard, a French physician, physiologist, and creative thinker.[13] He described the two kinds of people that exist in the scientific world: the observers and the experimenters.

The observers are the spectators who witness and record what is occurring, like the astronomers studying the stars. They observe nature as it happens.

The experimenters are those who start with a bias or theory for what is happening, create the needed conditions to test their position, and then do a study to see whether their prediction is valid.

Interestingly, when you perform that study, you must become an observer again — as nature provides the answer. Only then can the experimenter learn if their hypothesis is correct. This pattern of moving from an observer to experimenter and back to observer guides the researcher throughout his or her lifetime.

Science is served by both types of people. But difficulties can arise when someone is no longer an observer or a participant, but becomes a traditionalist who believes something can be only a certain way. Often it's because that is the way it has long been accepted, or it simply suits what makes sense to them. If they stubbornly hold on to that position, they'll always "succeed" in making their view the right one. They end up going nowhere, as their path is against nature. They want their own answer... rather than letting nature show hers.

Instead, a scientist must start with the idea that fueled their curiosity. But their theory must be tested, as we did when we simply combined the lowering of calcium and the raising of the pH. We found our premise *didn't* work. If I'd held fast onto our theory and kept trying to prove it true, we never would have moved beyond it to find the answer we did.

Science provided me with the answer, not my opinions.

Timing is Everything — Prevention or Treatment?

Creating our blood reperfusion solution seemed to be a great accomplishment. Persistence, hard work, and expansive thinking led to creating a solution that could *reverse the injury* that had been occurring during heart surgeries.

That got me thinking again. I wondered — if we can reverse the injury after the surgery — *could we prevent those injuries from happening in the first place?*

An epiphany can strike at the oddest time. Even finding a long-sought answer (like blood reperfusion) can usher in a *new* launching point for ideas.

Up until then, only a water-based (crystalloid) cardioplegia solution had been given to help protect the heart during surgery. ...But what about administering a *blood cardioplegic solution* as the operation started — similar to what we had developed for reperfusion — but instead now give this solution as the operation *is to begin?*

Birth of "Blood Cardioplegia"

Of course, our proposal to also use a controlled reperfusate at the beginning of the surgery had to be tested.

But before we would experiment with starting our blood cardioplegia as the operation began, I wanted to make sure we would be *maximizing the usefulness* of the solution. I started with a fundamental question: "Is only one dose of cardioplegia solution needed during surgery?" A single dose was the customary method at the time... but I had a good reason to speculate there might be a better approach.

When I had first returned to UCLA to join the faculty in 1971, Dr. Maloney's lab was also being used to study heart transplantation. Dr. Colin Bayliss, a research fellow from Canada, was conducting studies that showed a donor heart could be stopped with a cardioplegia solution before it was removed from the donor's body and stored cold (to lower metabolism) for up to 24 hours — before being placed into the recipient's body. The heart function was excellent after it was transplanted.

Dr. Bayliss concluded that he had discovered the ideal cardioplegic solution! Then something rather baffling occurred.

He tried this cardioplegic solution in a simulated cardiac operation in which he clamped the aorta for just 3 hours (versus the 24 hours without blood required for transplantation). This approach also differed in that the heart was not removed (as it is during transplantation). The result?

The three-hour heart *could not recover.*

You might expect the response to be *better* than with a transplant, since there is no trauma of removal from the body. Yet the substantially impaired heart function repeatedly occurred, making it impossible to consider using this cardioplegia solution in patients. Something was happening in the living heart that made the cardioplegia less effective.

I now believed that solving this riddle could help us improve our ability to protect the heart.

The sharing of ideas forms the foundation of research. Each Monday morning, I met with two or three of my research fellows, and Dr. Maloney when he was in town. I proposed my theory at one of these brainstorming sessions.

"It seems the difference between the successful heart function in a transplanted heart — and the failure during simulated surgery — means that the *cardioplegia solution was somehow no longer present* in the living subject's heart."

My research fellows looked puzzled. One spoke up: "With all due respect, we close the aorta before injecting the cardioplegia solution, so there is no incoming blood flow to wash it out of the living heart."

I responded, "That makes perfect sense, and is what everyone believes. But what if that's not correct?"

Again, puzzled looks.

I explained, "Obviously, the cardioplegic solution stays in the removed heart that is headed for transplant. But in the heart that stays in the body during open-heart surgery — could there be tiny vessels within the pericardium (the tissue sac immediately surrounding the heart), that could wash out our cardioplegic solution — despite the absence of any blood flow coming in through the coronary artery?"

Silence now blanketed our meeting room, as my usually animated colleagues let this theory sink in.

Fortunately, the tools to test this concept were in our hands. We designed a study using microspheres.

We experimentally mimicked open-heart surgery by stopping blood flow to the heart by clamping the aorta — and then injected microspheres into the body circulation via the heart-lung machine. This meant that any microsphere that reached the heart would have to come from collateral blood vessels in the pericardium.

As it turned out, they *did* reach the heart. The observed flow rate of 3 ml/minute was adequate enough to wash away any cardioplegic solutions![14]

We had uncovered something previously unknown (a cardioplegic solution would be constantly washed out of a heart) — that would impact how to deliver cardioplegic solutions to patients.

This led to our next study, built upon the simple principle: if it's gone, let's replace it.

Once is Good — More is Very Good

We could not avoid this flow that can wash away any cardioplegia solution, so we developed a plan to intermittently replenish it — to preserve its protective actions. We asked, "Would that be effective? And how often should the dose be repeated?"

We clamped the aorta for 60 minutes to simulate conditions during an aortic or mitral valve replacement. These studies were conducted by Roy Nelson, a cardiac resident surgeon from New York University who came to work with me for two years.[15] One group of test subjects received a standard, single dose, crystalloid (water-based) cardioplegic solution... while the other received repeated doses every 20 minutes.

Single-dose delivery led to a moderate decrease in heart function.

But the multi-dose cardioplegia resulted in *completely normal function*.

This was an extraordinary development that had clear implications for our patients!

It pointed out the problems with single-dose delivery, and opened the door to establishing a new, multi-dose protocol that may *avoid* the perplexing heart injuries that can still accompany technically perfect operations.

Though we wouldn't know it then, these findings became the seminal investigations for using multi-dose cardioplegia during open-heart surgery.

Blood is Thicker (*and Way Better*) than Water

We now knew our multi-dose method of delivering conventional crystalloid cardioplegic solutions was superior to the standard single dose. But we needed to take the next step: could our *blood cardioplegia* replace these water-based solutions in operations on our patients?

This seemed like a natural approach, since our bodies have blood running through their vessels, not water. Plus, excellent results had followed our giving a blood cardioplegia *reperfusion* solution after a prolonged period of ischemia. The question now was: would such superb recovery take place if this solution is delivered *throughout the period of aortic clamping?* Could it better prevent the heart from being injured?

A powerful test was needed, since this was a new concept, and if successful, would create a revolutionary shift in treating patients when the aorta is clamped during open-heart surgery.

An extended surgery was simulated by using *four hours of aortic clamping* with multi-doses of our blood cardioplegia solution. This four-hour length would account for the time needed for even the most prolonged operations.

But would it work?

In a nutshell, the results were spectacular.[16]

In fact, the outcomes mirrored those found in hearts that are simply left on the heart-lung machine and allowed to continue beating for four hours without aortic clamping. The findings were enthralling, because heart normality was preserved!

The Big Test

It was now time to take our discovery from "bench to bedside" by seeing how these new protocols worked on our patients.

The agenda was straightforward. There would be three protective phases during an operation. First, cardioplegia is introduced when we clamp the aorta. Second, there are maintenance doses every 20 minutes during clamping. Third, controlled reperfusion is administered before returning the body's own blood flow.

We tested this approach in 77 consecutive patients. The results were again outstanding![17]

The other UCLA cardiac surgeons were thrilled as we all came to a profound conclusion: "This will change the thinking about myocardial protection all over the world."

Welcome Acceptance

Our final step was to report these findings to the American Association of Thoracic Surgery. This was 1978, three years after I had presented to AATS when Rodewald from Germany marched up to the podium after me and opened my eyes to a new possibility for cardioplegia. It was time to present the results of what had sent me soaring in a new direction.

There was great sense of anticipation at the conference, as the immense potential of what we had found was evident to those that scheduled the order of presentations. They scheduled our paper to be presented first. I was pleased by this, though I wouldn't do the presentation myself. My name would be on the paper and that was all I needed. I was already known in the cardiac community. This was an opportunity for the research fellow to present it, as he had done the experimental and clinical analyses. In this case, David Follette.

I sat in the audience as David went up to the podium. He gave a wonderful presentation. The crowd of over 4,000 surgeons listened keenly. They recognized the impact that this discovery would yield.[17]

It would allow surgeons to no longer feel compelled to rush through procedures, in order to limit the time a heart would be stopped when its blood supply is interrupted. Cardiac surgery would be transformed as patients would survive and recover more fully than ever before. We had made operations much safer for them (and 40 years later… this innovation continues to be used).

This achievement was profoundly fulfilling. The ability to give to others, as encouraged by my mother and grandmother, now seemed to be within my grasp. Helping to ensure the success of cardiac surgery was a goal that exceeded what I'd imagined when my studies had begun several years earlier. Yet I also knew we still needed to await further testing before the full magnitude of this concept could be confirmed.

CHAPTER 7

Improvement: Cardioplegia Saves Lives

After observing and studying why the *heart was more hurt than helped* during open-heart surgery, we reported our new findings at the American Association of Thoracic Surgery. We described a successful approach that solved this universal problem.

You'd think I would be on top of the world.

The fact is, I nearly lost my job.

Although cardiac surgeons throughout the national and international community became early adopters of blood cardioplegia — because they now could have a safe and much longer operating environment in which to do their delicate work — the reality is that cardiac surgeons do not always have the final word in how a procedure will be performed. The patients' primary heart doctors are cardiologists, who act as gatekeepers. They refer patients and frequently try to prescribe the operative procedures.

I learned of this barrier initially at UCLA, where the cardiologists discarded our new treatment. They were angry and frustrated, and called for a joint meeting (of their group and the cardiac surgeons) to accuse the surgeons of experimenting on their patients.

They claimed our new blood cardioplegia procedure was "radical," and responsible for the "closures" of coronary artery bypass grafts that were occurring four months after the bypass procedures were performed. Yet they presented no evidence that blood cardioplegia had anything to do with these closures.

I responded to their questions by comparing our past use of intermittent ischemia (the periodic aortic clamping that *we* had also created) with the newly developed blood cardioplegia, and also provided the experimental results demonstrating its safety after four hours of aortic clamping, to justify why our clinical results with patients had improved with this new technique.

My presentation fell on deaf ears. The cardiologists were adamant about accounting for why some grafts closed four months after the operation. They could not find the cause, and they had to blame someone. That someone was us — me, in particular.

I wondered if I might be dismissed from the faculty. But a counterbalance also existed, as my fellow surgeons at UCLA embraced the new methodology, and it was being adopted by many surgeons that practiced outside our institution.

I was confounded and annoyed by the actions of my accusers. Who rejects proven science? Why would anyone dismiss procedures that have substantively shown improvement in the care of their patients? These were questions I could not yet answer. Unfortunately, it would not be the last time I would ask them.

I decided to spend no additional time on this conundrum. We had more work to do on our blood cardioplegia solution. My credo was that research is never completed. Instead, the process involves posing the next question that each discovery generates. The excitement and beauty of this pattern unfolds to involve observation, new questioning, and then testing to learn and grow. This unending thirst for understanding is what unveils the magnificence of science.

Our cardioplegia protocol was a major breakthrough — but could it be made better? I believed it could. I decided to explore how to magnify its usefulness by simplifying our method of its delivery.

Temperature — A Matter of Degree(s)

Aside from focusing upon how to use cardioplegia, I realized we needed to determine *the best temperature at which to deliver it* during different times of the surgical procedure.

A ripe area to explore. Hypothermia was a well-established added strategy to cool the heart when the aorta is clamped. Cooling lowers the heart's need for energy (metabolism), which falls 50% for every ten-degree drop in temperature. Conversely, the heartbeat is strengthened following warm cardioplegia delivery.[18]

To me, this observation suggested a balance might exist, whereby the blood cardioplegia solution could be delivered at different temperatures during the various phases of the procedure: starting the operation, throughout the procedure, and during reperfusion after it is complete.

With this in mind, I posed the following possibility to my team at one of our weekly meetings: "What if there wasn't *just one best temperature* to use with these solutions? Nature itself is commonly composed of blends, the most obvious being its alternating temperatures of day and night. What if it is better to use different temperatures during different parts of the operation?"

A radical idea, but the team was excited by how the world of free thinking had entered our research effort.

Testing with the Damaged Heart

While many of our studies began with a normal heart, we understood that normal hearts are uncommon in patients that need cardiac operations. Instead, their hearts are weakened and vulnerable to damage — they barely limp along. Protecting such damaged hearts was our mission, so we needed to do studies with a new experimental approach that mimicked the kinds of hearts we typically encountered.

To create such damage, we subjected pigs to 45 minutes of aortic clamping at normal temperature without any cardiac protection. It worked, as there was only 25% of ventricular performance recovery after the aortic clamp was removed. This mirrored the very vulnerable hearts that we cardiac surgeons commonly face.

Those hearts must then confront the added challenge of undergoing the prolonged period of aortic clamping (no blood supply) that cardiac surgeons will require to surgically correct the difficult underlying cardiac defect. These are termed *high-risk* patients, since recovery of such injured hearts may be precarious.

We simulated this experimentally by subjecting the animals having damaged hearts (due to their having undergone 45 minutes of aortic clamping without any effort to protect the heart) — to two more hours of aortic clamping with myocardial protection. This time frame mirrored the 120 minutes that we needed to correct a severe underlying heart problem. During this interval, we applied each of our new cardioplegic protection methods, as described below:

We started by delivering a five-minute introduction of warm blood cardioplegia, intending to improve nourishment to the damaged heart before its undergoing prolonged aortic clamping. Then gave four minutes of cold blood cardioplegia to limit damage during aortic clamping, repeating this cold solution every 20 minutes over two hours. Finally, a warm reperfusion was delivered just before removing the aortic clamp.

The outcomes were astonishing: cardiac performance in these vulnerable already damaged hearts *returned to 85% of normal!*[19] Just imagine: these high-risk hearts initially could only show 25% recovery. Yet our dramatically improved results (85% recovery) meant use of our cardioplegia method allowed us to "repair the heart metabolically," while at the same time to surgically "correct it mechanically."

Recognizing that the heart ended up *better* than when it started — made us appreciate that we had developed a very powerful new tool to prevent injury.

Oxygen Metabolism — Making Better Even Better

Understandably, we were thrilled. Our cardioplegia protocol *by itself* helped "an already hurt heart get better." When we informed Dr. Maloney, he was astounded and elated as well.

As always, our result — no matter how good it may be — does not only provide an answer. It also provides the next question, so we naturally asked, "Could its effectiveness be even further enhanced?"

This question brought me back to recognizing that the pursuit of scientific growth is often tightly linked to returning to the basic sciences. That attitude is usually absent in freshman medical school students. They often grow impatient with studying basic anatomy, biochemistry, and physiology. They want to "study sick patients, just like a real doctor." They don't understand that physicians must know these basics — especially about oxygen metabolism — to help them make effective decisions.

Yet little did I realize as a medical student, how these lessons about oxygen could subsequently help me learn to better protect a patient's heart from sustaining damage.

One magical gift of the laboratory environment is exposure to the ongoing thoughts of our research fellows. Their inquisitiveness inspires much of our progress. In 1986, Harold Lazar, a resident surgical fellow from the University of Michigan, spent two years in our research laboratory. He only studied damage after aortic clamping, and never did any cardioplegia research.

But Harold was very observant. He knew the healthy heart extracts about 75% of the oxygen from the blood that nourishes it. As a result, the blood that exits the heart (called venous blood) has a very dark blue color because nearly all of the oxygen (that gives its red color) is extracted in the healthy heart.

He came into my office one day with a troubled look on his face.

"What is it, Harold?" I asked.

"I have a question. Could the heart's metabolism be altered after we have stopped the blood flow?"

A curious question indeed. "What did you see, Harold?"

"When I've been restarting blood flow to the hearts of our sick animals after their own blood supply had been clamped off, I noticed the venous blood exiting the heart is red — rather than the dark blue it should be."

My eyes lit up. It was a striking observation.

"Red? So you're thinking that after they've had their blood supply removed for an interval of time… when it's restarted, these hearts are for some reason less able to extract oxygen from blood?"

"Exactly," Harold confirmed. "If they can't extract oxygen, maybe there's some damage to the mitochondria [tiny cellular structures] where energy metabolism takes place."

I took a moment to lean back in my chair, taking in this prospect.

Then Harold added, "I was also thinking — we know the amino acid glutamate is a key ingredient for the heart to metabolize oxygen. What if we simply add some glutamate into the reperfusion solution to see what happens?"

That suggestion triggered my memories of basic science classes in med school, and the roles that amino acids glutamate and aspartate played in heart metabolism.

I encouraged Harold, "If you can figure out how much glutamate to give it, please start the new experiment. I look forward to seeing the outcomes."

Harold did just that. He added glutamate into the blood at the end of the clamping period, and to his absolute delight, observed that the venous blood exiting the heart, which was previously red, now became blue! This meant the heart markedly enhanced its capacity to metabolize oxygen — most likely due to better mitochondria metabolism — and its performance substantially improved.[20]

Upon hearing his report, I said, "Harold, that is really amazing. How much glutamate did you add?"

"10.83 grams," he told me.

I was impressed with his precision in dose selection. "How did you arrive at exactly 10.83 grams?"

Harold hesitated a moment before answering. "Actually, I was searching the literature and the only thing I could find was that 10.83 grams was given to children with diarrhea."

"Diarrhea?"

"Yes. That was it."

"So Harold, you're essentially telling me it was a total shot in the dark."

"You could say that."

I began to laugh. Diarrhea was a pretty far cry from our exploring impaired cardiac metabolism. Sometimes discoveries are stumbled upon in the most unexpected ways.

Actually, I didn't know *how* unexpected until just last year — 31 years after Harold did this experiment.

I ran into Harold at an AATS meeting in Seattle, where I mentioned I was including his story in my memoir.

His amused response was, "Gerry, would you like to know how I *really* arrived at that figure of 10.83 grams of glutamate?"

"I thought I knew. It was a component of the diarrhea formula."

"No," Harold admitted. "I just told you that because it sounded more plausible than how it really occurred."

I stared at him. "The diarrhea story sounded *more plausible* than the method you really used? Harold... how *did* you arrive at that number?"

"I phoned up several Chinese restaurants and asked how much monosodium glutamate they put in their noodles. Then I used that information to calculate the amount of pure glutamate to use in our formula. And it worked — experimentally and in patients — and has continued to work for last 31 years."

Harold's prior story of determining glutamate dosage from studies of infants with diarrhea had been amusing. But his real explanation was hilarious. Who knew Chinese cooking would play such an historic role in cardiac medicine! I'm well aware that great revelations can come out of unusual events, but this had to be a first, strange as it was.

Harold then mischievously added, "By the way, my deep reasoning behind the Chinese restaurant query was that if it didn't make the customers sick and they came back for more, it would work on our patients."

I looked at Harold a moment and had to laugh out loud again. I've always encouraged my students to think outside the box *and* to maintain a good sense of humor about their work. Now 31 years later, I was reminded that one of the beauties of having students is their taking on the playful humor of their teacher, and then letting it fully blossom.

Despite how it came about, Harold's calculated addition of glutamate was successful, and his contribution proved to be a superb benefit that substantially improved recovery of injured hearts after their blood supply had been clamped off.

Although excellent results followed the use of glutamate in our cardioplegia solutions, we must always search for newer ways to make it even better. Sometimes a symphony already sounds great, but adding an extra violin or viola may make the music even sweeter.

Eliot Rosenkranz, a subsequent research fellow from UCLA that worked with me, wondered if the damaged heart was also deficient in aspartate, the other amino acid that plays a vital role in heart metabolism. He added this to the formula and found excellent results.[19] This enriched blood cardioplegic solution, with glutamate and aspartate, has been used ever since as a component of how we protect the heart during cardiac surgery.

The real beauty of our enhanced formula was that the cardiac surgeon now had the key tools to accomplish a dual purpose. First, we can fix the heart *mechanically* by the technical excellence of the operative procedure. Second, we can repair it *metabolically* by using our cardioplegia approach to help it at the cellular level. This combination allows us to provide the complete package of "repair and protection" to our patients.

A lesson became clear: basic biochemistry learned in medical school should not be dismissed. It furnishes the fundamental knowledge that is needed to uncover the critical stepping stones for solving clinical problems.

All Together Now....

I have enormous respect for the interdependency within a treatment protocol. Despite this vital interaction, I'm often asked by cardiac surgeons: "Of your entire cardioplegia protocol, which techniques have you found to be the most important?"

No doubt the inquiry was posed in the hopes they could select one or two items that are so highly effective that they could forgo the rest, giving them a shortcut to simplify their operations. But my answer always will compare cardioplegic techniques to a symphony. If the conductor were asked to identify the most important instrument, he would say it is the one that is not playing correctly. The harmony of an orchestra exists during myocardial protection, and intertwining the cardioplegic blood solution, its temperature, and route of delivery will define a critical and useful strategy for optimizing heart protection during cardiac procedures. All the instruments playing together are what make the music so powerful.

Going Backward is a Vital Step Forward

Our cardioplegia formulations became widely used, patients' lives were saved, and their post-operative health improved. While delighted, I also recognized our formulations can only fully protect the heart — if they are distributed to all the needy areas within it. Impediments to that existed, and they needed to be overcome.

For example, coronary artery bypass procedures were the most common cardiac surgical operation between the 1970s and 2000. These were done to correct narrowed coronary arteries, which obstruct blood flow to the heart muscle — and *will also restrict the cardioplegia solution* from getting into parts of the heart during the surgery. Stated most simply, it cannot work if it cannot be delivered.

This was the future challenge I alluded to back in chapter 2, citing that many years later I would adapt the cannula that I invented during my military service to deliver cardioplegia solutions *backward*. It was at UCLA in the late 1980s when we adapted this cannula to provide retrograde (backward) delivery by inserting the cannula through a tiny incision in the right atrium.

The benefit of this is that there is *no obstruction* when you give the cardioplegia solution from the reverse direction. The heart becomes wonderfully perfused, and this approach became a godsend for surgeons performing coronary bypass operations.

Becomes Universal Innovation

As so frequently occurs, our new development led to a fresh question: should *both* forward and backward delivery of cardioplegia be used in *any* operation, not just when there's a blockage with coronary artery disease?

The answer to this new inquiry became clear after we made a set of *unexpected observations* during an aortic valve replacement operation.

When we started giving blood cardioplegia forward (into the aorta), we sampled the venous blood exiting the heart and noted that it had the expected dark blue color. All was good — the heart was properly taking up the oxygen delivered by the blood cardioplegia. But after about two minutes, this exiting blood turned red again. To us, this meant we were giving more blood flow than the heart required — since its needs were low because it was decompressed and it had stopped contracting. It was natural for us to believe that all portions of the heart were receiving adequate flow, and that the heart did not need to take up any more oxygen.

But then our chief resident suggested, "Let's try delivering retrograde cardioplegia."

An interesting idea. So we gave the red (oxygenated) blood cardioplegic solution *backward...* and watched the color of the blood draining from the coronary artery openings. To our surprise, *it was blue blood draining from these vessels!* That meant the heart *still needed to take up more oxygen* from the blood than it was receiving from the normal forward cardioplegia — a possibility that only became apparent after we tried the backward delivery.

This unanticipated finding showed us that retrograde (backward) delivery entered areas that the forward flow did not adequately reach and nourish.

We realized this lack of full perfusion during forward blood cardioplegia delivery is true in *any* heart, and led us to develop *a new protocol* for forward *and* backward flow during all cardiac procedures.

This became the standard for cardioplegia delivery, and over 7 million of these modified cannulas have been used.

Life-Saving Erector Set

As a youngster, one of my favorite toys was the Erector Set, with which I spent hours in the solitude of my bedroom as I built new and exciting creations. Such innovative building tendencies — and our hunger for playful inventiveness — usually end as childhood stops. Yet I'm convinced that our minds retain the powerful desires associated with these innocent joys of accomplishment.

One of my most rewarding creations was the development of blood cardioplegia. Given the importance of what my team found, we pledged to translate our concepts into protocols — and devices — to deliver these treatments in simple, safe, and speedy ways so they could gain broad use.

Initial steps toward making this widely accessible began in 1980, when Shiley Inc. developed a blood cardioplegia device that could effectively administer its delivery. This device is shown alongside one that delivers cardioplegia in a water mixture that does not contain blood, in **Figure 1**.

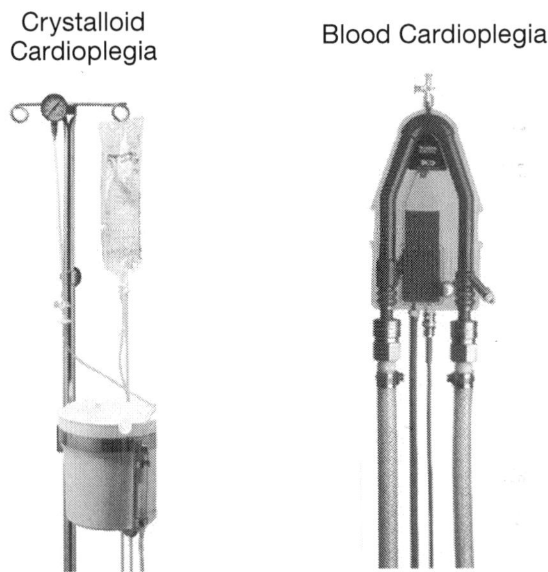

Figure 1: Original devices to deliver (on left) crystalloid (water-based) or (on right) blood cardioplegia that also can efficiently change the solution's temperature.

The next step was to develop a safe way to deliver the blood cardioplegic fluid, so that it could flow to the heart by either a forward path (via an artery) or a backward pathway (via a vein). Collaboration with Research Medical Industries yielded the development of a simple device that permitted delivery in either direction. (**Figure 2**)

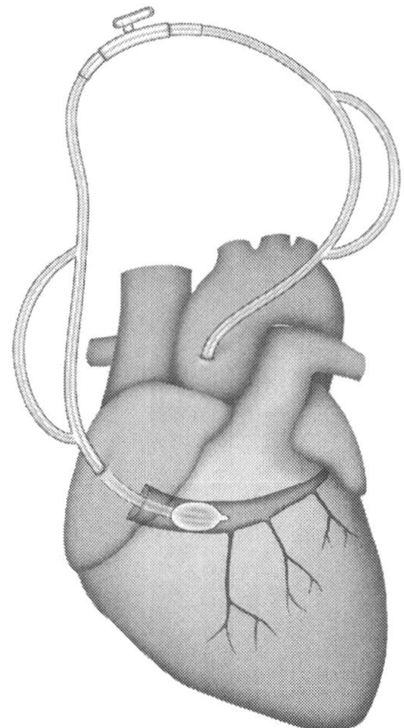

Figure 2: Integrated system to deliver blood cardioplegia antegrade (into aorta) or retrograde (via coronary vein), together with a simple stop cock to change the direction.

Of course, an effective and reliable cardioplegic solution needed to be affordably manufactured, stored, and distributed. Two pharmaceutical companies, CAPS and Koehler, came through and within a short time, the solution was widely available in the United States and Europe.

The development of this entire blood cardioplegia delivery system was a game-changer. Now the cardiac surgeon had the ability to enter the operating room and utilize his or her own Erector Set during every cardiac procedure. That included me, as the residents liked to jest, "Uncle Bucky is having fun operating with his own devices."

I felt gratified for having never let go of my child-like joy for innovation, and for now being able to share its fruits with others. In fact, in a moment of lightheartedness, I once teased a dear friend, Jim Barnard, who had made some playful observation about life, "Jim, when will you grow up?"

He paused a moment before he answered. "Bucky, I want to be just like you. I never want to grow up. I just want to grow old."

I had to laugh. As adults, I think we secretly yearn for ways to resurrect our youthful past. When a child is fortunate enough to become a cardiac surgeon, their greatest reward may well be entering the laboratory and the operating room. For my own operative procedures, I will admit it has been exhilarating to use the techniques I designed.

If It is Good, Let Others Tell the Story

From the beginnings of our success in development of blood cardioplegia, its use naturally began to spread to others who would report their own positive outcomes.

This included Floyd (Fred) Loop at the Cleveland Clinic, an open-minded person who welcomed the improvements our methods offered over conventional techniques of myocardial protection. As it would turn out, my association with Fred would prove very fortunate in forwarding the widespread clinical implementation of blood cardioplegia.

A change to treatment methods like ours comes with one additional consideration beyond their effectiveness: the ever-present concern of financial costs. This was true in our case since use of our novel devices added an initial cost of $250 per operative procedure when compared to crystalloid cardioplegia approaches — which are simpler as potassium chloride is simply added to a liter of clear solution and delivered into the aorta.

Instead, our technology required use of a blood cardioplegia delivery device, a special catheter in the aorta with another in the coronary sinus, and a cardioplegic solution that must be mixed with the blood in the heart-lung machine before delivery. Hence, the additional $250 expense.

While that hardly seems a significant figure, when multiplied by thousands of patients, it becomes a consideration for any institution — and was causing some to be hesitant.

Seeking a better perspective, Fred and I discussed the *whole cost* of hospitalization, rather than just operating room costs alone. Fred decided to conduct a more complete evaluation.

Fred operated on 819 consecutive patients with our techniques, and compared his results with those of five other experienced surgeons who used conventional crystalloid cardioplegia on 2,582 Cleveland Clinic patients. The resulting data showed that patients receiving our blood cardioplegia experienced one day less in the intensive care unit and one day less in the hospital. After his reporting these outcomes to me, I asked Fred if it was possible to summarize hospital costs. He did — and the results showed that overall costs were $2,200 higher for each patient receiving crystalloid cardioplegia.

Not only that, there was an entire additional group of patients called "outliers," whose conditions (having impaired recovery after surgery) required extended intensive care unit stays and longer hospitalizations, and were not considered in his first overall analysis. Overall costs for these "outlier patients" were up to fourfold higher. Interestingly, the number of outliers who had received crystalloid cardioplegia was *three times* the number of those who got blood cardioplegia.

Consequently, even though our innovative changes in myocardial protection added $250 per patient in operating costs — it saved the Cleveland Clinic over $10 million per year (they did 5,000 operations) when you factor in follow-up care in the intensive care unit and overall hospital stay.[21]

Fred Loop's analysis predicted that general acceptance of our innovative approach would save around $650 million annually, basing this savings on the 300,000 U.S. patients undergoing cardiac surgery each year at the time. Today, over 1 million cardiac procedures are done every year nationally and internationally, so these cost savings are amplified significantly more.

This financial analysis accelerated the adoption of our new methodology. The impact of our discoveries has only flourished in the 40 years since their beginnings. Today, 80% of surgeons worldwide use blood cardioplegia. Of those patients receiving blood cardioplegia, 6 million procedures were done with our blood cardioplegic delivery device, while 19 million patients received blood cardioplegia with comparable devices — such that over 25 million patients have now received blood cardioplegia. Additionally, over 4 million operations have been done with our retrograde catheter, and well over 4 million patients have received our specific cardioplegic formula during their operations.

While it is hard to calculate all the hearts that have been protected and how many lives have been saved from injury over the years, knowing that our work has expanded the safety and success level for the patient and for their surgeon provides me with the finest reward I could ever imagine.

The Investigator's Path

Throughout my career, my research has always begun with the observation of a problem. But the path to finding a solution to each problem continually varies and is filled with fortuitous encounters, surprising outcomes, and unintended benefits.

For the discovery of blood cardioplegia, my journey began simply by listening to Dr. Kirklin's observation of a heart that became stiff after receiving reperfusion to restore its blood flow. This led me to discoveries *and* a laboratory test where blending our two winning strategies of reducing calcium and raising pH in our reperfusion created *worse* results. Recognizing that this failure was based on an incorrect observation of ventricular fibrillation, led to our adding potassium that solved the true underlying problem, which created a protocol of multiple doses of blood cardioplegia. We then progressed to delivering them at different temperatures at various stages, in both forward and backward flows. My education came full circle as I even became a medical student again. I needed to relearn basic biochemistry in order to properly realize the value of understanding, and then using, amino acids to resolve a fundamental heart problem.

It was a series of many steps leading to a treatment method that is now nearly universally used as the primary form of cardiac protection. I have been extremely gratified by our accomplishment, which came nearly 20 years after I first observed the "heart more hurt than healed" during my internship at Johns Hopkins.

I would continue this pattern throughout my career: looking at a problem, taking three to six years to solve it, then moving onto the next problem.

I eagerly expected that our future discoveries, just like blood cardioplegia, would be equally embraced by the medical community to benefit the lives of patients.

I would find I was mistaken.

CHAPTER 8

You Don't Have to Die of a Heart Attack

My maternal grandfather, Zelig Levitt, had seven children and even more grandchildren. Grandpa was deeply religious and spoke mostly Yiddish. Yet none of us had trouble understanding him as he telegraphed his meaning through gestures, eye contact, and warmth.

He worked in the garment industry and had an ever-present twinkle in his eyes. Grandpa possessed grace and dignity, and was a role model whose lifelong dedication to hard work and persistence reflected his immigrant background.

Throughout my childhood, we celebrated Shabbat every Friday night with Grandma's delicious old-world cooking. Grandpa sat at the head of the table, cracking jokes and making observations, all in Yiddish. He groaned with pleasure as he ate Grandma's scrumptious kosher meals. His joy made us giggle and glad to be together.

His strength and vitality never waned, until the day I came home from school and found my mother crying on the phone. Grandpa was in the hospital. He had suffered a myocardial infarction. In layman's terms: a heart attack. As a 14-year-old who knew nothing about the human heart, I struggled to understand how this could have happened so suddenly. There were no warning signs. One day, he was hard at work and the next he was in the hospital, hanging on by a thread.

We raced to the hospital to see him. His doctors met us in the lobby and told us the hard truth: it didn't look good. "When a heart attack comes on suddenly," said a man in a white lab coat, "25% of people don't survive."

Tragically, the doctor was right. Grandpa died in the hospital two days later. The man who was larger than life, always so full of strength and vitality, died in a narrow white hospital bed. He never knew what hit him.

Family Affliction

Sadly, this was not the last brush with heart disease in my family. Many years later, I received a call from my father, who by this time was living in Florida.

"Hi Gerald," he said, his voice as bright as ever. But I knew something was wrong immediately. My father hated talking on the phone, so his calls came only in times of need or emergency. By now I was an adult, and an M.D. My father wasn't just calling his son; he was calling his physician.

"Dad, how are you?" I asked, deeply concerned.

"Oh fine. Listen, I just had something happen that Mom wanted me to share with you. I was out on one of my walks, enjoying the evening, and all of a sudden I got a very strong sense of...." He cleared his throat. "Well, it was a crushing pain right in the middle of my chest. Like an elephant sitting on my breastbone. Couldn't breathe. Funniest thing. Totally stopped me in my tracks. Do you have any idea what that might have been?"

I did. I asked him to describe if he had experienced any involuntary movements in reaction to the pain.

"Well, as a matter of fact, as pain shot down my arm — my arm raised and my hand just came up over my chest, clenched like a fist."

"Which hand?"

"My left one."

Dad had just described a textbook example of angina, or heart pain, which comes from impaired blood supply to the heart. While I had the natural concerns that a son would have for his father, I needed to keep on my doctor's hat. I sent him to promptly see a cardiologist. They found he had a classic case of atherosclerosis — a substantial narrowing of his coronary arteries.

I wanted to make sure no additional heart damage occurred before his symptoms could be addressed. He was admitted to a Florida hospital. I called the surgeons at that facility to learn if they were considering operating on my dad. I wanted to know how they would protect the heart during his cardiac procedure. From their answers, I was not confident they would conduct the operation using the guidelines I had established. So as soon as my father was stable, I flew down there and brought him back on a plane to UCLA where he would be cared for by my colleagues if a coronary bypass became necessary, using the intermittent ischemia techniques we described at the AATS (this problem with Dad happened before we had created our cardioplegia approaches). It turned out that a coronary artery bypass was needed, and so three vein conduits were grafted (transplanted) from his leg onto his coronary arteries. These conduits detoured blood flow around the blockages within his coronary arteries to restore blood supply to his struggling heart.

Fortunately, tests afterward gave us good news. They showed his heart still had excellent function. We'd avoided the heart attack that would have inevitably followed if he'd been left untreated, and caught the symptoms early enough that he suffered no permanent heart muscle damage.

Fifteen years later, Dad wasn't so lucky. My parents had retired to Tamarack, Florida and were enjoying a new life of leisure when Dad's chest pain came back. He went in for more tests, which showed that two of the three grafts had closed. More importantly, several sections of the heart muscle were no longer functioning properly and the heart was dilated. Another coronary bypass procedure was performed and he had another good recovery. But it was clear that at some point, he had suffered a "silent" heart attack and the permanent damage to his heart was severe.

The term "silent" means there are no warning signs and the heart attack happens without chest pain. Unfortunately, the dark legacy left behind by a heart attack unfolds over time, as damaged heart muscle dilates (stretches beyond normal size) to cause the late symptom of heart failure.

Soon after, they discovered a tumor on his colon and admitted him for an abdominal procedure. In a patient with heart problems, even the simplest surgery can be life threatening. I caught the next flight and joined my worried mom. Early on the morning of the planned procedure, the nurse called to tell us that the procedure had been delayed because Dad was having difficulty breathing.

Mom and I drove to the hospital in silence. I'm sure we were both thinking of Grandpa Zelig and how we had rushed to the hospital all those years ago; how our worlds were rocked by his untimely death two days later. Together, we hurried down the halls to Dad's room where we found him awake and aware, but struggling miserably to take a deep breath. I grasped his shaking hand and reassured him that everything would be okay. He believed and trusted my judgment... but I knew that the damage to his heart wouldn't heal this time. Dad had congestive heart failure.

Congestive heart failure occurs when the heart has healed from the heart attack, but the tissue remains damaged. The injured heart muscle is so dysfunctional that the heart isn't an efficient pump anymore. It can no longer get a good blood supply to the liver, kidneys, legs, and feet. Heart contraction is inefficient, and the blood in the heart backs up into the lungs. This makes it hard to breathe or perform physical activities.

It turned Dad into a cardiac cripple. His heart had been so damaged that the muscle had stretched and weakened. He maintained his mental acuity, but lost his physical vitality. He was a shell of the man I had known. It seemed like he spent more time in the hospital than at home. Grappling with the ongoing symptoms of heart failure became nearly unbearable.

Soon after, he broke his hip. He went in for an operation to have hip replacement, but the surgeon came out after to tell us that Dad wasn't waking from the surgery. Initially they thought it was a stroke, but it became clear that Dad's problem was an overdose of anesthesia.

The surgeon in me immediately began planning a course of care and strategies to save him. "Okay, Mom," I said, attempting to rally my mother with forced optimism. "This isn't permanent. He's going to wake up, and there are a number of issues we'll need to immediately address. First we have to...."

My mother laid her hand softly over mine. "No, Gerald. We can't. It's time to stop. Ever since Dad's heart failure, he hasn't been living the life he wants. He goes in the emergency room now every two weeks. He can't do anything. It's deprived him of all the joys of life. It's over."

"*Over?*" The word echoed in my mind. For once, my busy brain stopped and I had no plan or response. I felt empty as my mother acknowledged what I couldn't: this was the end.

"Hospice," she said quietly.

Dad passed away six days later.

It had been many years since my father's passing when I turned the attention of our team toward heart attacks. I no longer felt the loss merely as a son; it was also impacting me as a doctor. Tracing my father's journey was proof that when not treated proactively, the health of a heart attack survivor can go from good to bad to ugly in a relatively short time. Dad's experience went like this:

1. acute chest pains (angina)
2. coronary artery grafting (weeks later)
3. loss of muscle from silent heart attack
4. devastating heart failure develops after the damaged heart dilates
5. death

It happened over a period of years, but for me and everyone else who loved my dad, the end still came way too fast.

If anything keeps me up at night, it's the memories of my grandfather and father when they were hearty and hale, interrupted by their premature decline. For many, the grim reaper appears as an acute heart attack, like it did for my Grandpa Zelig. It strikes without warning, as half of its victims have had no prior symptoms.

Yet even those who survive a heart attack, like my dad, rarely escape unscathed. Damaged heart muscle may severely curtail activities, joys, and pleasures while it gravely shortens lives. I never will forget holding my Dad's hand during his final moments in hospice when we said goodbye, watching life slowly leave his face as he drifted away.

Over a million people suffer heart attacks every year.

My family had to go through the loss of loved ones due to limited options for treating heart attacks and the secondary complication of congestive heart failure. I found this entirely unacceptable. I became determined to find a way for physicians to intervene in this process so others wouldn't have to suffer as our family and so many others had.

I found a new mission.

The Weakened Heart

Many people believe that if you survive a heart attack, you're one of the lucky ones. You might make some changes to your diet, begin exercising more, take better care of yourself, but you have your life back.

But the truth is hardly that simple... nor is your future that encouraging.

Heart attacks *cause the death of the muscle region* supplied by that closed artery. When your heart pumps too weakly, as it will commonly do after a substantial heart attack, no matter how much you improve health habits, it can cause ongoing inescapable fatigue. You may develop abnormal heart rhythms (called arrhythmia, where the heart beats irregularly, too fast, or too slow). What starts out as a nuisance all too often progresses to a debilitated heart that significantly impairs your life. It can become overwhelming, like in my father's experience, where you have very little energy and the least amount of activity or exercise exhausts you. Where you have to rest all the time and can't breathe unless you sit up in bed. Where your swelling is so bad that you cannot even put on your shoes and must go to the emergency room every two weeks to have fluid drained. Essentially, you're incapacitated.

Frankly, the remaining life expectancy of patients in advanced stages of congestive heart failure is worse than those with terminal cancers — with a 50% chance of dying in one year and a 75% chance of dying in two years.

Dual Objectives

To counter such grim prognoses, I would develop two distinct goals. My first, the focus of this and the next chapter, was to offset these effects of heart attacks by returning function to the damaged muscle, ensuring that patients remain well until the natural end of their lives. The premise is that preventing the injured muscle from dying will prevent heart failure from developing after a heart attack.

I would later pursue another goal — to correct congestive heart failure in patients whose heart attack was not initially treated correctly. This will be the subject of subsequent chapters.

But at this point — I was directing all our efforts toward discovering a way to prevent heart damage from ever occurring in the heart attack victim. To do this, we needed to cast aside conventional views that heart muscle cannot be saved if treated more than two hours after a heart attack. Instead, we would consider something that had never been examined before: providing the injured area with a controlled reperfusion, rather than only delivering normal blood reflow after the attack.

Though not consciously aware of it, my driving force was knowing that if I had developed such a successful approach ten years earlier, it could have made all the difference for my dad, and, if it was available when I was age 14... would have helped my Grandpa Zelig.

While I was aware that was no longer possible, it wasn't too late for the countless others who suffer from heart attacks every year. My hope was to catalyze a systemic change that ultimately could save many lives. We simply *had* to do better... because the adverse aftermath of conventional treatment was far too great.

More Than Observer

Our profession's code, the Hippocratic Oath, states "Do no harm." But it is often misused by today's medical community, and unknowingly creates our greatest obstacles to making discoveries.

Why?

Hippocrates was an observer. To the ancient Greeks, disease was as much a normal part of life as health. From his perspective, the job of a physician was to understand and describe disease with as much precision as health. He didn't believe that interventions could improve the patient's standard of life.

But today, disease and disability are not for us merely to observe and certainly not to accept. Hippocrates would be at a loss in a modern hospital, where so much of what we do is in direct contradiction to his basic observational philosophy. His enormous contributions have formed the cornerstone for how we interact with patients, but as with all hallmarks, it was simply the first step. Therapeutic approaches and health care advances have allowed us to utilize a whole modern universe of ideas on our patients, taking us far beyond anything Hippocrates could have ever imagined.

Yet some conventional thinking has taken up his view that certain circumstances are inevitable and simply part of the disease process. Such has been the case with treating heart attacks. The lasting damage accompanying them was believed unavoidable — that the primary goal was to keep the patient from dying from the heart attack — and was not aimed toward circumvention of the consequences that often came later.

Normality: The Shape of Things to Come

As Hippocrates wisely observed many centuries ago, disease is a departure from normality. I have stated in this book that in order to comprehend the abnormal heart, it is critical for us to first fully understand the proper functioning normal heart — *which is linked to its proper shape.*

Most physicians, and the general population itself, believe the heart simply squeezes (like closing a clenched fist) to circulate blood. But as we would discover — both in this study and later with even greater clarity (described in subsequent chapters) — a healthy heart has an *elliptical shape*, like a football, and actually *twists* to eject blood — and then recoils to fill efficiently.

This is important to know because one of the biggest problems with heart attacks is *they change the geometry of the heart*. This change in shape alters its ability to function — and not for the better.

As you read this, realize that you are about to know more about heart attacks than most people — including many cardiologists and heart surgeons who treat them.

With the heart, geometry is everything. Like so many of nature's beautiful creations, the heart has a helical (spiral) formation, which is responsible for the twisting actions. While many people mistakenly think the normal heart is a pump that simply compresses (squeezes) to circulate blood and then dilates (expands) to fill — that motion is only the case for patients suffering from congestive heart failure. When the diseased heart stretches abnormally and its helix (spiral) shape becomes deformed, it appears and reacts more like a rotating basketball rather than an efficient spiraling football.

That's a problem, because the spiral shape is the essence of efficiency in nature. Furthering the athletic analogy helps illustrate this process: a high school quarterback can throw an accurate 50-yard football pass, but even the best NBA guard cannot throw a basketball 20 yards with the same precision.

So how does this fundamental change in shape occur?

Anatomy of a Heart Attack

Heart attacks begin with narrowing of arteries — the large coronary blood vessels that nourish the heart muscle. They can narrow for a number of reasons. It can be from cholesterol and fatty deposits called plaque building up on their inner arterial walls (hardening of the arteries), which reduce the opening and restrict blood flow. This plaque can also develop a crack (or ulcer) that becomes an opening to allow blood to enter the inner surface of this arterial wall and become trapped, so a blood clot forms, obstructing the vessel. These sequences cause restriction of the blood supply to the muscular region of the heart. When the coronary artery is completely closed, a heart attack occurs.

After a heart attack, modern treatments employ different approaches to resolve the problem of a completely closed artery.

Cardiologists use drugs to dissolve the clots in the arteries, or open the artery with a catheter and balloon (angioplasty) to restore normal blood flow.

Alternatively, cardiac surgeons may perform a bypass graft, like the one my dad had, to carry the normal blood supply around the blockage. This is done by taking a portion of a healthy artery or vein from elsewhere in the body — and inserting one end into the healthy artery or aorta that exists before the stoppage, and inserting the other end into the *unobstructed* part of that vessel beyond the narrowing — so that it *passes by* the blocked segment to provide unrestricted flow.

To appreciate the value — *and limitations* — of these approaches, it helps to understand what typically occurs when someone is brought in with a heart attack.

It is not what most people believe (including many cardiologists and cardiac surgeons).

Customarily, sirens are blaring as the heart attack victim is rushed to the hospital in an ambulance or paramedic's van. The doors of the Emergency Room burst open as a team of paramedics wheel in a gurney carrying a prone man, his face awash in fear, as the EMT rattles off all known information about the patient to the attending physician: patient is in his 60s, slightly overweight; he has severe chest pain and shortness of breath, rapid heart rate, with a blood pressure of 100/80 (normal being 120/80).

The patient is evaluated and then hurried into the cath lab. A catheter is placed into his pulmonary artery to find that his heart-filling pressures are elevated and the amount of blood ejected by the heart is lower than normal. The *ejection fraction* (the percentage of blood in his heart getting pumped out to the body per beat) is reduced from a normal 60% down to 35%.

This is what they can measure.

What is *occurring inside* is that the damaged heart muscle area immediately loses its capacity to pump. *This causes the heart's structural anatomy to change*. Every time the heart contracts, this injured region of the ventricle will expand and thin — as some of the blood in the chamber does not pump out, but rather stretches or billows the damaged region, making the heart shape look like it has a blister. This bulge is called an aneurysm.

In addition to the pain felt by the patient, this bigger ventricle may develop arrhythmias (abnormal heart rhythms) — or it may contract inefficiently.

To counteract the dysfunction of this now bulging region, the remaining still-functioning muscle areas (called the "remote muscle" — away from the damaged muscle) must also stretch or expand to help the heart pump more forcibly — to ensure the body has adequate circulation.

The result is that as the dead heart attack region develops its new bulging form, the heart's overall shape becomes more circular — like a basketball — instead of its natural elliptical or football-like appearance.

So what treatment will counter these effects?

At first glance, coronary angioplasty seems like a perfect remedy, since blockage of blood flow caused the heart attack in the first place. Cardiologists insert a catheter into the artery, push it beyond the blockages, and then deploy a balloon to stretch the narrowed vessels... a maneuver that will dramatically provide the patient with new blood supply. To assess this, the monitors are promptly checked by the treatment team:

"His blood pressure is back to 120 over 80."

"Pulse rate has dropped from 110 to 80 beats per minute."

"His pulmonary blood pressure is down... his cardiac output is better... his ejection fraction has increased from 35% to 50%."

The conscious patient chimes in by reporting, "Thanks, my chest pain is gone."

With his vessels once again cleared and his heart action improved, the patient is sent to the cardiac ward for observation and recovery. The treatment team congratulates themselves on another life saved.

What Really Happened

Without question, the initial results support the conclusion that this patient's life has been preserved. His chest pain is immediately relieved. His blood pressure increases, heart rate falls, and heart-filling pressures decrease. Everything looks good.

Indeed, these modern treatments have reduced the overall mortality that immediately follows a heart attack — due to abnormal heart rhythms (which can lead to dangerous ventricular fibrillation), or due to heart failure (causing lung congestion) — from around 20% down to about 5%. A powerful confirmation.

But it is essential to understand *why* the heart has improved — and after the patient leaves the hospital — how this "improvement" alters their future.

When the angioplasty restores blood flow, the bulging dead muscle in the heart attack region *shrinks* to a smaller, thickened — *though still non-contracting* region. (**Figure 1**) This heart changes shape in response to the now smaller size of the ventricle, so that the still-functioning (also called "viable" or "living") remote muscle no longer needs to stretch as much to compensate for diminished function. The bulge disappears, and the now smaller heart size begins to reflect a more normal shape.

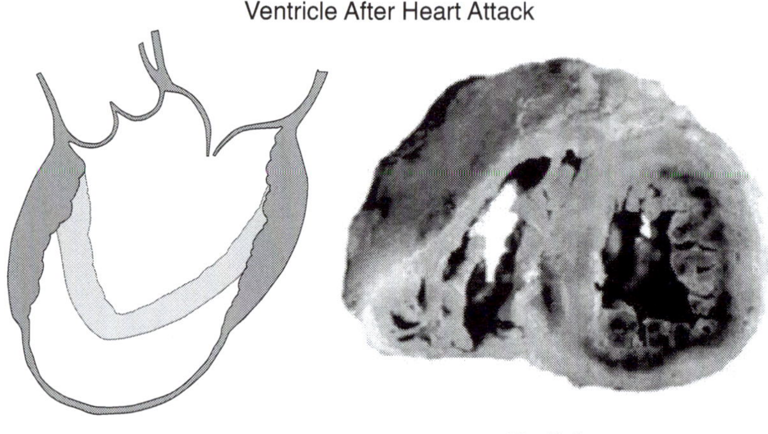

Figure 1: On left: cardiac shape of the normal heart in lighter gray color, showing its natural elliptical or V shape before a heart attack. The circular outer form (darker shading) displays the effects of a heart attack where the injured muscle becomes spherical.

On right: cross section of heart attack region after angioplasty has successfully restored blood reflow. Note extensive damage (toward the right side) shown by the darkened area in the inner shell of deeper muscle. The outer muscle shell is undamaged so that the heart surface appears normal, yet this entire region does not function.

Everything seems better. The treatment appears to have offset the heart attack. *But this conclusion is incorrect.*

The reality is it hasn't helped the heart attack area's ability to contract, since it remains non-functional. It has just helped the remote muscle (the muscle portion away from the damaged region). Things got better *because the heart's geometry improved* — the reduced size of the bulging muscle (now smaller and thicker, instead of bulging and thin) permits the functioning remote muscle to get smaller. That is the *only reason* the heart recovered its performance.

But the injured (now rigid and thicker) heart attack muscle is still not squeezing. The inner half of the heart attack muscle has been damaged — yet *the whole heart muscle simply cannot recover function if even 50% of its muscle is lifeless.*[22] As a result, the dead muscle that existed before returning new blood flow — *remains dead* after blood flow is restored — and non-functional. The principal goal of returning this damaged heart muscle's capacity to contract has simply not been achieved.

Consequently, the still-contracting remote muscle is *now totally responsible* for heart function. This responsibility began the instant the heart attack started — and it continues despite a successful angioplasty.

Now, cardiologists and surgeons know this inner half of the heart attack muscle has been damaged — yet nobody believes it can be helped. It is considered an unfortunate, but unavoidable *and unfixable* aspect of having a heart attack. This *fait accompli* conclusion has prevented progress toward finding another approach to treatment... *but they don't see the future.*

Looking Toward Tomorrow

While everyone celebrates the fact that opening the closed artery reduces the immediate loss of life from 20% to 5% after a heart attack... these treatments *often only postpone the mortality.* The patient may not die right away or in the first year, but a 1993 report documented that about 20% of them with substantial muscle damage will develop congestive heart failure, and succumb earlier than otherwise expected.[23] This conclusion is now amplified, as recent reports from England (in 896 patients),[24] the Mayo Clinic (1992 patients),[25] and Italy (284 patients)[26] demonstrate that delayed heart failure develops in about 30% of patients sustaining an acute heart attack. Each study clarifies that successful angioplasty does not prevent this disastrous complication.

This is because today's treatments don't save the *entire* heart muscle. They simply limit the extent of injury and cell death to the inner and mid-regions of the heart. Although the area of muscle damaged by the heart attack is not contracting, its surface appearance appears normal. In fact, cardiac surgeons believe that the region is healthy because its surface looks normal in the operating room. Yet this unmarked exterior camouflages a severe underlying internal injury. This deeper injury is the basic cause behind heart failure, the world's leading cause of death. (This problem will be further described *and solved* in subsequent chapters).

Conversely, because of traditional acceptance that the heart attack damaged muscle cannot be mended, all efforts are directed toward preserving and improving the remote muscle performance, since that is now the patient's lifeline. The key to this is that the remote muscle must be well-nourished by blood. Yet it is not uncommon for the arteries feeding it to be narrowed as well. Thus, the remote muscle is vulnerable to sustaining further damage because its need for increased blood flow may not be met. The aftermath of such injury is the triggering of glaring consequences: the heart will develop a drastic complication called cardiogenic shock, leading to its acute failure. A tragedy that is not pleasant to behold.

Stealing Away Life

As a surgeon who is asked to see patients in the coronary care unit, I vividly recall a prominent and influential businessman in his early 60s who'd had a severe heart attack and was suffering from cardiogenic shock.

When I approached his bed, his breathing was rapid and shallow. His skin had a blue hue and was cool and clammy — symptoms of impaired blood flow to the extremities. Why such symptoms? Because the body is spectacularly struggling to stay alive. Adrenaline is released to raise blood pressure to try to ensure flow to crucial organs, and in doing so, it constricts the small arteries leading to the skin, explaining its blue color and cool and damp appearance.

My patient had intended to hold a standard business "power meeting" with me in which he would be in control at all times. Yet cardiogenic shock restricted blood flow to all body organs... including the brain. This resulting poor body nourishment eroded his normally strong personality, thinking, and health. His forceful demands never surfaced and he became quiet, bewildered by how his body refused to cooperate. He had morphed from a leader into a suffering patient, leaving his wife to explain the dreadful nature of his illness to the cardiology team. He sat uncomfortably upright due to his congested lungs, while the team administered a range of cardiac support drugs to try to improve performance of the remote muscle... but all to no avail.

Treatment options are very limited for people in cardiogenic shock. That's why the intent is to keep anyone from reaching such a severely debilitated state. Otherwise, the only options available to cardiologists are administering drugs to make the remote muscle beat more efficiently, and possibly use pacemakers to ensure a normal heartbeat is retained.

But these approaches are often inadequate, because the remote muscle's own ability to function is again often limited due to obstructions in the coronary arteries that nourish it. What typically happens is there is 100% closure of the artery in the heart attack region, with 75% narrowing of arteries supplying the remote muscle. This limitation of flow will undermine the remote muscle's capacity to compensate for the *non-functional* damaged heart region.

While cardiologists won't typically perform angioplasty on remote muscle, surgeons are asked to perform coronary grafts on it to try to fortify its compensating function. But undertaking this task introduces significant new problems and risks.

The life of such a heart attack patient is totally dependent on the function of the remote muscle, but it is in a very vulnerable state. If there is inadequate *cardiac protection* while surgically completing coronary grafts, remote muscle damage will worsen and recovery may not be possible. As a result, cardiogenic shock will continue, even though the remote muscle now receives unobstructed blood flow from the newly placed graft.

The outcome was that the mortality for coronary graft surgery in these cardiogenic shock patients was as high as 50% in many centers — principally because insufficient cardiac protection resulted in damage to the heart's only functioning region — its remote muscle. Because of this, surgeons did not want to operate while the heart was still in its weakened state, and recommended delaying coronary grafting until four to six weeks later. Unfortunately, that postponement would be too late to help the fragile remote muscles causing cardiogenic shock, like in our businessman, where mortality is over 75% without surgical treatment (and still 50% with an operation).

Saving the Remote Muscle — Safely

I agreed that while coronary grafting could solve the issues with weakened and undernourished remote muscles, it was simply too risky to perform using conventional heart protection methods. However, I believed we could solve this.

This became our first goal toward improving patient survivability from heart attacks: exploring whether the protective methods that we developed for open-heart procedures (as reported in the prior two chapters) could offset these risks.

We began by mimicking the same adverse conditions in the hearts of animal test subjects as found in heart attack victims, and then conducted coronary grafting on the remote muscles. So what happened?

Our cardioplegia protocols found immediate success.[19]

We then moved from bench to bedside, using our novel techniques in 80 consecutive patients. Remote muscle was successfully protected in these heart attack victims! *Mortality was only 10%* — plunging down from the standard 50 to 70% — if we operated within 18 hours after cardiogenic shock developed.[27] What's more, we would later find that five years afterward — these patients still had a 70% survival rate.

So we not only avoided early mortality, we were also able to significantly reduce later mortality. We established that even though the remote muscle was a stress-vulnerable area, if you protect it well, it does beautifully. In fact, while others were afraid to operate on people already in cardiogenic shock, we firmly believed in our strategies. They were used in the businessman I described earlier. He recovered promptly and became a long-time survivor, recapturing his gusto for life and leadership as well!

Next Step: Saving *More* than Remote Muscle

While our protective methods were successful in saving high-risk patients, our ability to treat all heart attacks was still markedly limited — since the remote muscle was all that we could save.

So the intense frustration continued, as many heart attack patients experienced long-term decline as they later developed heart failure and lethal arrhythmias.

As I have described, the patient's long-term future must only rely upon the performance of the living remote muscle, since the dead muscle from the heart attack did not resume contracting. Later follow up is essential, since successful angioplasty does not prevent about 30% of patients from going on to develop congestive heart failure. Drug treatments will lengthen the patient's survival, but they do not substantially reverse the heart dilation (stretching) that causes heart failure.

As a result, a troubling scenario develops. The unsuspecting former heart attack patient could be out golfing, enjoying a beach vacation with his wife, or watching his granddaughter's school play... and all the while his remote muscle is stretching, setting the stage for heart failure, much as it did for my dad.

But with no known way to restore function to the *non-contracting muscle* region, the cardiologist's typical response to a heart attack continues: efforts remain focused upon restoring blood flow as fast as possible. *It does not solve the deeper issue, as the dead muscle portion still has no function.* Yet that reality is disregarded and urgent reperfusion (in this case, opening vessels to return flow) remains the Accepted Wisdom of cardiology strategies.

That's when it dawned on me: our prior work on reperfusion injury during cardiac surgery could also be applicable after a heart attack.

Our mission to immediately save lives must not be our only goal. We must aim toward having patients walk out of the hospital and welcome a lengthy future. That can only occur if we can make the heart attack region recover its ability to function.

Yet no one was doing this, because the heart attack region was considered dead.

At least... that's what everyone believed.

Searching for a New Reality

This is the challenge that launched our research in 1981: to see if near-normal function could be returned to the damaged heart attack muscle.

I believed this damage reflected an ischemic reperfusion injury. That is, the closed artery causes ischemia (no blood to the heart), and returning normal blood reflow to the heart attack region (as done by treating it with angioplasty) causes a reperfusion injury. From everything we had learned previously, as described in prior chapters, I thought we *should* be able to fix this.

I knew this approach would directly confront the traditional adamant belief that the "perceived" death of the injured heart region cannot be remedied.

But such beliefs must be confronted and tested.

Welcome to our new scientific quest.

CHAPTER 9

Restoring Life to a "Dead" Heart

"Miracles" can happen.

As described in the last chapter, the conventional medical view was that since an absence of blood supply caused the heart attack, immediately opening the artery to give new blood supply (reperfusion) should be the right treatment. Yes, it relieves the dire symptoms of the heart attack (improved blood pressure, cardiac output, filling pressure, heart rate), and favorably brings the dilated (stretched) basketball shape of the heart back toward its elliptical form like a football.

But while a sense of optimism is buoyed as the *seemingly* unscathed patient leaves the hospital a few days later... a very different future can unfold that reveals the more complete story (congestive heart failure).

The reason?

The primary function of the heart muscle is to contract to nourish the body. Yet returning normal blood reperfusion after a heart attack fails to restore this vital action — as part of the heart remains dead.

Sitting at my desk, determined to find a way to remedy these acute heart attacks... what initially came to mind was how we used blood cardioplegia to offset the reperfusion injury that follows the temporary absence of blood flow during cardiac surgery. I suddenly suspected that *the same type of injury may happen when normal blood flow is returned to the ischemic (blood deprived) region after a heart attack.*

What I knew was this: cardiac contraction cannot recover when even only 50% of the muscle is terminally injured[22] — the damage doesn't have to be 100%. Yet such an extent of muscle loss (50% or more) is common when regular blood is used for reflow after a heart attack.

As I considered this, a new light began to shine. The delivery of controlled reperfusion itself is straightforward because only two primary factors are involved. The first is the "composition" of the blood being returned, where substances would be added to normal blood to protect the heart, much like the gasoline additives to make your car's engine run more smoothly. The second is controlling the "conditions" of the reperfusion by adjusting pressure, ventricular volume or stretch, temperature, and flow rate.

But treating an acute heart attack was a new challenge — since many believed the muscle had sustained irreversible damage. Overcoming this conventional belief could be done in only one way: *by proving that using controlled reperfusion (instead of normal blood) could restore contraction to the heart attack region that was presumed to be dead.*

At the same time, I also knew there would be staunch opposition from cardiology teams to adopt the newer method of controlled reperfusion being used in cardiac surgery, since it takes longer to administer, and they believe their principal mission is to *quickly deliver regular blood reperfusion*. Their rallying cry, "The longer the heart goes without a blood supply, the greater the muscle death will be," seemed set in stone. But I believed the best yardstick for patient recovery must be finding an approach that restores the heart attack muscle's ability to contract again, rather than focusing upon a battle against the clock. *Angioplasty — with normal blood reperfusion — simply cannot achieve this goal of ensuring the heart attack muscle's recovery.*

In order to tackle this problem, I needed to more deeply explore the concept of presumed "irreversible damage" after an acute heart attack. I knew that despite the advantages of controlled reperfusion, it *can never make a dead muscle resume beating.*

But what if it *did* make it beat?

Diving Deeper

There were two accepted methods for determining irreversible damage (to document death of heart tissue) and both were conducted during postmortem (autopsy) examination. Researchers would place the injured heart segment in a tissue-staining fluid to perform a TTC (*triphenyl tetrazolium chloride) stain.* If the muscle sample stained a yellow color, it was deemed to have become necrotic (dead). The other method was to get a microscopic analysis of the mitochondria (tiny cellular structures) — which as you may recall from high school biology, control energy production in the heart. If they were disrupted, that meant the muscle had died, and it would foreshadow the patient's demise.

These methods had been used to verify irreversible damage in experiments by others, in which the blood supply to a region of a heart was stopped for 40 minutes, and then flow was returned. The functional findings showed the injured muscle did not squeeze, and became thickened and rigid ("contracture"). This complication was most severe in the heart's inner shell — and was triggered by the abundance of calcium that accumulated in damaged muscle cells, together with a disruption of the fragile mitochondria that use oxygen to produce energy.

These severe changes in performance, and associated lab results, were consistent. Yet that did not deter us from asking: *Was this injured region truly dead?*

An Accidental Breakthrough

As investigators, we wanted to first match what others reported. So we reproduced the 40 minutes of no blood supply in a test animal's heart, and noted the heart just sat there after the reflow was started. Not squeezing, like it was dead.

But just as we had concluded the procedure, an unexpected and new adventure unfolded.

My hand accidently touched the heart when I reached for something.

That's when it happened.

I stood straight up, taken aback. "What the...? Did you see that?"

"See what?" asked one of the team.

"Touch the heart."

"Excuse me? Why do you want us to..."

"Just touch the heart," I insisted.

He did. It happened again. "Wow — astounding! It moved!"

I smiled. "I know. This dead muscle — isn't dead. It may not be beating, but it sure ain't dead."

No one could believe it... yet there was no denying what we saw. As you might imagine, the observation raised an exciting new question:

"So if it's not dead — then what is it?"

We knew it was still injured. In a sense, it was stunned, but it could be temporarily aroused. I subsequently would learn that others had described this "stimulated" beat, but I was unaware of this when it happened in our study. What we were witnessing was not a normal heartbeat. It would only move when poked and only once each time. It's what would be called an ectopic heartbeat, which means this portion of the heart develops its own periodic beat that doesn't coordinate with the rest of the heart beating normally. It's not a useful beat as the heart does not pump, but there is no escaping that a contracting motion came from living muscle in a region thought to be dead.

This observation was vital — because dead regions never move. A cardiology friend of mine, Jan Tillisch, put this into colorful perspective by observing, "Steak does not beat."

But how could such a contradiction to conventional thinking occur?

Collaborative Endeavor

A unique benefit of working at a university is the ability to meet individuals with extensive experience in common areas of interest. We encounter each other at staff meetings, conferences, or through friends. We speak of our work with passion, looking for ways to support shared aims, always hoping to find a companion to tread with us on a newly forged trail.

It was just such an encounter that introduced me to Fritiof Sjöstrand, a Swedish physician and histologist (one who studies microscopic structure of tissue) at UCLA who was a pioneer in his field. Aside from a deep mutual interest in the heart, Fritiof was a marathon runner (at 75 years old) and I was a marathon swimmer. Focus, persistence, and overcoming obstacles were scientific and athletic qualities we shared — traits I liked to believe my Grandpa Zelig would be proud of, if he were alive to see them.

Fritiof agreed to join forces with my team during our experimental studies of acute heart attacks. We were both eager to bring new information to light on the effects of prolonged ischemia (lack of blood flow to the heart) and its treatment. Our aim was to blend his new method of ultrastructure tissue analysis with our innovative functional treatment of hearts undergoing a heart attack.

Fritiof was identifying the basic ultrastructure essential for cell metabolism, using an extremely high-powered (electron) microscope. This differed from many other histologists that viewed the basic cardiac structure with regular microscopes. He was delving deeper than most, looking at the structures responsible for the biochemical reactions that were the keystones of life. He was able to look at the causes of cell metabolism *within* the mitochondria. It was a perfect fit with our work.

The blend between what Fritiof could analyze, and what we saw clinically, was remarkable. One day he showed us ultrastructure images of where the amino acids are used in the heart tissues.

"Really?" I marveled at the images.

"Yes, that's where the amino acids sit. Why the strong interest? "

I replied, "Because part of our cardioplegia formulation includes giving the amino acids glutamate and aspartate to help the heart metabolize oxygen."

Fritiof was literally showing me where the glutamate and aspartate work. He provided visual and other documentation of what we were doing. It was phenomenal.

Furthermore, and to everyone's surprise, Fritiof discovered something quite startling and important to our work: he believed that the conventional and accepted testing methods to determine muscle tissue being dead *were flawed.*[28]

His pictures showed that the traditional testing technique *itself* caused the mitochondria to be destroyed. These vital structures were found to be *entirely normal* when his method of tissue preparation was used.[28] It took a world-renowned electron microscopist to explain this to us. A cohesive team took form, as he worked on the histology (structural) and we worked on the muscle (functional).

A terrific collaboration.

Most importantly, beyond finding that the technique of preparing conventional staining methods themselves can produce mitochondrial disruption, Fritiof discovered that the *mitochondria were normal after prolonged ischemia* — a finding previously thought to be impossible. Yet such normality indeed existed. Simply stated, a look was worth a thousand words — and their normalcy was fully evident after viewing the images on his slides.

Consequently, if the mitochondria are normal — they can produce energy after a heart attack — which verifies there is continuing life within a damaged region! This landmark finding became the foundation behind our search to discover if the injured portion could recover its function. We were excited to move forward.

Turning Surviving into Reviving

Our next and most vital step was correlating Fritiof's findings with our study that aimed to recover this heart region's function (its ability to contract). His pioneering methods would document what was happening in the heart structure, while we looked at its performance, much like Julien Hoffman and I were able to do when we used microspheres to verify blood flow inside the heart.

If we were successful, this unequivocal evidence would show that standard beliefs are wrong... a persuasive finding that might open the door to a whole new way to approach treating heart attacks.

We were acting as rebels and renegades, dissenters, and heretics. But we would not be stopped. *Unless the science stopped us.*

In our experiments, we would obstruct a large branch of the anterior descending artery (which supplies the front of the ventricle and septum) for time intervals that ranged from 40 minutes... to two hours... to four hours and beyond. Our intent was to use controlled reperfusion, as described in the cardioplegia chapters, and determine if the heart could remain alive. Until this time, no other experimental study had ever shown that myocardial cells could survive after lengthy periods without blood flow.

Yet we knew that even this profound accomplishment would not be enough. Our journey needed to lead us further down an uncharted path. So we began *a series of studies* that would go far beyond showing the heart was still alive after these long periods of no blood. We would create new protocols to test if the injured muscle — previously thought to be irreversibly damaged (as by a heart attack) — could regain function.

A daunting endeavor. To accomplish it, we knew we'd need to resolve many as yet unanswered questions. For example, one fundamental issue is...

Oxygen Demand

Critical to keeping a heart alive is making sure it is sufficiently nourished. We knew the oxygen requirements of the beating heart, the fibrillating heart, and the arrested (stopped) heart. But what about a heart that has had a heart attack? What were the requirements of the bulging muscle that's not squeezing? To our knowledge, no one had ever measured this before.

With our research fellows, Fumiyuki Okamoto and Brad Allen, we recreated a bulging segment in a working animal heart by nourishing this region with an infusion of blood containing high potassium — essentially mirroring what happens structurally during a heart attack (except this bulging region would be pink due to ongoing perfusion, instead of blue as it is during a heart attack).

What we discovered next was entirely unexpected.

The oxygen requirements of the *non-contracting bulging segment* were nearly as high (70%) as a fully working heart!

Fortunately, we found we could immediately lower those demands to almost negligible levels (10%), by decompressing (venting) the heart with the heart-lung machine (to mimic what is done in cardiac operations). This provided much greater protection against further damage, and venting following a heart attack became another critical component of restoring the heart.[29]

However, solving these oxygen needs was *only one of 16 studies* that we did during our four-year journey, during which we discovered piece after piece after piece of what was needed to protect and restore the muscle damaged during a heart attack.[30] These many individual aspects would work together to solve a huge problem. It is much like what we had to do to solve cardioplegia and everything else that I describe in this book. It is never one simple step to resolve these critical issues. If it was, somebody else would have already solved them.

Who would pursue something like this? Only crazy "Uncle Bucky" does that.

For us, however, it was tremendously exciting. We kept finding all the hidden pieces to each wild puzzle. Once you do that, suddenly you have solved problems that were deemed unsolvable. Then you can create solutions to medical issues, whose implementation may affect massive numbers of individuals and their families.

Collaborative Components

Our 16 studies established new principles for treating heart attacks.[30] The approaches crossed over between the specialties of cardiology and surgery. We were not proprietary about *who* did what — our goal was to define *what* could be done. Our new protocols would intertwine with one another, requiring an orderly choreography to implement them together. The surgeons and cardiologists involved in our tests were no longer simply doctors; they were dancers in an exquisitely orchestrated, life-saving ballet.

While understanding the importance of each of our new findings may be beyond the realm of the non-medical reader, the milestones of this voyage need to be acknowledged in this memoir. As each one was met, another challenge presented itself — until we had found all the parts to the riddle.

This is a partial list of what we uncovered:

- Using the heart-lung machine together with controlled reperfusion initially expanded the window during which we could regain recovery of heart muscle from 40 minutes to two hours.
- Those vital tiny mitochondria that control energy production were *still intact after six hours* without blood flow — and remained alive and functional after controlled reperfusion.
- Lowering calcium levels in the reflow blood prevented movement of calcium into the heart attack cells, which then avoids impairing mitochondria function.

- The damaged non-contracting muscle bulging from a heart attack *needed 70%* of the oxygen required by a normal beating heart. Yet when decompressed (vented) as during surgery, it required only 10%.
- Using a gentle reperfusion pressure of near 50 mm Hg prevented the edema (swelling in tissues) that would result from higher reflow pressures.
- Identified proper concentrations of high glucose (to include in the blood reflow) needed for nutrition and increased osmolarity (number of particles in blood) to avoid water accumulation in the tissue.
- 20 minutes of controlled reflow was required to achieve maximum recovery. (Shorter intervals achieve less functional improvement.)
- Muscle injured by the closed coronary artery sustains four to five times more damage if the heart is not decompressed during medical procedures.
- Decompression by venting is essential.
- These new methods worked equally well in the experimental surgical operating room *and* the experimental catheterization lab.[31]

The last discovery deserves special emphasis since we found that our approaches could be used in the cardiologist's catheterization lab or in the operating room. The common objective is to follow the new principles of how reperfusion is delivered. Typically there is a debate whether the cardiologist should do their procedure or should the surgeon perform an operation. But the reality is the heart muscle does not care how blood gets back into it. It can come through an angioplasty catheter or via a surgical graft. *The shared aim of returning function to the heart attack area is the only significant goal,* not territorial disputes between cardiologist and surgeon.

The New World is Finally Reached

Once we had our recipe down, it was time to begin the final set of studies. We subjected the heart to prolonged durations of no blood supply, in order to create the inevitable cell death that would result from an injury that was believed to be inescapable.

The results?

During this experimental investigative process, we found the heart was much more vibrant than its "presumed counterpart" (thought to be a dead steak) — despite several hours of ischemia (no blood flow). At every stage, Fritiof's documenting that the heart sustained only negligible cell damage served to counter what had previously been established as Accepted Wisdom. The heart was still kicking — *and could still function* — thanks to our novel controlled reperfusion treatment.

We then tested our procedure in the most challenging of circumstances: when the heart muscle region experiences *six hours* of ischemia. If this was successful, it would more than meet the need for developing a treatment that could help a heart attack victim who had been untreated for a prolonged period.

This approach was also completely unheard of. No heart could survive six hours without nourishment… *or so it was believed.*

This was a critical stage for us. With all that we learned, if our methods didn't work for such extended periods of time, their use would be limited. A great deal was at stake. We faced a powerful test of our credibility.

The validity of our approach was confirmed.

Our use of controlled reperfusion consistently made cardiac regions that had received no blood flow for six hours… *recover their ability to contract!*[32]

What's more, Fritiof's ultrastructure analysis confirmed what we had observed functionally: the mitochondria responsible for producing energy were not disrupted. It was amazing!

Better yet, we still didn't know the limits to how long a heart could survive using our protocols. Might the heart survive eight hours… or ten hours… twelve hours? In a sense, we had no idea how long it would be before the heart was truly dead.

Going Public

We felt what we had established would create nothing less than a revolution in conventional thinking. It was a game-changer. We hoped our colleagues in the medical community would pay more attention to these results than they had to our prior reporting of early findings when we recovered function after two hours of an acute heart attack. In 1981, I had watched as Jake Vinten-Johansen, the research fellow conducting our study then, presented our preliminary results at the American Heart Association in a session about novel techniques. After he finished, not a single question was asked, nor any interest expressed.[33]

But now it was several years later and we had every reason to believe people would be excited about our newest findings. Nobody had ever before accomplished getting the muscle damaged in a heart attack to function again — let alone after six hours![34] Our team showed it could be done.

...Yet once again, to our great disappointment, this demonstration of recovery of muscle previously thought to be dead — had absolutely no impact upon the cardiology community.

They seemed wholly indifferent.

Although potentially demoralizing, I didn't take it as a low point. I don't function that way. As the composer Phillip Glass observed, "If you do not worry about people that do not care about you, it is the passage to freedom."

You keep on working. The high point for me is when we find the answer, and progress is only furthered when you keep making your understanding of it better and more useful and meaningful.

The truth will eventually win....

Leaping from Theory to Practice

Even though the larger medical community ignored our initial findings, the events of one night showed me that some of my colleagues at UCLA had taken note of our research... and gave me an unexpected opportunity to turn theory into practice.

It was far after my normal UCLA office hours when a knock on my door lifted my head from my notes.

"Yes?" I called out.

"Doctor Buckberg?" a man asked in a soft voice. "I am Nobi Kawata, recently appointed clinical cardiologist in the medical center. I am sorry that I do not have an academic appointment. So I apologize if this interruption is inappropriate."

"That's fine, Doctor Kawata. Welcome to UCLA. How can I help you?"

"Time is short. I have a patient — a man who's had a massive heart attack and is at great risk of dying."

This caught my attention.

"Frankly," Doctor Kawata added gravely, "I have nowhere else to turn."

That got my full attention. He explained the patient had no chance given the normal procedures. His heart attack occurred 11 hours ago.

"Eleven hours?" My maximum experience up until this point was six hours. This was a big jump... and would present a powerful test of our concepts. I had never tried my procedures on any patient, let alone someone after 11 hours of ischemia.

Big jump indeed.

Dr. Kawata had heard about my research on controlled reperfusion and hoped it might work on his patient. The region undergoing damage was large, and the problem of early death was compounded by his likely developing heart failure in the long term, if he survived.

I knew we needed to try. "Please take me to meet him."

My office was a short distance from the medical center and we rushed over. The patient was in the cardiology cath lab. I quickly accessed the situation and called the operating room.

"This is Dr. Buckberg, I have a red-line case."

A red-line means ultra emergency. You are put ahead of anyone else into the first room available. They immediately got a message to the perfusionist on emergency call to come in while I reached the chief resident. "We have a patient with an acute infarction and need to proceed now."

The patient was moved into the operating room and all was ready to go within 30 minutes. Everyone assembled (nurses, residents, anesthesiologists, perfusionists) knew what to do. Once we began the operation, I was able to look at the heart. Sure enough, the part affected by the heart attack was bulging and blue (no blood supply). We immediately put him on the heart-lung machine and decompressed the ventricle to shrink it down and diminish its oxygen needs.

While no one said anything, I could tell from their eyes that several were wondering just what the heck we were doing. No one had ever done anything like this before on someone 11 hours after the heart attack.

Everyone had operated on heart attack victims in cardiogenic shock, where the focus was taking care of the remote muscle to keep the person alive. But they'd never done our protocols for treating the "dead area" of the heart to restore it. In fact, I'd never discussed this with the house staff at all. But I now told them we had a way of dealing with this.

So we began.

One of the first things I did after we started the heart-lung machine was to feel the heart. To my delight, the damaged region of the heart was soft.

"Thank goodness — the heart is still soft. The calcium hasn't flooded into the muscle cells and impacted mitochondrial function." It was hopeful news.

We first performed the necessary grafts to open the narrowed arteries to supply blood to the functioning remote muscles — the part of the heart keeping the man alive. We wanted to give it the best possible protection.

Then we did a graft on the artery feeding the heart attack region. We infused our cardioplegia solution into the damaged area (about 50 cc a minute, making sure the pressure wasn't too high) for 20 minutes.

I utilized everything we had learned from our 16 studies. It was all coming together under the most demanding of circumstances.

All of this went perfectly. The operating team followed each instruction, even if they didn't always know the purpose of each task. Then came the moment of truth. Time to remove the clamp and restore the blood supply.

We did. The *whole* heart started beating, including the heart attack region.

I was ecstatic. "You see it. That's incredible!"

Everybody was thrilled and stunned. What we had done was unheard of. It was truly extraordinary. Yet based upon our experimental background, it was predictable!

Dr. Kawata's patient recovered in smooth fashion, and imaging studies verified the region undergoing acute myocardial infarction had indeed regained normal function. Dr. Kawata was very excited and grateful.

I was delighted that UCLA cardiologists would now know what we could do clinically with patients. I expected streams of patients to soon come our way.

But that did not happen. Old mindsets are hard to change. We had very few patients referred to us even after we had shown what we could do and the much greater prospects that we offered, for both short- and long-term recovery.

Still, I was undaunted. For someone forging a new trail over the course of several years, this experience showed we had reached the next mountaintop.

I ultimately operated on 16 acute heart attack patients at UCLA using our new method. We achieved significant recovery of contractile function (the "so-called dead muscle" contracting and functioning again) in 15 of them. Most important, there were no deaths.

Once again, I was out of the lab and making use of our results. My experience differed from that of many practitioners who repeatedly perform the same job as everyone around them, rather than welcoming revolutionary procedures that may challenge the status quo.

But when you have an advance in treating heart attacks this dramatic, the status quo *has* to change. The process of constantly growing and doing things better is needed to form the future.

Making the Unknown Known

The time had come for us to report our bench to bedside data. We submitted this four-year package of experimental and now clinical findings (with patients) to the *Journal of Cardiothoracic Surgery* in 1986.

My choice to wait before publishing any findings for our studies illustrated my belief in Julien Hoffman's credo "to withhold data until all bases were covered." Aside from our preliminary report of experimentally restoring heart function after two hours of ischemia and my reporting our experimental successes after six hours (both at American Heart Association), I refrained from publicizing results to any of our sixteen studies, even though any one of them was worthy of reporting since each was a new finding. But I don't pursue research to publish papers. I do research to provide concepts, and you can't provide complete concepts if you have one study reported in journal A and another study reported in journal B, etc. You want to have them all published together.

Our submission package was closely reviewed by the *Journal of Thoracic and Cardiovascular Surgery*. Their evaluation process was extensive, as I needed to answer questions from 3 reviewers of each paper (48 different responses) that resulted in my writing 126 single-spaced pages of replies, and revising the papers to meet each request for improving clarity. All were accepted as I successfully met their challenge. The importance of this novel data was clear, as the entire study was placed into a special supplemental issue. A grand surprise, since over the past 66 years, the only other such Journal supplement was one that recognized C. Walton Lillehei, who was called the Father of Modern Cardiac Surgery.

While the team and I were gratified to have our work published, action needs reaction. The power of our efforts ultimately resides not in publication, but rather in their use to help sick patients. This starts with the crucial step of educating the cardiology community that it was now possible to recover the damaged heart muscle and ventricle after a heart attack. That treatment could be done either by surgeons using grafts in the operating room or by cardiologists performing angioplasties in the cath lab. In either case, you put the patient on full bypass, vent the ventricle to decompress it, and place a catheter beyond the obstruction to give a controlled reperfusion.

But for that to be adopted — the entire medical field first needed to acknowledge the limitations for the patient when normal blood is used as the reperfusate. In particular, the cardiologists must recognize that our treatment works, since they are the gatekeepers that allow the emergence of new developments, and their acceptance will then become the starting place for the initial testing of a new pathway by their cardiac surgeons.

The Three-Step Process

This new way to treat heart attacks does not introduce a competition or turf war between cardiologists and surgeons. Instead there must be a collaborative evolution of treatment that requires three steps.

- First, the cardiologist must recognize the limitations of traditional angioplasty, and be open to a way to deliver controlled reperfusion surgically.
- Second, surgeons in those same hospitals must learn to perform a new reflow method on acute heart attack victims. Their successes would show their cardiologists that this treatment works.
- Third, the cardiologists must then adapt new strategies allowing them to use these approaches in their own catheterization labs.

Fulfillment of this cooperative process will initiate a new treatment for the heart attack patient, the true beneficiary.

Challenging Road

Despite having a clear roadmap for change, I knew altering commonly held beliefs is not easy to do, even with concrete evidence demonstrating that substantial advances are now possible. Battle lines are drawn by members of the medical community who are well-accustomed to practicing in a certain way. Such alterations always take many years to become reality, but there must be a steady forward movement of ideas to push against the status quo.

To help put forward this change, I organized a group of national and international colleagues of cardiac surgeons in 1992 to agree to test the effects of controlled reperfusion on heart attacks in their clinics. This was done to further the credibility of our early results that were reported in the 16 studies, and to encourage the medical community to consider this dynamic new protocol to treat acute heart attacks.

At UCLA, we only had 16 patients.[35] But now participating surgeons and cardiologists were not limited to only our UCLA staff, but included surgical colleagues from prominent centers in the United States, France, and Germany. There would be 156 patients.[36]

Results were excellent.

The average duration of time between the heart attack and treatment was 6.7 hours, with one patient experiencing *23 hours* of no blood flow to the damaged heart region. Using our controlled reperfusion methods, the overall mortality for the 156 patients was 3.7%. (Deaths only occurred in 6 of 66 patients in cardiogenic shock, which included 12 patients with sudden death.)

Further, we compared our findings against 1,200 traditional angioplasty patients who underwent only 3.9 hours of ischemia — and who had 8.7% mortality.

Yet most importantly — the surgeons *were able to restore contraction* (squeezing capacity) in the region undergoing a heart attack in 87% of patients. Something that had never happened before with angioplasty. Ever.

The positive outcomes of our controlled reperfusion patients were clear, as they had a short hospitalization, and the dangers of them developing arrhythmias and heart failure were minimized or eliminated. All members of our team believed this accomplishment would lead to widespread acceptance and success of our new treatment for heart attacks.

So what happened next?

Our results for 156 consecutive patients with acute myocardial infarction were presented at an international meeting of the American Association of Thoracic Surgeons (AATS) in 1992 — and were met with a deafening silence.[36]

There was only marginal discussion by the surgeons after our presentation. Yet what we put forward was amazing — solid evidence that our techniques had helped hearts recover the ability to contract again following acute heart attacks in 156 patients from three different countries.

Echoes of the Past

Though frustrating at the time, I now realize that the absence of audience response following my presentation of a new way to treat heart attacks reflected an unending dilemma.

My recent attendance at the Centennial Anniversary Meeting of AATS was revealing, as I learned the classic adage of "history repeats itself" was integral to the organization's inception. In 1913, Willy Meyer (who would later become our second president) attended the American Medical Association meeting in Minneapolis, where he was to describe the first successful treatment of cancer of the esophagus. Until then, this was considered a universally fatal disease. The AMA meeting was attended by 3,246 physicians (matching the 3,000 to 4,000 that attend our meetings), and Meyer's talk followed papers by four established leaders, like Charles Mayo. They described traditional surgical problems like use of bone clamps, elbow trauma, thyroid operations, and foot gangrene management. Considerable discussion followed each speech, as these heated debates generated a buzz of excitement that went on for three hours.

Willy Meyer finally took his turn to introduce his groundbreaking solution to a dreaded disease. Yet his anticipation of a bright new future was not fulfilled. He was met with stony silence. The zeal had disappeared. No questions were asked and there was no discussion. His remarkable findings were met by utter apathy from the AMA general surgeons. Yet Meyer was not dejected. This rigidity simply sparked his drive to ignite a new society in 1917, and the American Association for Thoracic Surgeons just celebrated our 2017 Centennial Meeting.

Unfortunately, unyielding opposition to new ideas was not alleviated by the new organization's creation. Echoes of the past rang again for our new treatment of an *acute heart attack*. Resistance now came from cardiac surgeons, not general surgeons, as the evidence that acute heart attack muscle can recover function — despite treatment occurring six or more hours after the coronary vessel closed — was discarded.

The irony is that the AATS was formed because nobody listened to Willie Meyer, yet such a barrier has continued to persist for 100 years.

In truth, this blockade reflects an eternal counterforce against new approaches. Resistance to our new treatment for heart attacks isn't due to differences between cardiologists vs. surgeons, or surgeons vs. surgeons. It is the disparity between the rigid mind and the open mind. This goes beyond just the world of medicine.

My understanding of this behavior pattern became clearer after reading Spencer Johnson's 1998 book, *Who Moved My Cheese?* This internationally best-selling volume sold over 10 million copies and deals with resistance to change.

The book describes that while the world is constantly transforming, many people fiercely hold onto wanting things to stay as they have been. Yet the book proposes: "If you don't change... you will become extinct." Such fates of decline or disappearance have certainly befallen major companies like Kodak, Circuit City, and Tower Records — all of whom had resisted change.

People are apprehensive of what dramatic change might demand of them. Yet the book poses the profound question:

What would you do if you were not afraid?

It is a far-reaching question about life as well as about science.

This query also parallels the guidance offered in 1865 by Claude Bernard, the previously mentioned French physiologist and my "historical" mentor. The search for a new answer must involve acceptance of the possibility of failure — and what it may reveal. That differs greatly from the inflexible stance of "excluding contradictions" because of your wanting the answer to be what you already believe.

Ultimately proof, not rigidity, always win. The solution to the devastating problem of acute heart attacks is never determined by canvassing a vote from the medical or surgical audience. Instead, validation comes from the recovery of the heart attack muscle's ability to contract, following application of a new innovative treatment.

Acceptance has not yet come... *but it will.*

The Fear Factor

One might well have expected a much better response from cardiac surgeons. But another factor came into play: most of the surgeons had never operated on heart attacks.

The accepted protocol was that heart attack patients are cared for by the cardiologists. Very few surgeons operated on acute heart attacks, because mortality was higher in these patients than when using just angioplasty (at least prior to our protection methods), and given what was known, they believed the heart attack area itself could not be helped. They could only improve reflow to the remote muscle. But as I described earlier, remote muscle is very vulnerable right after an attack, and could be easily injured when performing a bypass graft to improve blood flow to it. Such damage would impair heart function and jeopardize survival.

Because of this concern, surgeons did not usually operate on heart attacks for fear of losing their patients. Such deaths raise their operative mortality report card and will substantially hamper referrals. Consequently, in order to lower risk, a five-to-six-week waiting period was customary before operating on a patient with a heart attack.

So the cardiac surgeons ignored our results, even though we reported for the first time in history that 87% of patients had recovered full heart function in muscle that was without blood flow for over 6 hours, and had demonstrated an extremely low rate of mortality (3.7%).

The result was a lack of acknowledgement for these findings in *both* the cardiology and surgical communities — even though most recognized that angioplasty *does not* provide recovery of function. The patient bears the brunt of this impasse, since about 20% to 30% of them will develop heart failure over time.

Unfortunately, this distressing situation remains just as true today as it did in 1992. This disinterest continues despite our showing that the use of controlled reperfusion "does not pit cardiac surgery against cardiology" — since these techniques can be used equally well when the surgeons perform grafts or the cardiologists conduct angioplasty.

Resisting Change: To Preserve What Has Always Been Done

Part of the reason the medical community resists these findings is that adopting them will require a fundamental shift in methods of treatment. Our approach would dramatically alter catheterization lab procedures, as cardiologists would need to learn a new skill set as they must adopt and use different types of technologies and instrumentation. Their routine and established cath lab approaches would further be amended by adding perfusionists to run a portable heart-lung machine (which is available). The costs would increase, but markedly superior clinical outcomes could result from this innovative treatment.

Ideally, hospitals might construct a single integrated treatment room that houses both a catheterization laboratory and an operating room, perhaps locating such rooms in the ER to maximize coordinated efforts. A fresh series of protocols would naturally develop around these hub areas, enabling their cath lab to work as smoothly as our operating rooms.

The bottom line is, at the time of this writing, none of these changes have been either contemplated or achieved. It is as if our findings had never been discovered.

Certainly there are costs associated with the modifications I've described. But what is the *real price* of this resistance to change? In the nearly 30 years since our breakthroughs, millions of heart attack patients have been admitted to hospitals across the world. Thousands upon thousands have died of either the heart attack, or they developed heart failure at a later date due to the damaged muscle not being saved.

Unfortunately, these avoidable patterns of patient suffering and early death mimic the sad pattern of my father and grandfather. While the incidence of cardiovascular disease has been reduced by around 30% using today's standard

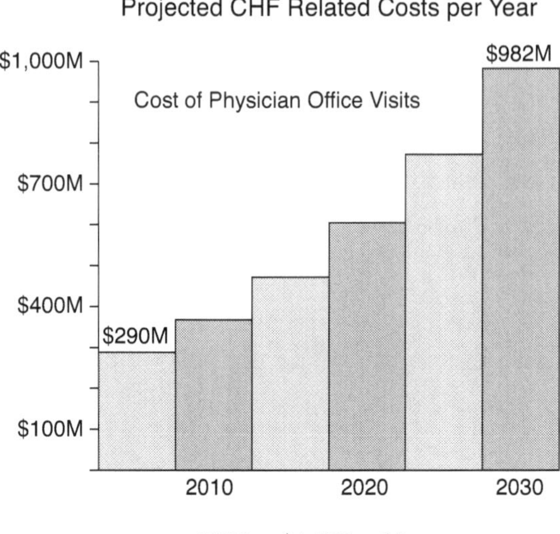

Figure 1: Projected costs for office visits to treat heart failure between 2005 and 2030.

treatments... *the death rate from heart failure has remained unchanged* between 1995 and 2009 (latest figures reported).[37] Plus the estimated financial cost in 2030 to care for these patients — will be $1 trillion.[38] (**Figure 1**)

The Challenge of New Ideas

Though startled by the medical community's resistance to our new life-saving knowledge revealed in this chapter, this would not prove to be an isolated case.

I have often wondered why so many surgeons readily welcomed the innovative ideas for protecting the heart during a cardiac operation (blood cardioplegia) that I developed at the initiation of my career — while others within our cardiovascular profession almost automatically and fiercely oppose implementation of the other new solutions to the major cardiac problems addressed during the next 45 years of my career — including treatments for heart failure and sudden death (cardiac arrest). All of these (and more) will be described in the following chapters.

Is it complacency — believing that what you already do is sufficient? A fear of failure — afraid to try new things that depart from what's familiar?

Erring on the side of caution by continuing what's been done before is always easiest and creates less risk (even if that path may fairly consistently create an unsuccessful result for many patients).

So why was there such an enthusiastic acceptance of blood cardioplegia?

I realized it comes down to a simple truth: if the heart's performance is severely impaired after an operation has corrected the underlying defect, the surgeons feel at fault. In other words, the heart was more hurt by the procedure than it was helped. They recognized their actions had a detrimental impact — as they were *active participants* in the problem — which fosters an eagerness to embrace new fundamental solutions that will improve treatment.

In contrast, patients afflicted with a heart attack, heart failure, or sudden death are often looked upon as being affected by "natural events." It is not the physician's fault if they don't recover. *The problem is the disease.* The comment that "our treatment is what everyone does all the time" is commonplace. In such cases, it seems to me that the cardiologist may become an *observing participant,* perhaps passive as they monitor pharmaceutical approaches to see how they produce positive changes to the patient's symptoms (the role angioplasty plays will be discussed later).

Still, I cannot be certain. These observations are personal reflections, and have not been evaluated for validation.

The Road Before Us

As I've said, even with the opposition I would repeatedly experience to my discoveries, I never become discouraged. I believe my task is to find the answers and to make them known. In the same way that my grandfather found a way to telegraph his intent even while speaking only Yiddish, I must continue to find ways to get the message out — even to those who don't want to hear it — *as well as to those* who may not speak the scientific language of researchers or the medical vernacular of cardiologists... *you.* As I mentioned, part of the intent for telling my story here is for the public to become aware that we have ways to counter the all-too-frequent misery and early death that still accompanies heart attacks, as well as ways to resolve the other conditions described in this book.

As acclaimed astrophysicist, author, and recipient of the NASA Distinguished Public Service Medal, Neil de-Grasse Tyson, once said: "The good thing about science is that it's true whether or not you believe in it."

The truth is, treatments solving these problems exist.

Readers of this book may add their voices to mine and those of my colleagues who continue to push the rock up the hill, trying to encourage the larger medical community to transform. Frankly, we owe it to our patients, our colleagues, our loved ones, and the world at large to advance this long-overdue shift. Change and evolvement are inevitable. The answers are already here.

How long do we wait before we embrace them?

CHAPTER 10

Re-oxygenation Injury: If a Little Oxygen Is Good, Is a Lot Better?

We learn the importance of oxygen at a young age. It becomes apparent the first time we try to hold our breath or discover how far we can swim underwater. Our understanding expands in grammar school when we learn that room air contains about 21% oxygen, and later, that "green tanks" of pure oxygen (100%) are used to supplement breathing, as in the oxygen tents shown in old movies.

Yet we generally take oxygen for granted.

Until we don't have it.

From the moment a newborn's bottom is lightly spanked in the delivery room to initiate breathing outside the womb for the first time, to the hearty pink color of babies in the nursery, eyes open in animated wonder... we witness the marvel of how breathing room air, containing normal oxygen, contributes to their healthy appearance.

Conversely, a world of sorrow emerges when these children fail to get enough oxygen. They appear dusky and blue, languishing rather than exhibiting the normal activities that characterize healthy infants.

The causes of this can relate to heart as well as to lung conditions, and the history of cardiac surgery includes developing excellent ways to correct this problem to allow "blue babies" (called cyanotic) to become oxygenated.

Yet among these worthy accomplishments, I would discover something startling. Though helping these babies receive increased levels of oxygen would seem a viable way to offset this problem — sometimes it made things worse. Much worse.

My first exposure to the dilemma of oxygen being a problem rather than a cure happened when I was asked by the pediatricians to express my thoughts about an infant who had a deep blue color because her lungs were immature and had become congested. The heart itself was beating fast, but working well.

The solution seemed straightforward. The pediatric cardiac surgeons could easily take over for the lungs and heart by using a miniature heart-lung machine. In this way, they could provide her sufficient oxygen so her stressed lungs would not have to work — they could rest, allowing them to heal.

This was done by inserting two small tubes into the infant's blood vessels. These tubes were connected to the small heart-lung machine, which administered its usual high levels of oxygen. Newly oxygenated red blood was pumped back into the proper artery to be distributed to the body. The infant's coloring improved and became pink. All appeared better.

Then to everyone's surprise, things were *not* better. This child's lungs suddenly grew more swollen from fluid accumulation (water in tissues), and the heart began *not* working well, contracting poorly.

The child's condition deteriorated despite our having delivered a treatment that takes care of what was wrong. Even though the heart and lungs were put at rest so there could be healing, their condition became worse than before treatment was started. The supposedly wonderful thing I had learned of in school that came from those miraculous green oxygen tanks — now appeared to be causing terrible harm.

This wasn't what we expected. It wasn't what the parents were expecting. Obviously, they and their physicians were distressed. "How do you explain this?"

I couldn't.

They had done nothing incorrectly. I could only say, "Something is occurring that we don't understand."

Unfortunately, I would discover this experience was not unique. Oftentimes, when others treated blue babies in this same way, these children would develop swollen lungs, and most importantly, their hearts became "stunned" — their contraction diminished — and sometimes would completely stop beating.

An Even Bigger Dilemma

As it would turn out, this dire situation wasn't the only circumstance in which providing supplemental oxygen became a problem.

Brad Allen, chief resident of cardiac surgery at UCLA, visited my office looking preoccupied and perplexed.

I asked, "Brad, what is troubling you?"

He seemed frustrated as he related stories of treating children that were blue from a congenital heart defect whose hearts were then superbly corrected in surgery... only to have them develop poor heart performance, sometimes succumbing from cardiac failure. Brad recounted his painful exchanges with distraught parents whose infant now had a corrected heart, but faced uncertain survival. Brad's question was clear.

"What happened to twist this technical success into a potentially tragic outcome?"

Brad had been helping to correct underlying heart defects in infants and children — both those who were blue (cyanotic, from too little oxygen), or others that were pink (having normal amounts of oxygen). But he was baffled. The duration of the operations were similar... with each infant receiving the same cardioplegic solution to prevent damage when the heart's blood supply was temporarily interrupted... *and* each receiving the same elevated concentrations of oxygen on the heart-lung machine. Yet while the pink babies thrived... some blue babies were experiencing the tragedy that he described.

Though adding a surgical operation differed from our first example of only helping the blue baby's lungs since the heart was normal, there was one striking similarity:

These blue babies always experienced heart damage when oxygen was delivered in high concentrations.

The sleuthing needed to begin.

Probing the Riddle

As I only performed adult cardiac surgery, listening to Brad describing these problems about pediatric surgery was eye-opening. The pink children, in whom surgeons closed a hole in the ventricle, had a smooth course: heart action was normal, their lungs remained clear with normal breathing patterns, and no body swelling occurred.

In contrast, substantial problems developed in some of the blue (cyanotic) children. Their procedures often fixed a poorly developed left ventricle, or corrected the positions of the aorta and pulmonary arteries that were in the wrong hookup position to the ventricles. The reasons for their cyanosis were corrected by a technically successful operation. But despite such benefit, the infants' lungs became stiff (not stretching or functioning normally), and the heart and other tissue areas became swollen.

This led to the awful situation where the child's chest sometimes had to remain open after surgery, because closing it would put too much pressure on the already swollen, poorly contracting heart. This meant the child would remain in the ICU under careful watch, with a biologic dressing on the surface of the heart, while the organs and tissues dried out for two to three days before the chest could be closed. As you might imagine, this was a very intense and stressful situation for the surgical staff — and especially for the parents. Unfortunately, this drama was almost predictable if the infant was cyanotic before the surgical procedure.

In every case, the child's procedure had required the use of the heart-lung machine. Could this miraculous technology — that had literally transformed heart surgeries and helped save countless lives since the 1950s — somehow be the source of the problem?

A Walk Through Surgical History

The role of oxygen in modern cardiac surgery began in the 1940s, as the first operative procedures were done to improve blood oxygenation in blue babies.

The major cause for cyanosis is birth defects in which there are holes or flaws within the heart, whereby *blue blood* (which has had its oxygen depleted after being used by the body) becomes improperly redirected into the arteries of the body's circulation *where red oxygen-rich blood is meant to be circulated.* Because of this, cyanotic (oxygen depleted) blood goes to body organs, instead of normally first going to the lungs to take up oxygen. This was a dreadful problem, as you can imagine.

Cardiologists and surgeons could only use the tools that were available at that time; they did not have sophisticated modern X-rays, angiograms, and echograms. Yet their intuitive wisdom and sage diagnostic abilities determined there was too little oxygen in these babies. The most common defect was called *tetralogy of Fallot* (TOF). It was comprised of several primary defects: a hole in the septum (the muscular curtain between the left and right ventricles), a narrowing of the pulmonary artery supplying the lungs, and the thickening of the right ventricle (due to its having to now work harder.) Unfortunately, the prognosis was grim for these cyanotic children, and the pediatric community felt tremendous grief for their plight.

But in 1944, a groundbreaking surgical approach to improve oxygenation for these children was developed at Johns Hopkins Hospital, and it overcame these limitations.

There was a unique cast of cardiac pioneers at Hopkins during this time. This breakthrough started with Helen Taussig, a cardiologist and one of the giants of cardiovascular disease, who cared for cyanotic children that no one could help. She was desperate to figure out what was happening inside them, since all would perish at a very early age.

Dr. Taussig's thirst for knowledge overcame her own limitations, including dyslexia, and a hearing difficulty that prevented her from using a stethoscope, one of the most potent diagnostic tools for a cardiologist as they could listen to the beating heart. Her unstoppable creative drive was her forte, and this led her to come up with innovative ways to understand and then help these desperately ill children.

Since these defects were genetic, she knew nature itself created the causes behind what was happening in these children, and so she did something extremely remarkable: she analyzed the baby's evolution in the womb. This included recognizing that before they were born, the lungs of children are collapsed and do not receive blood flow to gain oxygen, since oxygen is supplied by the mother. The mother essentially becomes the baby's heart-lung machine, because her oxygen-rich blood is diverted or *shunted* into the embryo's body through a tube called the *patent ductus arteriosus*. Dr. Taussig properly reasoned that these infants did fine in the womb — until this *ductus* would naturally close after birth — at which point the baby became cyanotic.

The baby's own lungs were to take over at this time, but because of anatomical defects, this was not happening sufficiently. Dr. Taussig surmised that cyanosis would not have developed if the infant's ductus had remained open, since it would have provided an alternative path for blood flow between its body and lungs that would have compensated for the baby's defect. That was not possible because the ductus closed at birth, certifying that nature didn't intend it to remain open.

Dr. Taussig asked, "Is there a way medical science can make a substitute?"

As I've always appreciated, the beauty of the university is that within its walls lives an abundance of innovative, dedicated people, whose individual talents may blossom further through interaction with colleagues from another field of study. This marvelous blending of gifts existed at Hopkins, where the Chief of Cardiac Surgery was Alfred Blalock. He possessed a creative intellect and was a titan in his field, and I would later have the good fortune to learn from him when I came to Hopkins in the 1960s.

Before arriving at Hopkins, Dr. Blalock had done experiments at Vanderbilt University where he created a shunt (hookup) that connected a branch of the aorta (the body's main artery) to the pulmonary artery (which normally carries oxygen-depleted blood to the lungs). He was trying to increase the lung blood pressure. But even though the operation worked well technically, his hookup couldn't raise blood pressure in the lungs. This was due to a natural adaptive mechanism in the body in which, under normal conditions, only the lower part of the lung receives blood flow. This sets the stage for exercise, during which increased blood flow would enter the whole lung, and not burden the lungs with high pressure. This natural adaptation for allowing an amplified blood flow in the lung, prevented Blalock from achieving his expected results and caused him to abandon this pursuit.

At Hopkins, Dr. Taussig came to Dr. Blalock with her theory about what was happening with her cyanotic children, hoping a surgical solution to the problem could be found. After listening to her observations, Dr. Blalock said, "Helen, it sounds to me like you're looking for a substitute ductus to replace the one that nature closed. It so happens that I have made such a ductus. While it did not increase blood pressure in the lungs as I had intended... *it did significantly increase blood flow to the lungs.*"

The First-Ever Innovative Procedure

The reader needs to appreciate that until this time — ten years before the invention of the heart-lung machine — *no one was operating on hearts.* It was believed to be impossible. At the same time, one couldn't help but become terribly saddened upon seeing the suffering of the many blue babies under Dr. Taussig's care. These children had no reprieve from a death sentence due to their defects.

Dr. Blalock took on the challenge.

Before conducting this trailblazing surgery on a patient, there needed to be experimental evidence that this shunt could work in a cyanotic subject. Yet this task of creating cyanosis in an animal test subject had never been accomplished.

This assignment fell onto the shoulders of Dr. Blalock's highly gifted lab technician and colleague, Vivien Thomas. Thomas was himself a pioneer, having demonstrated phenomenal insight and surgical abilities despite having never gone to medical school, and during a time when such opportunities in the lab did not exist for African Americans. In fact, the splendor of the relationship between these two colleagues was highlighted many years later in the television movie, *Something the Lord Made,* which received great acclaim (including nine Emmy Award nominations and the win for Outstanding TV Movie).

After numerous frustrating attempts, Thomas finally managed to make an animal subject develop cyanosis, and together, he and Dr. Blalock showed that this shunt *could* counteract the cyanotic condition.

It finally came time to perform the operation on a baby.

The first infant underwent the operation in 1944, but the road to success was not smooth, as the administrators at Hopkins denied all African Americans access to the operating rooms. Dr. Blalock cast aside these "social traditions" and demanded that Vivien stand alongside him to oversee the technical aspects of this procedure.

Meanwhile, some of the Hopkins staff in attendance to observe the procedure voiced skepticism, holding fast to the conventional belief that surgery on the heart was simply not feasible.

Yet it was the surgical team's actions — not the rigid conceptual barriers — that took center stage. The drama of success was instantaneous, as opening the shunt made the baby's blue color immediately change to pink!

This extraordinary procedure was named the Blalock-Taussig shunt and it initiated the modern era of cardiac surgery.[39] The world welcomed the chance to learn this stunning approach, and Dr. Blalock traveled the globe to teach it to others.

Building on Their History

Many years after this breakthrough event, I remember donning my "white suit" to start my medical life as an intern at Johns Hopkins Hospital. On that first day in 1961, I was awed to enter the Center for Surgical Sciences building (today called the Blalock Building). It represented a magical world to this 26-year-old. The elegant lobby displayed beautifully framed photos of past chief residents, a historical panorama that included the most famous heart surgeons in America, who had started at this very place where heart surgery originated. Certainly, this kid from the Bronx could have been intimidated, questioning if his abilities would ever match theirs. Could I carry on their legacy? But mostly I was hungry for learning, feeling fortunate and grateful to be at one of the world's preeminent hospitals! Walking through these hallowed halls was exhilarating.

From here, I went upstairs to the floor above the operating room, where interns and residents would take lunch. The menu was simple: saltine crackers, peanut butter and jelly, and soup. We were paid $45 per month. Across from me at the luncheon table was an English resident in orthopedics, who was perplexed by the traditions of Hopkins. Quenton said, "Gerry, I do not understand this place with its 150-year history and heritage displayed by a bevy of paintings of past pioneers. My English hospital is 750 years old, yet we do not tarnish the walls with such graphics." An interesting perspective, but it overlooked the importance of honoring those who had laid down stepping stones toward the future; the paintings were not simply there to provide a stroll down memory lane.

The impact of being at Hopkins at this time was profound. I remember my first impression of Helen Taussig. She appeared grumpy and did not communicate with surgical residents. But when she walked the halls of Harriet Lane (where pediatric patients were cared for at Hopkins), she was surrounded by a concert of cardiology residents and fellows hanging onto her every word.

Yet the truth of a person is not always visible from such external visual clues, just as the surface of the heart does not always reveal what is occurring within it. That truth is borne of performance. Dr. Taussig's clinical analysis of cyanotic children changed their lives and changed history, and her actions launched the field of pediatric cardiology. Her unyielding passion to create an innovative treatment let her cross the "impassable aisle" between cardiologists and surgeons to jointly champion the Blalock-Taussig procedure.

Equally impactful is that my internship at Johns Hopkins Hospital occurred while the Chief of Surgery was Alfred Blalock. Inspiring, logical, and wise, Dr. Blalock became a role model who had an enormous influence on my career.

For me, history and tradition became dramatically fused during an early experience in the operating room. As a young intern, it was astounding to have the chance to scrub in and stand alongside of Dr. Blalock, one of the greatest surgeons in the world, as he was about to perform his renowned shunt procedure on a blue baby. Traditionally, everyone in the operating room wears green scrub suits, but upon entering the OR, I saw the anesthesiologist was an elderly, frail lady dressed entirely in white. I wondered, "Who is she and why the white uniform?" I was told she was Olive Berger — who had performed the very same task, also while wearing white — when Dr. Blalock first conducted the procedure in 1944.

I held retractors as I watched Dr. Blalock guide his chief resident through each motion of the Blalock-Taussig shunt procedure. I was standing shoulder-to-shoulder with the "giant of heart surgery," drinking in each thoughtful comment while he tutored the next generation in the procedure that launched the field of cardiac surgery. The pinnacle came when Olive Berger peered at the blue features of the cyanotic child and remarked, just as she had that first time, how pink this child's appearance became as the shunt was opened and oxygen-rich blood nourished the body.

Though I didn't realize it then, that historical first surgery would hold additional resonance for me later, as Dr. Blalock's first assistant in that original operation was William Longmire, who would be my Chief of Surgery at UCLA from 1964–67.

Folklore in Hopkins' Hallowed Halls

Dr. Blalock's renown made him a legend at Hopkins, and naturally placed him at the center of many classic stories. These included tales of chief residents being overwhelmed when they first operated with him. In one story, a chief resident had been assisting Dr. Blalock in a procedure that aimed at enlarging the opening of the mitral valve (a structure between the left atrium and ventricle) that had become narrowed because of rheumatic fever.

In performing this operation, Dr. Blalock put a suture (stitch) encircling the top of the appendage of the atrium. He then placed his finger into the appendage to manually widen the thickened mitral valve, while tightly closing this suture around his finger to prevent any bleeding.

But he still noted bleeding after closing the suture. Dr. Blalock was from Georgia and spoke with a southern accent. As he couldn't use his one hand with its finger in the atrium, he quickly instructed, "Hep me, Hep me, Hep me" to the resident — meaning "Help me, Help me, Help me." The resident was unsure what to do, until Dr. Blalock stated, "Suck, Suck, Suck" — which meant to place a suction tip at the site of the bleeding. But the flustered resident thrust the sucker past Dr. Blalock's fingers and pushed it into the left atrium, essentially sucking out all the patient's blood! Dr. Blalock instantly commanded, "Step on it, Step on it, Step on it" — meaning the resident should immediately stop the suction by stepping on the tubing that ran across the floor. The resident promptly responded and there was a resounding *thud* as his foot hit the floor. Dr. Blalock winced and stoically declared, "That's maa foot" — his attention never wavering from the surgery he was performing.

Of course, all was corrected.

This oft-repeated tale revealed the straightforward nature of Dr. Blalock, who was also our leader of cardiac surgery. It made me further appreciate how fortunate I was to have the chance to satisfy my hunger *to learn* while at Johns Hopkins, a unique institution.

Unexpected Lesson

New ideas face criticism, and resistance to innovative change is not limited just to the world of medicine. Ironically, one of the first times I became aware of this rigidity was at a social event at Hopkins.

As was custom, the Hopkins surgical faculty would periodically invite interns and residents to a gathering at their homes, perhaps to make up for the usual saltines, peanut butter and jelly, and soup that we could afford on our meager salaries. While this was a gracious invitation, I soon discovered that the societal traditionalism at Hopkins was markedly different than its pioneering scientific advances.

One such event occurred at an elegant house with a swimming pool. I'd brought a date, Ingeborg. In 1961, women wore one-piece swimsuits that went from their thighs up to their shoulders. So when Ingeborg walked out looking gorgeous in her usual bikini, it set the conservatives aflutter. Women were aghast. "How can she dare do that?"

Though Ingeborg's swimwear would eventually become the norm, this showed me early on what happens when people are confronted with something new.

In her own way, Ingeborg was presenting the future, as I would later do with my work.

Naturally, I married her.

Arrival of the Revolutionary Heart-Lung Machine

After Dr. Blalock's original operation in 1944, the newly created Blalock-Taussig shunts were used universally, their success opening the door toward the future expansion of cardiac surgery. Still, while they improved the amount of oxygen to the body tissues of these blue children, they only provided a temporary solution since the underlying cardiac problem was not corrected by these hookups. As the baby grew, the evolving child needed more and more blood going through this fixed artery. To remedy the problem, we needed to get inside the heart and correct the tetralogy of Fallot defects, or other causes of cyanosis.

This goal would not be possible until 1953, when John Gibbon, a Philadelphia surgeon, invented the heart-lung machine.[40] This astounding contribution transformed the field of cardiac surgery by taking over for the heart and lungs. The surgeon could now open the heart and fix the cause of its symptoms. Our legendary Professor Blalock never tried to use the heart-lung machine, yet he dramatically showed the power of his mentorship by passing this torch of leadership to his students, who subsequently became worldwide leaders.

With Great Progress Comes Great Responsibility

How lucky I was to have been at Hopkins near the beginnings of open-heart surgery. I got to be part of a generation of surgeons whose toolbox now included the heart-lung machine, which advanced cardiac surgery in ways previously unimaginable.

Yet here I was, many years later at UCLA in 1992, trying to discover a possible flaw in the usage of this same miraculous development.

While I am an ardent advocate of *building on* tradition, I also believe it is our absolute responsibility to question if any of what we consistently do is always the correct choice.

Physicians, and especially surgeons, know that their actions will affect a patient's health and possibly their life. We meet this enormous obligation by using the best tools at our disposal to remedy an illness. The creation of the heart-lung machine placed a new set of accountabilities upon both the surgeons and the perfusionists (who actually operate them), as this device takes over the patient's breathing and oxygenation of their blood. But we must make critical choices about how we adjust this device to deliver the proper amounts of oxygen, as well as adjustments to flow, blood pressure, temperature, and other factors.

Nature makes these decisions when the patient's heart and lungs are functioning normally. But... *it is up to us* the minute we begin the heart-lung machine. We become "The Ultimate Decision Maker," and our judgments can powerfully influence surgical outcomes — and impact the patient's future.

My search to understand the problems we encountered in blue babies led me to ask, "Could the heart-lung machine suddenly shift from a friend to a culprit when we use it in efforts to cure their *hypoxia* (too little oxygen)?

This new responsibility of controlling the delivery of oxygenated blood to compensate for the baby's own lack of oxygen... reminded me of our studies with cardioplegia and the development of "controlled reperfusion" following a lack of blood flow to the heart. In those cases, we adjusted the composition and conditions of the first reflow of blood to offset the damage that the return of normal blood supply would cause during open-heart surgery (Chapter 6) or after an acute heart attack (previous two chapters). Now the task was delivering new oxygen after it has been deficient.

This brought up a new question: Could *we be causing* the surgical problems we were encountering in blue babes?

Airing Out the Issues

Conventional guidelines have been established for how the heart-lung machine is used. The traditional protocol includes administering oxygen at 400 to 500 mm Hg "PaO_2" — a term that describes *oxygen tension* or how much oxygen is dissolved in the blood plasma. These are much higher levels of dissolved oxygen than what we normally have in our blood after breathing room air, where PaO_2 is 150. The use of elevated levels is based upon making certain there's adequate tissue oxygen for body nourishment. No one was looking to alter this globally accepted reasoning because results were good.

Yet an intriguing dilemma confronts a medical team, who must ask: Should we simply do what we *believe* is good... or follow what we can *test and prove*?

We needed to look deeper into the role of oxygen to answer this question.

Oxygen, the Double-Edged Sword

The vital benefits of adequate blood oxygen are widely recognized. But oxygen may *also* cause damage when delivered in excessive amounts. These lessons about this dual role of oxygen are well known, yet sometimes we hear them *without listening.*

For example, long before the development of open-heart surgery, it was well-documented that premature infants, when exposed to high concentrations of oxygen therapy, may develop serious damage in the retina of their eye, sometimes becoming blind. This complication would ultimately lead to the lowering of oxygen concentrations in treating immature infants. Yet even this change was not initially embraced. Concerned by the use of these high concentrations, renowned pediatrician Arnold Patz applied for a grant to the NIH (National Institutes for Health, the main U.S. government agency for funding health research) to study the issue.[41] But his concerns were rebuffed and cast away with an admonishment by their expert committee that said, "Everyone knows premature babies need high oxygen concentrations."

It was a classic example by leaders at the NIH of how *conventional knowledge* is simply accepted even though no one had even considered or tested Patz's concept.

As he found (as have I on many occasions), experts are rarely receptive to having their cherished viewpoints challenged. Fortunately, Patz was not deterred. He found other funding, did his study, and his findings showed a dramatic reduction of baby blindness followed his lowering of oxygen concentrations.

Patz's conclusions have since been accepted and his guidelines are now used in premature infants in every nursery. But *cardiovascular practitioners* have not learned, established, or adopted them.

The benefits of oxygen are clear, but adverse consequences of its use in high concentrations have emerged. Increased oxygen can give rise to creating detrimental chemicals called *oxygen radicals* (also called *reactive oxygen species,* or ROS) — that destroy tissue by disrupting cellular structure and function, damaging DNA, and by igniting a cascade of other problems.

Fortunately, one of the many marvels of nature is that our "body fortress" contains elements that protect us against different types of stress. Antioxidant substances are produced to offset the damaging effects of increased oxygen tension and combat ROS. Yet this natural defense mechanism does not fully develop in the premature infant. Their body's antioxidant concentrations are low, which weakens their oxygen protective mechanisms, and accounts for them developing blindness after too much oxygen is delivered.

But here's the reality: cyanotic children have this *same* diminished defense against *hyperoxia* (too much oxygen).[42] For this reason, they may suffer enhanced injury when their low blood oxygen levels (only 25 to 30 mm Hg) — are routinely and dramatically enhanced to 400 to 500 mm Hg during an open-heart operation.

Looking Where No One Was Looking

Everything I have described was known at that time, yet no one had tried to examine if the heart-lung machine might play a negative role when used in the treatment of blue babies that undergo the surgical repair to correct the cause of their cyanosis.

In order to see if different guidelines were necessary, I realized we needed to learn more about oxygen. This revealed some information that was pivotal — *and fascinating.*

First, a normal level of blood oxygen, obtained as we breathe ordinary air, is called *normoxia* (normal oxygenation). In this circumstance, the oxygen saturation in the blood is about 98% — with *nearly all of the oxygen* carried in the red blood cells, which transport the bulk of oxygen to tissues.

The remaining oxygen is called *dissolved oxygen*, which floats in the blood plasma (the fluid in which blood cells and platelets are suspended). Breathing room air provides the 150 mm Hg oxygen level that is normally dissolved in the blood plasma, which actually yields negligible benefit to body function compared to the major contribution of oxygen in red blood cells.

Since normoxia (the oxygen level in room air — 150 mm Hg) causes 98% saturation of red blood cells, one might ask: "If a little bit of oxygen is good, is a lot better?"

Now, one *might assume* more is better, as had long been believed. But in reality, raising the oxygen level to 400 or 500 mm Hg as is typically done, cannot increase the oxygen saturation level to much more than the 98% level achieved by breathing room air. *But it does dissolve more oxygen into the blood plasma.* In fact, the heart-lung machine makes this occur very directly because its oxygenator is exceedingly efficient: if the oxygen setting is at 400 mm Hg — then 400 mm Hg of oxygen is dissolved in the blood. Yet the oxygen saturation within blood rises to only 99% — not a significant difference.

Intriguing information. But it remained unresolved about *how much oxygen should be administered* to blue babies.

Just raising such a question to traditionalists will garner vehement rejection, and stimulate their counterargument about keeping oxygen levels high — a strategy that they believe has "proven" itself over many decades since not all blue babies suffer damage from such operations. They perceive the greater risk is losing the baby because of "insufficient amounts of oxygen" from the heart-lung machine, and so the possibility of hyperoxic damage is not acknowledged. This prevailing attitude precisely matches the thrust of the NIH experts' comments as they denied the grant application of Patz, thinking his study of lowering oxygen levels to prevent blindness in premature infants was foolhardy.

Yet conclusive answers cannot be gained by adhering to past beliefs — or by assuming that what seems logical is valid. The answer is *only revealed through investigation.* While the results may be surprising, they are always true. The challenge is to uncover the underlying reasons for them.

Welcome to the job of the researcher.

Initial Investigating Step: Confirm What Is Known

In order to prove if conventional re-oxygenation could harm blue babies, we had to start by showing we could produce this damage in animal test subjects that had been made cyanotic and then treated with sudden hyperoxia (elevated oxygen concentrations).

There was precedent for the preparation of this task, as Vivien Thomas had done the same thing to set the stage for Dr. Blalock's experimental shunt procedure. Our infant piglets were made cyanotic by either lowering oxygen levels in a ventilator (a device that supplies air for breathing), or with a heart-lung machine.

Once we had created our cyanotic piglets, we first confirmed that these low levels of oxygen did not cause damage (since no injury existed in blue baby heart muscle before re-oxygenation). Our findings showed their hearts had no injury.

That led us to our next step: having the heart-lung machine introduce hyperoxic (excess oxygen) re-oxygenation.

The results were glaringly apparent: *oxidant damage consistently developed* during the first 5-minute interval in which a traditional 400 mm Hg oxygen level was delivered! Heart performance deteriorated and antioxidant reserves fell.[43]

This established there was an inherent problem with the use of high re-oxygenation levels in cyanotic infants with lung problems. That is exactly what happened to the blue baby (described at the beginning of this chapter) that surprisingly developed heart failure — the unexpected observation that ignited my search into finding why this tragedy occurred.

While gratified that we had found the reason for this unexpected deterioration, I remained troubled that physicians did not appreciate or understand why this extensive damage may happen. The result is that blue babies continue to receive high-oxygen re-oxygenation protocols in major centers around the world.

Our goal became clear. We needed to uncover solutions.

Closing In!

We knew that cyanotic babies don't have a strong reserve capacity of antioxidants (those natural substances that combat toxic oxygen) and have limited ability to produce them. Consequently, these babies are unable to neutralize the damaging agents that surplus oxygen will produce. So we thought to first see if a treatment that *added antioxidants* might offset this damage.

We tried various types of antioxidants, using different amounts of each. Though met with failure many times, we were tenacious in our pursuit.

We finally found the adverse oxygen-related changes could nearly be avoided by adding any one of four specific types of antioxidants — provided they were given *before* hyperoxia was caused by the heart-lung machine.

Then we took a different step. Instead of finding a way to counter administering high levels of oxygen, we confronted our suspected culprit *head on* and lowered the amounts of oxygen administered.

The result was both elegantly simple and profound:

Re-oxygenation injury did not happen if normal oxygen levels (100–150 mm Hg) was used, and hyperoxic levels (400 mm Hg) were avoided. This assumption was what we had hoped to be true — the proof is always in the pudding — *and now we had proven it*. Everyone on the team was delighted that we had found a solution to this terrible global problem.

But we were not done yet. The most critical and challenging part needed to be solved.

Re-oxygenation and Heart Surgery

So far, we had only done trials on animal subjects that did not experience the open-heart surgery that would be needed to help these cyanotic babies. Our next step involved confirming whether re-oxygenation damage will develop as the congenital defect causing cyanosis was corrected.

The battle plan was clear: we would mimic what occurs in a typical operative procedure. The heart-lung machine delivering typically high oxygen (400 mm Hg) levels was started for our test subjects. Five minutes later, the aorta was clamped and our cardioplegic solution (which we had shown to be safe in neonatal hearts) was used for protection during the cardiac repair.

The outcomes mirrored what occurred in our prior hyperoxic re-oxygenation studies (those without a cardiac operation), as the same glaring injury reappeared. Remarkably, only five minutes of the 400 mm Hg re-oxygenation were needed again to cause severe oxidant damage and impaired heart function.

These findings *confirmed* our expectations of the damaging role that traditional re-oxygenation played in blue baby's hearts that undergo a technically perfect surgical repair of the reason behind their cyanosis.

Our next crucial step was to explore if our newly discovered antioxidants could avoid such toxic re-oxygenation damage.

We had high expectations.

But they weren't met.

Though superb success occurred previously (when we did not stop the heart's blood supply since we were not recreating an operation), only 50% recovery followed the antioxidant use during cardiac surgery. While we had hoped for a "magic pill," reality set in, as these drugs fell short.

Though disappointed, we still had one other arrow in our quiver. We would vary the amount of oxygen delivered.

It certainly made sense to us. But would it work?

Indeed it did.

Nearly complete avoidance of oxidant and functional damage followed our keeping the oxygen level at 100 mm Hg (versus the conventional 400 to 500 mm Hg)! We were on the road toward success. A rewarding outcome was achieved!

But could we do even better?

Taking a lead from our studies on "controlled reperfusion," we now developed a strategy called "controlled re-oxygenation." In colorful terms, this means "You dance with the same guy who brought ya." That is, we would begin the procedure by *matching the low oxygen level* that our cyanotic babies had when they came to us.

So we started the heart-lung machine at the same hypoxic level (too little oxygen) *that had already existed* in the cyanotic test animal — about 25 mm Hg — and maintained this hypoxic level for the initial five minutes before clamping the aorta to start the repair.

The oxygen level was then made normoxic (100 mm Hg) and kept there throughout the period of clamping.

The outcome?

Complete recovery of normal heart performance and antioxidant reserve capacity!

We were elated!

I felt both gratified and reassured that this sequence of *controlled re-oxygenation* "paralleled" our earlier victories with controlled reperfusion after acute heart attacks.

Time to Go Public

The design, implementation, and completion of this study's many steps required three years of laboratory research. Yet an astounding and simple conclusion was reached: *hyperoxia (O_2 at 400–500 mm Hg) should not be used in cyanotic children.*

All of our data on re-oxygenation injury was accumulated before publishing any of it, echoing the previous tactic I used in reporting reperfusion injury. In 1995, this new research was submitted to the Journal of Thoracic and Cardiovascular Surgery, the field's most prestigious and well-read journal.[43] The journal's editor was John Kirklin, who previously had provided my first career invitation to be a guest speaker at the University of Alabama 20 years earlier, and whose astute observations kindled my controlled reperfusion studies. He had deep interest in re-oxygenation injury because he had helped develop the initial heart-lung machines at the Mayo Clinic, where the earliest operations were performed on cyanotic infants. Kirklin was not a traditionalist. His focus was upon learning, improving, and solving problems related to this device.

Kirklin graciously helped me organize our report's contents. He challenged any ambiguities, as a tutor might do with a wayward scholar. I loved it! We shared the same aim: teaching the reader. Each of the 13 articles was evaluated by three reviewers and accepted. These studies were then published as a Supplement to the Journal — only the third time it had issued such an addendum. The second had been our study of reperfusion injury.[30, 43]

But Does It Work Where It Really Counts?

Now it was time for our final step: to apply our experimental findings from the lab to the clinical environment. Ultimately, the only true confirmation of this approach is if it will help our patients.

A pediatric cardiac surgeon was needed to make this natural progression from lab to patients (bench to bedside), as I did not operate on children. Brad Allen, who was cited earlier in this chapter, took on the role. He was working in Chicago at the time that we did our re-oxygenation studies, but always kept in touch. He was fascinated by our findings and wanted to test this approach in patients.

Armed with the new ideas we uncovered, he approached Michel Ilbawi, an eminent pediatric surgeon and head of Brad's department, and asked to implement a new study. It was admittedly pretty gutsy of Brad to suggest that the established master should consider changing his ways. But Ilbawi, like Kirklin, knew existing solutions were not perfect, and his open-minded attitude propelled our discoveries to be applied in his blue baby patients. A true leader, Ilbawi provided Brad with the confidence and support that sows the seeds of growth.

Brad set the oxygen levels in the heart-lung machine at 120–150 mm Hg, rather than the traditional 400–500 mm Hg levels... *and found substantial reduction in oxygen-related damage.* Simultaneously, he realized the road to success is often paved not only by the initial answers, but can also benefit from further steps. Brad recognized that another source of injury could be the white blood cell (WBC) component, which can plug capillaries, and invade injured cells to produce dangerous oxygen radicals. His route to counteracting this damage was to use a WBC filter.[44]

Brad Allen and Michel Ilbawi's results in blue babies matched our experimental findings — as improved heart function and greater antioxidant reserve capacity followed their combining lowered oxygen in the heart-lung machine with using a WBC filter.

Their approach was then used in 72 patients with severe cyanosis. Recovery of heart function was excellent, without lung swelling or body swelling from water accumulation. There was no need to leave a baby's chest open after surgery due to a swollen heart.[45, 46]

A dramatic change from their prior experience with conventional high-oxygen approaches.

Further Corroboration

Another UCLA alum played a significant role in confirming our initial findings. While a postdoctoral fellow with us at UCLA, Kiyozo Morita had conducted many of our experimental studies on re-oxygenation injury, along with Kai Ihnken from Germany. Kiyozo became a respected pediatric surgeon in Japan, and applied our protocols with great success on his patients.

In 2012, he was invited to write an overview about re-oxygenation injury in the *World Journal for Pediatric and Congenital Heart Surgery*.[47] Aside from recounting his prior experimental work at UCLA, and citing findings from his own practice, he summarized internationally published papers about cyanotic children that were successfully treated with controlled re-oxygenation. These reports came from the United States, England, Turkey, Germany, Japan, and China. Each verified that use of normal levels of oxygen in heart-lung machines had offset impairment of heart function and oxidative reserve capacity. Moreover, since re-oxygenation affects the *whole body* (it is not limited only to the heart and lungs), Kiyozo showed that reduction in brain damage also occurred in cardiac surgical patients.

I was elated by Kiyozo's achievement, and filled with pride as I watched how those whom I'd mentored in the laboratory evolve into leaders in their fields.

Now, we naturally expected there would be widespread changes in the re-oxygenation treatment of blue babies following this worldwide confirmation of our 1995 experimental findings.

This did not happen.

How could that be?

I do not have the answer, but know that many pediatric surgeons think our worldwide analysis of the role of oxygen injury is simply unimportant. They don't believe that the problems they see are related to re-oxygenation injury. Instead, they blame these unforeseen complications on other reasons. After all, they followed long-accepted traditions, so how could those actions create such a problem? Surprisingly, they adhere to this unyielding conclusion despite their need to sometimes keep a recovering baby's chest open for several days because the damaged heart swells after its injury... or need to use a temporary mini heart-lung machine because the baby's heart cannot support life.

As Frank Lloyd Wright, the renowned architectural genius, said, *"An expert is a man who has stopped thinking because 'he knows.'"*

CHAPTER 11

Back from the Dead: Sudden Death and the Lazarus Syndrome

The Bible tells the tale of Lazarus, who is returned to life from the dead. Though an ancient story, it still resonates today.

Nearly 400,000 times a year in the U.S., someone suffers an abrupt, unexpected death involving their heart. Called "sudden death" in medical reports, it is characterized by the immediate loss of consciousness that follows the loss of an "effective" heartbeat. This means the heart either stops completely or continues beating in such a way that it is ineffective at delivering blood to the brain. This is critical, as failure to pump sufficient blood to the brain will result in brain death after only four to five minutes.

Understanding this is important in order to differentiate between what's simply described as a "heart attack" from what is called "sudden death." In both cases, the heart may malfunction due to its receiving an inadequate supply of blood, most commonly the result of narrowing of its nourishing arteries, since about 70% of these sudden death patients have disease in their coronary arteries. The difference is while there is damage to the heart with a heart attack, it continues beating and supplying blood to the brain.

With sudden death (also known as "cardiac arrest"), the heart will either stop beating, or more commonly, develop an abnormal heart rhythm called ventricular fibrillation. This chaotic heartbeat prevents any meaningful contraction from the now quivering heart muscle. There is no blood pressure and this triggers sudden death.

This process is devastating, and has nearly always been fatal.

Beginning of Change

Things began to shift in 1961, when knowledge that sudden death led to 100% mortality without treatment spawned the emergence of two remarkable discoveries.

First, a defibrillator had been developed to electrically shock the heart and restore a normal rhythm. This is the type of device commonly seen on medical shows where paddles are placed on the patient's chest as "Clear!" is shouted to be sure no one is touching the patient. A precise electrical shock is administered to the body in the hopes of restarting the normal heartbeat.

Still, the problem remained as how to keep the heart pumping blood — especially to the brain — until a defibrillator could be brought to the patient and then applied (hopefully successfully), so that further treatment might then be used.

This led to the second discovery, a technique that would eventually be taught not only to doctors and nurses, but also to emergency medical technicians (EMTs), lifeguards, and eventually people in all walks of life: cardiopulmonary resuscitation, or CPR. This is accomplished by manual compression of the sternum by pressing down on the chest with two hands at a certain rate per minute. This external treatment physically compresses the heart to make it eject and pump blood through the body to deliver oxygen to the brain and other organs. CPR is always combined with artificial respiration to bring oxygen-containing air into the lungs.

The combination of these two new treatments allowed us to stimulate and maintain a heartbeat without opening the chest. They made a huge impact.

Now we *could* bring someone back from the dead. Lives would be saved.

Indeed, the development of CPR created a sea change in cardiology — which I know firsthand as I was fortunate enough to start my internship at Johns Hopkins Hospital in 1961 when these new protocols were introduced.[48] I felt very lucky to be part of this thrilling new advance.

Not only did I have the chance to meet two of the authors of this report (William Kouwenhoven, an electrical engineer, and James Jude, a cardiac surgeon), most importantly, I also had the opportunity to use these innovative methods when sudden death developed after cardiac surgery.

I recall my first experience. A post-surgical patient died from sudden death as he unexpectedly lost his heartbeat, stopped breathing, and sank into his bed unconscious. With no other physicians around, I called out to a nurse to alert the staff. I immediately checked for a heartbeat by feeling the patient's pulse: it was absent. I started chest compressions while another intern forced air into the patient's lungs by performing mouth-to-mouth breathing. This was done until a breathing tube could be placed, which allowed the ventilator to fill the lungs with oxygen and then empty them of carbon dioxide.

This was a very tense time for me — an intern — as I suddenly had full responsibility. My patient's life was at stake! It was no longer a training exercise.

I heard others wheeling in the defibrillator as we kept giving CPR. This was momentarily stopped so we could place the paddles on the patient's chest. After making sure everyone was clear of the patient, the button was pressed — creating the telltale *zap* as the device discharged an electrical current onto the chest that then reached the surface of the quivering heart.

The defibrillation worked on the first try! The heartbeat rhythm resumed, and a strong pulse could be felt. The drama was intense, but the patient revived. Even though colleagues congratulated me and the other intern for our actions, I was mostly relieved, and awed that this miraculous combination worked.

Those minutes were breathtaking. We witnessed a dead person magically recover to become a living one. How wonderful that these researchers could create such a treatment! Soon, I would be just one of many physicians worldwide whose ability to save lives became amplified by utilizing a novel treatment with a profound impact.

Experiencing this incredible contribution firsthand made me think about how wondrous it would be if I could someday come up with such a powerful new idea that others could use.

While I realized that CPR was still a small step forward since only 10% of patients receiving it at that time survived, the door seemed open toward learning why sudden death events occurred... and the important second step of designing new treatments to vastly improve success in resuscitating patients.

Surprisingly, that did not happen.

Today the Same as Yesterday

CPR is still used today, much as it was back then.

When other people are nearby to witness a person's sudden death after the heart stops beating — whether out in the world at large, or nestled within the hospital setting — we call this event a "witnessed arrest," and immediately starting CPR has become the international standard.

Yet despite what you may have been told or seen on television medical shows that glorify the heroic efforts of teams that use CPR to save a life... the sobering truth is that 90% of these patients succumb. Remarkably, this 10% survival mirrors the same rate that existed in 1961 when CPR was discovered.[49, 50]

This tragedy becomes compounded, as among the rare 10% of patient survivors, half of them (50%) suffer permanent brain damage because blood supply to the brain was inadequate.

This sad dilemma begs the question: *Why hasn't there been more progress?*

The Main Problem

The unfortunate reality is conventional medical wisdom considers that once sudden death occurs, there is little more we can do than what we already do. Yet this "established" belief is the nemesis to progress. It hinders the evolution of new approaches, and contradicts Einstein's fundamental concept of "nothing changes until something moves." What must move first is our thinking.

The plot thickens, as misleading statistical analyses compound the problem by providing illusions of "progress." In this case, subsequent improvement in survival from 10% to 15% was now considered a "50% enhancement of outcomes." Self-congratulatory praise is shared among the medical community, but this reaction departs from reality — as actual survival only rose by 5%.

To uncover elusive answers, investigators must frame their fundamental focus differently. The question must be, "Why do 85% of patients *still die* from an event that suddenly snatches life away from someone seemingly completely normal only moments before?"[50]

Minimal Movement

As described, minimal advancement between 1961 and 2018 has allowed the 85% mortality to continue. This 5% improvement was marginal as it resulted from only minor enhancements: how often to shock the heart to reverse ventricular fibrillation, and using body cooling to lower oxygen needs and reduce the inflammation from impaired circulation. This latter cooling technique came from clues gained through patients who revived better when they were found in cold water (for example, a driver losing consciousness after plummeting his car into a frozen lake), compared to patients suffering sudden death at normal temperature.

The absence of significant treatment improvements is due to the medical community's view of sudden death as a *disease*. Therefore, it aims its efforts at restoring an effective heartbeat. This total focus on how to administer the fewest shocks from the defibrillator, or learning if body organs should be colder or warmer, has resulted in the minimal 5% survival improvement over 50 years. The ongoing failure to reduce brain damage in the rare survivor has clearly exposed the profound limitations of adhering to traditional treatment.

An innovative approach is needed.

The first step requires *recognition that traditional methods have failed.* This appreciation must be coupled with a willingness to consider new approaches to counter these awful outcomes.

New View: Sudden Death as a Symptom, Not a Disease

The lack in understanding the causes behind these lethal occurrences is readily apparent from the actions occurring in hospital hallways. Sudden death is confronted by Code Blue teams that rush in with their crash carts. Their only goal is restoring normal heart rhythm. There is no consideration of why the heart stopped and how to remedy this.

So why is this short-sighted?

Because sudden death is not a disease, but *a symptom* of the disease that produced it. This implies that something else is needed beyond simply restoring a heartbeat.

While CPR would continue to be used to maintain critical brain nourishment during sudden death (since brain damage in the rare survivor will impair mental capacity and later cause their premature death) — I knew that developing a fresh strategy to discover and fix the underlying reason for the sudden death was also essential.

Brain is the Key

It has been common knowledge that "irreversible" brain death develops when blood flow is stopped for four to five minutes, so that the primary focus has been to nourish the brain (with CPR) while at the same time trying to return function to the stopped heart.

Yet it is also crucial to ensure that the brain continues to have adequate blood flow *after the patient's heart starts to beat again.* This is not an easy task, because most of the rare sudden death survivors develop a weakened cardiac function from their underlying damaged heart muscle. This accounts for much of the severe brain damage that develops in half of the 10% of surviving patients. It is why the conventional approach of "treating the heartbeat" instead of "treating the cause of the heart malfunction" creates the reason that brain damage occurs.

Until I realized this, my approach had been like that of others: to save the heart, but lose the brain. An unacceptable trade-off. But what else could we do?

Journey Begins

The path before us seemed clear. Our prior experimental and clinical studies on heart attacks documented that the heart can be fixed. While we clearly needed to do this, I believed it was also critical to find a way to sustain an adequate brain blood supply during — and after — the sudden death event.

This brought up the same enduring question that began when I was at Johns Hopkins: why did some patients survive, when most do not?

I remained perplexed. Could the answer to this mystery be the unattainable holy grail of cardiac medicine? The challenge to finding a solution seemed overwhelming. I was highly motivated, but it was still natural to question if a solution was possible.

Read on and you will find, just as I did — that answer is yes.

Changing the Study

At the time, we weren't studying sudden death, but rather, trying to find out what happens during an acute heart attack (caused by closing one artery)... under conditions where there is *also* narrowing in the artery that supplies the remote muscle. We used pigs as the test subjects, as their circulatory system is similar to ours (as mentioned before, pig heart valves are sometimes used to replace human valves).

Such conditions (one artery closed and another narrowed) imposed a severe affront to the circulation, and sudden death occurred in 80% of these pigs as they developed ventricular fibrillation. It was irreversible, despite our multiple attempts to defibrillate this quivering state. Their deaths mirrored the high mortality of patients who sustain sudden death.

A German research fellow, Friedhelm Beyersdorf, was the leader of our study. Very bright and inquisitive, he came to me with a new approach.

"We're studying the changes after a heart attack, but we're losing the animals. We know that controlled reperfusion will save the heart muscle after it has been without blood supply. So why not do that same treatment to pigs with a heart attack that develop the irreversible ventricular fibrillation that causes their sudden death? I think we can save them."

I looked at him a moment... and grinned. "That is a great idea. Let's do it!"

We weren't focused on sudden death until he raised that possibility. But I instantly recognized that it was a prime opportunity to try to address this almost untreatable clinical event — that causes a catastrophic 85 to 90% mortality.

As team members shared ideas, the excitement grew. Our collective pride blossomed as we designed a unique approach to this problem. But we still needed to take the second step.

We had to test it.

This pattern differs from traditionalists who might say, "I don't think that's possible and we're not going to spend time and deplete our precious funds on it."[50] But as I've said many times, conventional thinking is not my approach, for it creates a barrier to considering what might be attainable. Especially when a near fatal illness (85 to 90% mortality) may be conquered.

Perfect Conditions

The medical conditions we were creating in our test subjects as we studied acute heart attacks were perfectly suited for this new direction of research, as most sudden death patients also had narrowing of more than one coronary artery.

We worked out the details with Friedhelm after listening to everybody's ideas. Our underlying premise, based upon prior studies, was that damaged heart attack muscle can be saved and recover function. This approach "treated the heart," rather than followed the typical focus of simply "restoring the heartbeat." It differed from traditional attitudes, where the heart attack's cause that triggered the sudden death was not of immediate concern, since that could be corrected later in the rare survivor.

We were motivated to find a different approach that immediately dealt with the cause, since we knew the weakened heart would not function optimally even *after* the heartbeat was restored. Poor heart performance could cause death in the resuscitated patient in the hospital or soon thereafter. Even *if* it did not cause an early death, impaired heart function will still lead to brain undernourishment (and damage) in survivors.

The question now became: how could we treat the cause of the heart attack *while we were reversing sudden death?* This approach, if possible, would save the heart and the patient — and might avoid the all-too-frequent brain damage. In other words, our new target created a powerful dual goal: remedy the heart attack and avoid the brain damage at the same time.

Indeed, we were "outside the box" with this proposal. But that is the essential step in the evolution of dramatically new treatments.

Our New Study

I knew that reproducing real world clinical events was crucial to our designing and testing new treatments.

First, the brain needed to have adequate nourishment during the initial treatment of sudden death, so we made sure the CPR would keep blood pressure at or above 60 mm Hg. A key ingredient to this was having the blood pressure monitored through *every* stage of treatment. If the pressure ever went down, we sped up the frequency of compressions, raising the rate from the typical 60 compressions per minute up to 100 (100 is *now* the officially recommended CPR compression rate).

Step two was to recognize that CPR still does not ensure adequate blood flow to all the organs. So we believed the subject should be brought to the cath lab to be promptly placed on the heart-lung machine to fully take over pumping blood and lung ventilation. This intervention can be done without opening the chest, as we simply puncture the skin to access the blood vessel, much like one does with a needle and tube for an intravenous drip. This sequence exactly parallels how we treated acute heart attacks (Chapter 9), permitting us to directly treat the cardiac cause of sudden death.

Step three was to provide controlled reperfusion into the region that had undergone an acute heart attack, mirroring the approach we described in Chapter 9.

Reproducing Reality

To imitate the likely scenario that develops from these fatally fibrillating hearts, we induced sudden death conditions in animal test subjects. We first performed CPR for two hours to mirror the time needed to transfer a "patient" from the field to the hospital and directly to the catheterization lab to diagnose the cardiac reason for sudden death. The heart-lung machine is initiated in the cath lab and the diagnosis of the cardiac cause can be determined. An additional hour (using the heart-lung machine) is then added. This mirrors the transfer time to the operating room and the interval needed for delivering controlled reperfusion for the cardiac cause of sudden death. Blood reflow to overcome the remote muscle's narrowed artery is also done.

So the heart-lung machine was kept on for a total of two hours — the first for making the diagnosis and moving the patient to the operating room. The second hour represented the time we needed for delivering controlled reperfusion into the acute heart attack region and for bypassing the remote muscle's narrowed artery.

Success

Our findings tell the story.

There was 100% *survival* using the innovative method, which is in sharp contrast to the typical 85 to 90% *mortality* with conventional sudden death treatment. Heart function completely returned to normal, and each heart attack region recovered substantial function despite three hours without blood supply.[51]

This was stunning. *We had found a reproducible way to treat sudden death!* Our mood was euphoric and we congratulated each other.

As our focus centered on survival from sudden death, we did not evaluate neurological damage. We knew the brain received adequate blood pressure during CPR, and heart performance was similar to what is expected following a routine elective operation. We anticipated that brain function would be successfully retained because it always had flow at a high pressure (delivered by CPR), but realized that subsequent testing would be needed to make sure.

This great experimental triumph intensified our desire to apply this new treatment method to a patient with sudden death due to irreversible ventricular fibrillation — an event where anything more than just 15 minutes of CPR reduces the survival rate down to below 1% and there is consistent severe brain damage in those rare survivors. Essentially, we needed to see if our approach would save the life of someone whose survival was otherwise impossible.[50]

We didn't have to wait very long.

One morning, I had performed a routine valve replacement. The procedure went well. The new aortic valve was in place and heart function was excellent. The patient was to be moved back to the intensive care unit (ICU) and I returned to my office, satisfied that things had gone as planned.

Until I got a call: the patient's heart had developed ventricular fibrillation as he was wheeled back to the ICU — it caused sudden death!

"Doctor Buckberg, we've been doing CPR, but all attempts to restore his heartbeat have not yet...."

I didn't wait for further details. I hung up and rushed to see the patient, grabbing a member of my team along the way. We hurried to the hallway where interns and residents were administering chest compressions and supplying ventilation.

"Clear!"

Everyone stepped back as the defibrillator paddles were activated. The patient's body arched from the shock... but effective heart rhythm was not restored.

"Clear!"

They tried again. Again, no change. Seeing the resident who'd been giving CPR was tiring, I had my team member take over, while I checked the blood pressure reading on the monitor — it was barely 60 mmHg. My team member increased the rate of chest compressions to 100 per minute, as we wanted the pressure kept over 60.

I sent a message to others on my team that we needed to immediately go to the operating room and deliver controlled reperfusion. We were told all rooms were in use and they were not sure how long before one would be available.

More CPR and unsuccessful attempts at defibrillation continued as we waited for an operating room. It had already been 25 minutes and I saw the residents, interns, and nurses checking watches.

Remember, accepted conventional thought was that patients could not survive if receiving CPR longer than 15 minutes without restoring a heart rhythm.

I took over performing chest compressions from my tiring resident. We continued in vain to restore a heartbeat and waited for an OR. We were now at 45 minutes of CPR.

Finally one of the residents tentatively said, "Doctor B, I know he is one of your patients, but it's been over 45 minutes. There's very little chance of him recovering at this point. Really none."

"Well, I don't know that, not at all," I replied. "Here's what I do know — the heart is working because I'm compressing it. The brain is alive because we are maintaining a good blood pressure — it's never had lack of nourishment. I can fix the heart with controlled reperfusion, and I suspect the brain will be undamaged as long as we maintain a good blood pressure to perfuse it. *We just need an operating room."*

As you might imagine, they thought I was foolish. They didn't know of the successes we'd had in our lab... something I deeply hoped we could now duplicate.

Finally, an OR opened up and we brought our patient in. The rest of my team was ready and I put the patient on the heart-lung machine. I had already fixed his underlying cardiac problem. He had not suffered a heart attack, but we used controlled reperfusion to counter his ventricular fibrillation, just as we had in our test animals.

But would it work?

He responded beautifully! His heartbeat came back strongly, and we were able to take him off the heart-lung machine in routine fashion. His heart purred along!

Plus — he awakened promptly and there was no brain damage.

Suffice it to say, our whole team was ecstatic. We'd just done the impossible! Of course, the impossible is only impossible... until it isn't.

We applied our novel approach in 14 patients at UCLA. Thirteen patients had complete recovery of the heart (measured five to seven days later), while one patient succumbed to brain damage and death. These findings contrast sharply with results following conventional sudden death treatment (where brain damage develops in half of the 10 to 15% patients that recover cardiac function). By contrast, good brain function existed in 13 of our 14 patients.[52]

These were remarkable findings. We were thrilled!

Spreading the Word

I shared our findings with other surgeons — colleagues and friends I knew personally — as well as through presentations I gave at medical conferences. Indeed, these were the findings I shared with Connie Athanasuleas at the Duke University meeting, as described in the first chapter. I asserted that the traditional belief that there is 100% mortality of patients receiving CPR longer than 15 minutes *is simply not true*. I went on to explain that this innovative treatment involves three management principles:

- Make sure the brain doesn't die by giving CPR at a rapid rate to maintain sufficient blood pressure.
- Use the heart-lung machine to support the body and discover the underlying cause of the sudden death.
- Repair the heart region so it can function normally, followed by controlled reperfusion rather than using only normal blood supply.

Ours was a new approach that differed radically from the norm. And while I knew everyone was horrified by the high mortality normally associated with sudden death, I correctly anticipated there would also be enormous resistance to initiate a treatment that was so unlike what they were used to.

But that did not bar some who listened, were eager to learn, and applied the approach themselves. Subsequently, our integrated treatment would be used in 34 sudden death patients in different centers in the U.S. and Europe, with equally outstanding results. Patients underwent an average of 72 minutes of CPR (ranging from as short as 20 minutes to as long as 150 minutes in one of our own cases) and had a 79% survival rate — with only 5% developing brain damage.[53] As with our original test subjects, the patients' response in heart performance mirrored what would be expected from a routine heart operation. None of the typical complications expected with sudden death patients occurred.

Our approach, including a greatly extended use of CPR, was certainly novel. Yet the outcomes demonstrated that patient survival can occur after far longer time frames than those predicted by the traditional concept that "greater than 15 minutes of ventricular fibrillation is an irreversible condition."

Sometimes *much* longer.

I encountered such an extended duration in a patient of mine who experienced sudden death in the ICU. We had already repaired her underlying heart problem, and only needed to get her back to the operating room to give her controlled blood reperfusion to remedy the otherwise irreversible ventricular fibrillation.

Called to her bedside, I performed CPR, checking the wall monitor to ensure that my compressions provided the necessary blood pressure. We tried to defibrillate her heart multiple times, all without success. So I continued CPR, waiting for an OR to become available.

Finally, an intern reported the OR was ready. We could take her down right away.

Except I wouldn't. I wanted a transit monitor — a portable blood pressure monitor that could travel with us as we rolled her through the hall, to the elevator, and down to the operating room — so I could continue to make certain our CPR was adequately maintaining a higher blood pressure to nourish her brain.

Keep in mind that our approach was unusual, even in our own hospital. *Very* spirited discussions took place, as many staff members wanted to immediately go to the operating room.

"Why are we waiting, Dr. Buckberg? The OR is ready!"

"I'm not moving her until you get a transit monitor up here."

"She's dead. We tried to defibrillate her five times — she won't get better here. Let's get her into the operating room and work on her heart to fix it!"

But I was not budging. I needed that device to monitor blood pressure. For whatever reason, one wasn't forthcoming. Meanwhile, residents and nurses kept insisting we immediately head to the OR.

"Listen, I will not go to the operating room to treat her unless I know her brain blood flow is sufficient while we're transporting her there! If it's not, she'll die of brain death, even if I fix the heart. I'll wait over two hours if I have to!"

As it turned out, we did. Two and a half hours passed — 150 minutes.

The transit monitor finally arrived and we rushed her to the OR where her heart was given controlled reperfusion — and her neurological recovery was excellent.

This remains our best example, thus far, of recreating the Lazarus Syndrome.

Great Success... Has Gone Nowhere

The initial experiences in our 14 patients appeared in the *Journal of Thoracic and Cardiovascular Surgery*.[52] I received further feedback of its success during my travels to national and international conferences, as surgeons informed me of similar results after treating their post-operative cardiac arrest patients.

By 2006, we reported the 34 additional patients who had been successfully treated for sudden death with our methods by close colleagues.[53] This time I wanted the cardiology and resuscitation community to learn of this innovative and dramatically successful approach, since they generate the guidelines for treatment protocols of sudden death victims.

This did not happen. Our manuscript summarizing these never-before-seen international results was rejected by the two major cardiology journals.

"The pitfalls are unknown" was the reason they cited for rejection, though I suspect the truth was that we had incited an uneasiness. We had challenged the status quo by criticizing the limitations of current treatment. Perhaps their ire was raised by our asserting that "conventional approaches deal with the symptom of sudden death, but disregard its underlying cardiac cause."

We simply could not find a good source to publish our information in the cardiology journals. We ultimately did publish in the journal *Resuscitation*,[53] but it was not customarily read by the cardiology and cardiac surgical community. Frankly, it doesn't mean anything if one publishes... and nobody reads it.

So the death rate from sudden death remains at over 85% (minor improvement over the 90% observed in 1961 when CPR was developed), with brain damage still developing in 50% of rare survivors. Opposition to our innovative approach continues, despite these harrowing numbers.

In fact, the only improved methodology that's been embraced has been the induced topical cooling of the body — hypothermia — to lower the ventricle's and brain's energy requirements. The ability to decrease brain damage by cooling exists, yet this technique can only be used in the rare survivor (less than 10% of patients), and devastating brain injury still persists.[54]

In a sense, this focus on cooling reflects a step backward in the development of more advanced techniques for sudden death. Our prior research of heart damage showed that hypothermia is only one little part of the process, and that much more is needed to be done,[55] which is what motivated our use of controlled reperfusion.[19]

This large gulf between the understanding that others have, and the actions that must be taken... must somehow be bridged in order to make current treatment of sudden death successful.

Imagining a Better Tomorrow

The future seemed bright — because we had found and proved the solution. Yet new ideas must be turned into practice. The medical community must change its thinking by welcoming the freedom to adopt innovative and effective treatments that have been tested experimentally and proven in sudden death patients.

The approach remains three-pronged. CPR is first used to maintain brain blood flow. The heart-lung machine is then employed to stabilize the circulation and diagnose the underlying heart issue. Finally, the cardiac problem is corrected and controlled reperfusion is administered to remedy the reason behind development of sudden death. The tools to achieve all this are now available.

With present technologies, EMTs and other emergency personnel performing CPR can monitor blood pressure levels to make sure they are protecting the brain during retrieval and transportation of the body, allowing for much longer time periods than previously thought possible.

Portable heart-lung machines that are now available can be utilized by simply puncturing the skin with a needle to access the blood vessel — something that emergency personnel are also capable of doing, even while in the ambulance, and en route to the hospital!

The cardiac catheterization lab is capable of diagnosing the underlying cardiac problem, and must either learn to do the corrective treatment there, or send the patient to the operating room. Use of the heart-lung machine to protect the heart and brain can be done in either location, with controlled reperfusion given for heart recovery.

These are not new ideas. Our innovative approach exactly parallels techniques already used to treat patients sustaining heart attacks. The only difference is that heart attack patients have not died. CPR is not needed because they are alive. But most everything else done for the sudden death victim exactly mimics the way we treat heart attacks. Of great significance is that this approach adds a new dual treatment goal: *save the heart and the brain.*

The answers are here, as our 80% survival rate from sudden death, and the avoidance of nearly all brain damage, has been confirmed in patients treated at other major international centers.[53]

While such a positive future is within our grasps, the seeds for this change have not grown, as there is only marginal funding for sudden death by the National Institutes of Health (NIH), the chief U.S. agency devoted to health research. This inequitable deficiency is shown dramatically in a recent survey of NIH allocation of funds — that compares the number of deaths from a particular illness with the funding that NIH provides "per death" for that disease. For example, 750,000 patients with cancer died in one year, with NIH spending the equivalent of about $7,000 per deceased patient on research. Cardiovascular disease resulted in 500,000 patient deaths (except stroke), with approximately $4,000 spent per each of those patients by the NIH on research in cardiovascular disease.

Sudden death (cardiac arrest) occurred in 400,000 patients and the per-patient expenditure was $75. (**Figure 1**)

Disease	Deaths/yr	NIH Investment	$/Per Death
Cancer	750,000	5.2 *Billion*	$6,933
Cardiovascular	500,000	2 *Billion*	$4,000
Cardiac Arrest	400,000	30 ***Million***	$75

Figure 1: Funding from NIH to treat disease / patient deaths. Note comparisons between cancer, heart disease (excluding stroke), and sudden death. (Funding totals for 2013; downloaded from NIH August 4, 2014)

Amazingly, the situation has only gotten worse. The recent AHA update shows *further reduction* in allocations: 2017 funding for cardiac arrest (a disease with 85 to 90% mortality) is expected to fall to $63 per deceased patient!

So you have a disease (cardiac arrest) that *we can correct* (80% survival and minimal brain damage) — and practically no money is allocated for it. While immense funding is directed toward two other disease categories *they cannot correct.*

Astoundingly, this shortsightedness continues despite our international report documenting the success of these innovative methods. I suspect commitment to reverse the extremely high death rate from sudden death has not taken hold because they still believe there is no solution. We have one, but they don't want to hear it. That's because the solution means one must accept failure, and recognize it is essential to change the traditional approach to treatment.

I realize our approach radically alters what has been the norm for decades. Significant modifications would be needed in both methods and facilities. Cardiologists must use a heart-lung machine and learn to insert tubes for its use through the skin. New teams will need to join the cath lab for the heart-lung machine to be used there, and cath labs would need to be re-equipped. Both of these hurdles must be overcome to allow controlled reperfusion to take place. Resistance to these initial increased costs and training must be quashed, when weighed against the vastly improved patient outcomes that can be expected.

The key motivator is that many lives can be saved. Not the 10 to 15% as is the case now, but the 80% that have very little accompanying brain damage. This stunning impact becomes clear when we consider how many of the 400,000 patients in the U.S. experiencing sudden death can be returned to normal fruitful lives.

Signs of Progress

Despite the disappointing lack of acceptance of these methods, there are encouraging signs.

Recent experiences in Japan for treating sudden death have included extended periods of CPR and a rapid set up of the heart-lung bypass using the skin puncturing method. But they didn't follow all our protocols, as they used normal blood rather than controlled reperfusion in treating the underlying heart attack and did not decompress the heart... which led to only limited survival improvement (raising survival from 10% to 30%) and did not prevent brain injury.[56]

Yet this limitation does not diminish the enormous importance of their findings, as their promptly initiating a heart-lung bypass by skin puncturing methods can serve as a guidepost for others. These same methods were duplicated by medical teams in Korea and Taiwan, showing that rapid heart-lung bypass can be done in sudden death patients within just a 15-minute interval.[57, 58] Such innovative efforts have not yet been undertaken by the leading centers in the United States and Europe.

Still, sporadic feedback of success continues, as with the surgeon who came up to introduce himself after I gave a lecture in Bakersfield, California, and said he'd heard me present my findings at an earlier conference.

"We've done your protocols on ten patients. It's been unbelievable! Everything worked out just as you said it would. It all went beautifully."

Truth Wins

Our efforts to educate are never ending, as we pass along our findings in written and oral presentations in journals and meetings... *and now through this book.* I want the huge numbers of people that could be affected by sudden death, as well as their loving families, to realize this tragedy can be avoided.

Regrettably, the failures of the past will persist until the Lazarus Syndrome is revisited. Yet I remain confident these protocols will find their way into mainstream cardiac care... hopefully sooner rather than later.

CHAPTER 12

Unwitnessed Arrest

Part I: The Never Taken Pathway

Conventional wisdom states that brain death happens after four to five minutes of no brain blood flow.

But is that true?

I was in my office during the late afternoon when I got the call from Brad Allen in the lab. I knew this was the day he was conducting the long-awaited procedure on our first test subject. His words were cryptic.

"You better get down here."

"What's wrong?" I asked.

"You just need to get down here."

I hurried through the hall, to the elevator, and then down to where the procedure was done.

Upon entering the lab, I noticed how quiet it was. No usual bustle of activity. Everyone standing around, waiting for me.

I glanced past a lab table and onto the floor. There, a pig was walking and sniffing around.

"Is *that* the test subject?"

Brad's reply was a big smile. The entire team broke into grins.

The impossible had been achieved. They had administered controlled reperfusion following *30 minutes* of no blood flow to the brain — and this pig demonstrated full recovery.

It was absolutely unbelievable.

Previously, a brain without blood flow for just four to five minutes was thought to be irreversibly damaged. Yet here we had shown that an absence of blood flow *for 30 minutes* was remedied by our treatment protocol. The implications of this were far reaching and game-changing. We were thrilled!

But then... our next four test subjects did *not* have this same great recovery. In fact, each suffered significant brain damage.

We went from monumental and exhilarating success... to posing unexpected new questions: what could have gone wrong and where do we go from here?

A gauntlet had been dropped before us. It introduced a challenge we must meet. If we could.

Yet to fully appreciate where we were at this point, we need to go back to the beginning of this story....

New Outlook on Perpetual Problem

The previous chapter focused on *sudden death* under circumstances that we call "witnessed arrest." When observers "witness" someone collapse as their heart stops, they quickly perform the traditional treatments of CPR and defibrillation, and blood flow to the brain is maintained as best as possible. It is a serious event that can occur in hospitals, airports, stores, homes, and many other locations. As pointed out, even with such conventional life-saving efforts, 85 to 90% of people do not survive and brain injury develops in half of the rare few that do.

The chapter also revealed how this problem is offset by using controlled reperfusion to protect the heart, while maintaining adequate brain blood flow during resuscitation.

While we waited for the world to embrace our new life-saving approach (and I continued writing articles, letters, and having conversations to help forward that shift), we came to recognize there was another related and very serious challenge that needed to be considered.

Unwitnessed Sudden Death

We've all heard the classic philosophical query: "If a tree falls in a forest and no one is around to hear it, does it make a sound?"

While this question has no simple answer, it relates to another question that might: If someone suffers cardiac arrest (sudden death) and no one is immediately nearby — *can they possibly survive it?*

Such a grim scenario had been given a new term in cardiac medicine: "unwitnessed arrest."

Unwitnessed arrest describes a sudden death event where there is a *time lag before treatment can be started*. It may be that sudden death is observed, as might happen when someone looks out of their window to see a person collapse in the distance, leading to a 5-to-15 minute delay before CPR is started while 911 is called. Similarly, someone in normal condition at home or in an office enters a room… and is later found dead when the closed door is reopened, perhaps after a similar 15-minute time frame.

As you might expect, the results for this are even more dreadful than with observed sudden death. The mortality rate for unwitnessed arrest is essentially 100%, with severe brain damage in the *ultra*-rare survivor.

Such circumstances create an almost inconceivable challenge to the arriving emergency medical team, who knows the bleak mortality rate for someone dead for 15 minutes without CPR administered. They may even ask, Why start? Gone is gone.

It is a desperate situation without a solution.

Or is it?

The Impossible Dream

Conventional knowledge accepts this tragedy as inescapable. As a result, no one attempts to solve it. But these appalling consequences were unacceptable to me. Instead, they became the ignition key to spark a new voyage for my research.

This endeavor made me think of the way Miguel de Cervantes described how Don Quixote confronted the windmills. Quixote's intent was to bring justice to the world by reviving chivalry and undoing wrongs. While I don't compare my own actions to the fanciful imaginations of Don Quixote, our pursuits do share an implausibility and boldness.

Quixote envisioned his opponents to be the solid, rigid, never-changing windmill structures. He reasoned that he had chosen a worthy foe as he imagined them to be giants. But instead, the spinning blades of the windmill proved to be his greatest obstacles. While they served a valued purpose by turning millstones to grind grain, they broke Quixote's lance as he made his gallant charge on his opponents.

I could easily imagine these windmills to mirror the diseases we confronted. Solid, unyielding, and seemingly impossible to counteract. I would devote all my energy and resources to do battle with them. Yet an almost equal obstacle was the "whirling blades" of conventional medical beliefs. They were every bit as obstinate as the diseases themselves. They formed a shield that prevented the penetration of new ideas.

While the actions of those practicing modern medicine deliver enormous value, their prevailing rigid adherence to the past has thwarted the introduction of novel ways to overcome diseases we all confront.

Many would think it was irrational that I would even try to recover brain function after it had been absent a blood supply for an extended period. But most of my accomplishments — and those of many others before me — faced similar skepticism in their early phases. While these barriers make our pathway more arduous, the pursuit is never abandoned because of them. Our only chance to overcome certain death after unwitnessed arrest is to attack these windmills.

Our Past Opens Doors to our Future

From my perspective, this clinical problem with unwitnessed arrest reflected the ischemic reperfusion injury that we had previously approached in the heart (restoring blood flow after it had been absent). Now, something similar was occurring in the brain. I believed this biologic response might happen in all body organs, not just one.

The next step was to test if this conviction was true.

But how could we adapt what we successfully learned in treating witnessed arrest — to the even greater challenging circumstances of *unwitnessed arrest?*

Here the victim sustains severe damage — because no CPR is given during the 15 or more minutes before help arrives.

Nature taught us a significant biology lesson in allowing us to demonstrate that controlled reperfusion after a heart attack — will completely overturn the cell death that conventional thinking believes to be terminal. This principle now needed to be tested in a new way — as we switched the organ in question from the heart to the brain.

While the study and events cited in this and the next chapter took place from 2008 to 2011... I introduce them now because this concept's presentation should follow sudden death, our previous chapter.

A Focus on the Brain

All organs suffer damage when deprived of blood supply. The extent of injury varies from organ to organ, and depends upon how long the blood flow is absent. The heart will still function without flow for 45 minutes, but it is damaged. Lungs show injury after two hours, as does the liver.

I recognized these adverse changes become more dramatic in the brain, where brain death is traditionally expected after as little as four to five minutes without oxygen nourishment. This belief sets the stage for an anticipated terminal brain injury if there is a delay of 15 or more minutes before restarting the circulation in sudden death patients.

This reminded me of another traditionally-presumed conclusion: that when a lack of blood flow has caused a heart attack, returning (normal) blood after a period as long as six hours was considered futile. Yet our controlled reperfusion (which uses a specific composition and delivery of reflow blood) *prevented this predicted damage and provided recovery.* We would test this concept again, as our first task would now be to determine if CPR — which, in effect, restarts flow with normal blood — would produce a similar injury to the brain. Then we'd need to find out if controlled reperfusion would once more prevent this tragedy.

Our first step was to freshly evaluate and appreciate the positive role that CPR plays in witnessed arrest... and then to inquire if it could also play a very different role — becoming *the culprit that prevents recovery in unwitnessed arrest*. This was a critical question, since giving CPR is the first thing done when coming upon someone whose heart has stopped, even if a lapse of time has passed. Our studies had documented that delivery of normal blood was the *enemy* after extended ischemia (absence of blood flow) — and CPR may start that same process since it will deliver normal blood reflow following the extended ischemia that occurs in unwitnessed arrest patients.

Most importantly, should our theory be true, our conclusion would not be helpful unless we could provide a better alternative. That requirement ignited the second step of our study. We believed that controlled reperfusion *could* be the answer. So an unprecedented opportunity for a solution was now before us. But it was one that could only be successful *if controlled reperfusion successfully protects the brain.*

Why Nobody Was Looking

Two opposing issues existed for determining proper medical guidelines for starting recovery after the blood supply is interrupted.

First, conventional belief is that *ischemia itself* is the lone problem. Speed then becomes the overriding imperative, spurring all efforts to deliver new blood supply as quickly as possible to stop the damage. Thoughts about *how* the reperfusion process itself can prevent (or cause) tissue damage are never even considered.

Yet our accumulated studies had shown an entirely different reality.

Which brings us to the second issue: the process of reperfusion. My fascination with controlling reperfusion launched from my understanding that normality is "organized" and it becomes disrupted by disease. This concept first captivated me when I observed the frog's cardiovascular system at Ohio State University, just as it catalyzed my interest in medicine. I subsequently realized that such organization is everywhere, as nature's orderliness is revealed in countless examples: the intricate design of a leaf as viewed under a microscope, the patterns of a spider's web, the spirals of the cosmos — such examples never end. This beauty creates the orchestra of life, whose melody is wonderfully smooth and efficient.

Conversely, *disorder* is created when nourishment to an organ is taken away by a stoppage in blood flow. Beauty is replaced by chaos within the physical components of the cells in the deprived tissue. And as we discovered, these adverse events are not completely reversed when normal blood is delivered to the previously ischemic heart. We observed that such a disorder will create an imbalance of calcium levels that causes muscle rigidity... leads to an acid accumulation that stifles metabolism... promotes loss of amino acids that will impair oxygen uptake... and causes an inability to prevent water from accumulating in the cells. Recognition of these negative outcomes led us to deliver controlled reperfusion to correct these deficiencies. We lowered the calcium, gave a buffer to offset acidity, provided amino acids, and gave a drug (mannitol) to remove the excess water.

Controlled reperfusion became the answer to the problems caused by normal blood reperfusion. Its track record is remarkable, as it returned normal heart function and avoided irreversible changes even after six hours of no blood flow to the heart in both experimental subjects and patients.

This knowledge established the framework for designing how to approach an unwitnessed arrest patient — when the patient is encountered ten to fifteen minutes after experiencing sudden death.

We set aside the conventional belief that all efforts should be totally directed toward delivering new blood supply as quickly as possible, since such an approach yielded complete failure: 99% mortality, with the ultra-rare survivor experiencing terrible neurologic damage. A revolutionary approach was needed to treat what is, in effect, a universally fatal disease.

We found data corroborating the theory that after an absence of blood flow, use of CPR *would* induce brain damage, since each time the chest was compressed, the brain would receive *normal blood*. Such awful real-life results were confirmed in experimental studies done by others: survival was unlikely if more than *ten minutes of ischemia (no blood flow) had elapsed before CPR was initiated*[47]... and even in those that did survive, severe brain damage occurred if CPR was not started within four to five minutes after sudden death.[50]

These dire findings only pushed us harder to answer the question: "If delivering normal blood by CPR generates a neurological reperfusion injury — *would delivering controlled reperfusion to the brain prevent it?*"

A significant question, as we knew a positive answer could have vast implications.

Visions Beyond Unwitnessed Arrest — Strokes!

This last question was the one I brought to my team, which now included Brad Allen, who had been instrumental in our studies of controlled reperfusion after a heart attack as well as in our approaches to re-oxygenate blue babies. He had returned to Los Angeles from Chicago to become a visiting UCLA faculty member, and I was happy to have him aboard.

Interacting with others is one of the great joys of being part of a research team, and new ideas emerge from such interchange. We came upon a major realization as we discussed this project.

I said to Brad, "What we're really studying here is how to protect and heal the brain after it has been ischemic… *regardless of how it got that way.*"

Brad recognized where I was going. "Gerry, what I think you're suggesting is immense. We both know that unwitnessed arrest, while tragic, isn't nearly as common of an occurrence as…"

"Stroke," I said emphatically, finishing his sentence. Brad and I were on the same page. "The same extended ischemic period of insufficient blood flow to the brain that exists in unwitnessed arrest *happens with stroke as well.*"

The ramifications truly were gigantic. Even though the lack of brain blood flow causing a stroke is due to a blocked brain artery, our remedy of controlled reperfusion had the same potential with it as with *sudden death*. Just imagine: there are over 700,000 stroke victims annually in the United States alone.

Our growing anticipation and excitement were palpable.

Daring to Defy the Past

Though eager about ultimately exploring the possibility of addressing strokes, our initial focus remained on unwitnessed arrest. Toward that end, an added hurdle quickly became apparent to one of our new team members, who said, “You realize, even if we can find the answer to treating unwitnessed arrest, our protocol to avoid using CPR will meet great opposition.”

“You mean more opposition than we usually face?” I countered, laughing. He had not yet experienced the entrenched resistance that develops when the status quo of medicine might change.

But I told him he was right. “A dramatic change in thinking would emerge from our approach, since our belief is that restarting normal blood flow by CPR is why unwitnessed sudden death victims do so poorly.”

Indeed, this new concept might change the response by everyone — from the EMTs called to the scene — or a bystander or loved one who makes it to the person. We’d advise *them to do nothing*, because we’d have a different protocol.

The challenge was enormous, and as another resident chimed in, “It’s going to be a tough sell.”

But an indisputable reality framed my response. “Today’s treatment causes 99% mortality and severe brain damage in the rare survivor. Please explain to me why everyone keeps doing something that they know does not help?”

I reminded them that our approach does not impugn CPR, as it is a vital component of *witnessed arrest*. It maintains brain blood flow from the outset of cardiac arrest. But CPR may be detrimental — if its start is delayed for more than five minutes after blood flow has stopped.

At this point in my team’s discussion, our approach was only conceptual — a theory. It had still to be tested. The task before us was clear, as we needed to develop a game plan to save both the heart and brain by applying controlled reperfusion after unwitnessed arrest. Equally important, we needed to clearly demonstrate the adverse consequences of applying CPR in unwitnessed arrest.

It was time to begin. We had to build a solid case to stimulate a change in thinking.

Current Approach Recreates Current Results

This was to be a joint project with Friedhelm Beyersdorf, our German research fellow who had made the keen observations that stimulated our clinical (witnessed) sudden death studies. Friedhelm was now Professor of Cardiac Surgery in Freiburg, Germany, and did this collaborative experimental research with us. We would work closely together again, as the 6,000 miles of land and ocean between us did not limit our tight connection.

First, we needed to document experimentally why conventional treatments after unwitnessed arrest caused a very significant problem. At UCLA, we caused unwitnessed arrest in animal test subjects by inducing ventricular fibrillation after passing a wire into the heart through a vein and delivering an electrical current. No treatment was given during the first 15 minutes.

CPR was then started, and the heart-lung machine initiated ten minutes later to provide the body with adequate flow of regular blood. Two of six piglets died, and though the four survivors recovered adequate heart performance, each sustained significant brain injury.[59] We had saved the heart, but lost the brain.

In contrast, Friedhelm's team induced the same 15-minute period of cardiac arrest *without CPR.*[60] But when treatment was started, the heart-lung machine delivered a *controlled reperfusion solution* to the whole body. A dramatic difference, as the brain and body *never received regular blood reflow during initial resuscitation.*

Each pig survived with superb heart function. But most importantly, neurological recovery (brain function) was excellent. His team and our group were thrilled because this extraordinary outcome had never been previously achieved. An example of this unheard of recovery is shown in **Video 1.**

To view videos online, type the address link shown below each video image into the search bar of your web browser. eBook readers can click directly on the link below each video.

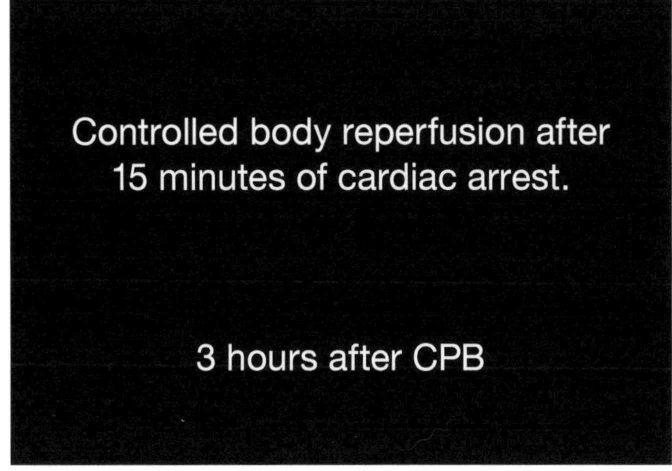

Video 1

www.vimeo.com/buckberg/15-minute-recovery

Our excitement was tremendous, as these findings substantiated our theory! Simultaneously, they opened the door toward evolving a meaningful and unique treatment of an otherwise devastating disease. This collaborative effort first validated the expected severe neurologic reperfusion damage caused by CPR when it was the primary treatment of unwitnessed arrest — and then dramatically certified that delivering controlled reperfusion is a powerful tool to return superb heart and brain function.

It was a life-preserving finding that had never before been accomplished following an injury that the world thinks is lethal.

However, while these results were captivating, they were also unrealistic. This 15-minute time frame would not account for the amount of time needed for a reperfusion team to be called *and* then set up and use the heart-lung machine in a sudden death patient.

Yet simultaneously, we had learned from our colleagues in Japan, Korea, and Taiwan that it only took an added 15 minutes of set-up time to start the heart-lung machine — using the simple method of inserting a needle into the artery from the groin (a straightforward approach that made it unnecessary to open the chest to begin the heart-lung machine). This knowledge let us evolve a new game plan to test an extended period of unwitnessed arrest of

30 minutes — to mimic a real-world scenario in which we take advantage of incorporating their proven shortened set-up times for beginning the portable heart-lung machine.

Marching Orders (and Disorder)

Before we launch into the next stage of our study to see if controlled reperfusion can offset brain damage after *a longer period* of ischemia, I want to provide a simple non-medical parallel to help the reader understand the havoc that ensues in the body when ischemia is "remedied" by normal blood reperfusion — and alternatively when treated by controlled reperfusion — by comparing it to a marching band.

Imagine the participants all marching in unison. A marvelous sight. The beauty of the body's natural order in metabolic, cellular, and structural forms — within an organ and between all the organs as they work in harmony.

But this majesty disintegrates when the band is ordered to halt and is dismissed. Now all the marchers move in different directions — forward, backward, sideways. The prior coherent march disintegrates into disunity, a dysfunction that mirrors what happens when blood flow stops to the organs during ischemia.

This uncoordinated action is *accentuated* if the band members are then abruptly ordered to begin marching again. This sudden attempt to return order is comparable to restoring *normal* blood flow after unwitnessed arrest. Each marcher tries futilely to restart from a different place, but chaos reigns. It is impossible to synchronize their motions with those of the other band members.

A "reshuffling period" is needed to transition the marchers from chaos to regaining alignment. This regrouping period parallels delivering *controlled reperfusion* after ischemia. By supplying the selected ingredients to reverse the chaos within the organs, their "starting position" changes in a way that realigns the metabolic, cellular, and physiologic processes toward normal. Synchronization recovers and a "re-unified band" can now perform well again.

Diving into the Unknown — 30 Minutes of No Brain Blood!

Before we began the next stage of our study, I reviewed what we had already learned.

We knew the accepted perception that irreversible damage in the body follows periods of no blood flow... reflects a finding that is based upon the awful recovery that always follows reperfusion with *normal blood*. This nemesis has resulted in the time-honored belief that an irrevocable damage follows only four to five minutes of brain ischemia.

Yet this was powerfully contradicted by our findings that controlled reperfusion will successfully treat the brain after 15 minutes of sudden death. These revelations could open the door to developing new treatments to avoid the (previously believed) "inescapable" dilemma of permanent brain damage after unwitnessed arrest.

Further, the scope of our study on unwitnessed sudden death may be far reaching, since it might expand into an application for treating strokes — *the third leading cause of death in the U.S.* These high stakes inspired everyone, me most of all.

This compelled us to explore our next challenge: *could the brain recover from even longer periods with no blood flow?*

How privileged we were to launch the next phase of this "impossible dream" — as will be revealed in the following chapter.

CHAPTER 13

Unwitnessed Arrest

Part II: Expansion, Rejection, and Future Realities

The foundation for the next stage in our search had already been laid by Friedhelm's study, which showed that brain damage could be completely avoided after 15 minutes of unwitnessed cardiac arrest. We would now aim for 30 minutes as we expanded to evaluate longer ischemic time periods. This interval was lengthy enough to allow scrambling a resuscitation team to initiate the use of a heart-lung machine following unwitnessed arrest.

Our next stage would create an opportunity to study this for both unwitnessed arrest and potentially, for stroke treatment. Brad raised the question, "What if there was a way to treat the brain of a stroke victim by giving controlled reperfusion *directly into the obstructed artery*?"

A fascinating notion. With a stroke, the heart is working fine, so there is no inherent need for a heart-lung machine to take over the circulation.

I pointed out, "And if what you're suggesting were possible, it would provide a much quicker path to administering the controlled reperfusion. The question is, how can you do this?"

Brad considered that. "Let me think about it."

He first had to confront the dilemma of having no way to mimic a stroke, other than stopping all of the brain's blood supply — by sudden death. A big obstacle to overcome — if we were also going to study how to treat stroke victims without cardiac arrest.

Brad returned to my office a few days later.

"I've got it."

His innovative thinking led to an ingenious method to obstruct all of the brain's blood flow by blocking its blood vessels as they came from the aorta — by accessing them through a small incision into the breast bone. He would then use small simple neck incisions to access the carotid arteries that lead to the brain. While brain blood supply was interrupted for 30 minutes, catheters would be placed in them for delivering either normal blood or controlled reperfusion into the brain for our testing.

I had one word to describe Brad's plan: "Phenomenal." But my next words were: "Now prove it!"

We began our experiments.

Blood flow to the brain was stopped for 30 minutes in animal subjects, mimicking what happens after prolonged sudden death or in the early stages of a stroke. This was followed by delivery *of normal* blood reperfusion — to match how a typical brain injury is conventionally treated.

Immediate and irreversible brain damage was apparent, and vastly exceeded what we saw after 15-minute periods of brain ischemia (no blood flow to the brain). This reflected the real-world outcomes of patients that survive a stroke. They may develop paralysis on one side of the body, speech and language impairment, memory loss, vision issues, behavior changes, and have their lives shortened.

The next step was the most critical — as we now delivered *controlled brain reperfusion* after the same 30 minutes of brain ischemia. We knew that if this didn't work, we would have to rethink our approach, start over, or perhaps even abandon the pursuit.

The dramatic scene that was described at the beginning of the prior chapter — when I was urgently called by Brad to go down to the lab — told the story of the outcome in our first experimental piglet subject.

I shall never forget that moment....

Our team had administered our controlled reperfusion. Despite having just experienced 30 minutes of no blood flow, the piglet was conscious, walking, sniffing around, and looking normal in a natural mobile state.

We could barely contain ourselves.

This immediate recovery of the body and normal neurological function contradicted every traditional belief about ischemia and brain damage. *No one in the world had ever done this before*! It was simply unbelievable!

I commended our team, "This is so wonderful. Congratulations to all of you. It's just fabulous."

Since a picture is worth a thousand words, the reader can type the video link address into their computer's search engine, or eBook readers can click on the link to see the memorable video that tells an astounding story. (**Video 2**) Our thrill at this result was enormous, as it may benefit so many deserving people.

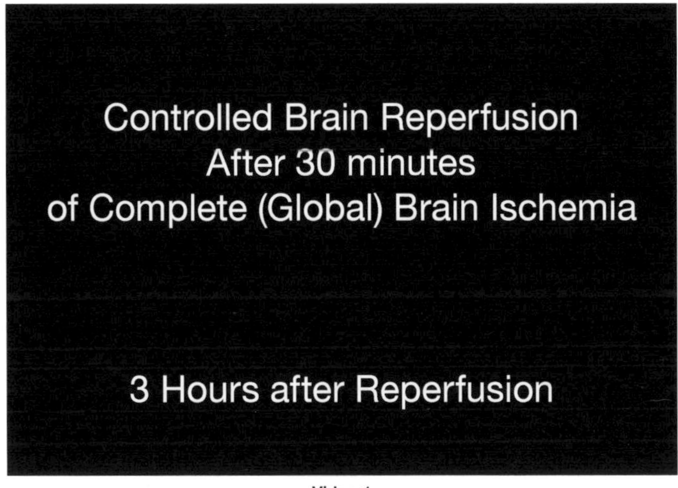

Video 1

www.vimeo.com/buckberg/30-minute-recovery

"Houston, We Have a Problem"

Unfortunately, our joy ride of success was not long-lived. An unexpected development occurred.

Our next four test subjects did *not* have this same terrific recovery. In fact, each of them suffered significant brain damage.

We went from the highest of highs to facing entirely new questions.

Our previously observed return of normal brain activity in the first piglet after 30 minutes of no blood flow was simply unheard of. This singular success could *never* have been by chance. Nature doesn't work that way. There was no "miracle." Instead, our initial triumph demonstrates how science can overturn a conceivably unsolvable problem. *What we did* made brain recovery happen, and our confidence was unshaken by the four subsequent failures.

We just had to find the mistakes that made us unable to reproduce recovery.

Racing Down the Rabbit Hole

The world of discovery is an electrifying voyage, one accompanied by hurdles that must be conquered.

This consistent challenge of research is not always acknowledged when final results are reported. The real journey is seldom a smooth one, since overcoming roadblocks requires innovation and persistence.

As stated before, my underlying credo is: "If something that you believe should work... *does not...* then either your idea is wrong or your study was done improperly." The ischemia/reperfusion concept is valid, so our failures could only mean that we did not do the next four studies correctly.

Our team would work doggedly to overcome the technical errors that had blocked our subsequent recoveries, much the same way a Schnauzer acts after he bites your leg. He never lets go without getting what he wanted.

We would spend the next two years looking for our answers.

Armed with a belief that truth is often hidden but waiting to be revealed, we proceeded to unravel the pitfalls of failure... as we re-entered the unique world of research.

Learn by Doing

A discerning and meaningful motto observes, *"Good judgment comes from experience, and experience comes from bad judgment."*

Seasoned researchers have good judgment because they've been wrong so often. It teaches them how to avoid future mistakes, while simultaneously giving them the tools to address the ones they cannot evade. They do not quit easily. They become agile by practicing, just as one does for sports or an art.

For this reason, we didn't give up after encountering negative results. I knew the answer was there, and our first objective was to scour through every piece of our technique to search for it.

It's (Always) in the Details

The drama of discovery evokes great excitement for the public. But the scientist is not certain of reaching this unique final result when he or she begins. Instead, it evolves along the winding pathway of the pursuit. Clues to the future answer emerge — but they must be identified, appreciated, and carefully followed.

Our reevaluations made us recognize we did not yet know how much blood to deliver during reflow. Could this be the consideration that prevented us from duplicating our initial success? We needed to establish these amounts, especially since they might set crucial guidelines.

Since our overriding goal was to have the brain nourished with sufficient oxygen, we began exploring what volume of blood flow was needed during reflow. This task was initiated by recording oxygen saturation on the brain surface. An electrode was placed on the scalp's skin that covers the underlying brain. It was a relatively simple technique commonly used in patients, which would tell us the saturation in the brain blood beneath.

Our belief, from previous studies that had been done in patients, was that flow is adequate if there is 55 to 70% saturation. But this was not true in our studies, since we had maintained those levels in all four piglets that developed serious brain injury.

Our next step toward solving this mystery would build upon drawing knowledge from our other prior experiences. In this case, we knew that the heart can have a *normal surface appearance* — while its inner shell is severely damaged — as we had observed during open-heart surgery or when normal blood reflow was given after a heart attack.

"Could such a discrepancy also occur in the brain?" we wondered. "Might measuring oxygen saturation throughout the brain better reflect what was occurring within it — and be a superior indicator than only monitoring the brain surface?"

That question led us to compare *brain surface oxygen measurements* against *total brain oxygen uptake* (which measures surface *and* deep regions). This could be done as we controlled brain blood flow — as we could readily measure the oxygen level in the blood going to the brain, and then in the venous blood leaving it (after it had extracted oxygen from its blood supply).

So what did we find?

The total brain oxygen uptake *differed from what we expected* from the surface measurements. The surface could receive abundant oxygen — while the inner portions remained undernourished. In fact, we observed an inverse relationship, meaning that *if the surface level was less, the whole was better.* (We would later learn the reasons behind this discrepancy.)

Before doing more studies... we first tested piglets that did not have any limitations to their circulation, and determined that delivering 750 ml/minute of brain blood flow was necessary to maintain normal healthy brain function.[61] This baseline flow became our gauge to ensure that the brain would receive an adequate reperfusion blood flow in our further experiments.

The fruits of this new knowledge led us to do six more controlled reperfusion studies, with fresh optimism that we'd solved the flow and oxygen nourishment problem.

But we did not fulfill these positive expectations.

Only two of six pigs recovered, despite receiving the normal brain blood flow rate. Again, we were stumped. This should have worked, especially since the controlled reperfusion avoided brain damage in two subjects. Apparently, normal flow wasn't the answer — at least not the only answer.

Again, we needed to pore over our protocols to find the flaw. We restudied the data, and indeed found that it spoke back to us.

We discovered that recovery only happened when average blood pressure was above 60 mm Hg. The four subjects that did not improve, had a lower pressure and developed severe injury, despite our providing the normal brain blood flow rate. We now understood a proper blood pressure was another part of the answer.

So defining how to achieve the desired pressure became the next impediment we needed to overcome — especially as several intertwining factors made this task difficult.

We already knew that stopping a brain's blood supply is always accompanied by a response in the body that generates a very high blood pressure — as adrenaline concentrations rise abruptly in the blood to excite the vascular system. But this could awaken the subject. To prevent that from happening, we had increased the inhaled anesthesia dose (from 1% to 3%). This lowered the blood pressure by relaxing blood vessels — and ensured the subject stayed unconscious.

But while we found that these higher doses did produce the desired reduction of blood pressure — they *also lowered* the total brain oxygen uptake — *while simultaneously raising* surface oxygen saturation! This taught us an unexpected, but important lesson: whole brain nourishment had been diverted *away* from the inner part of the brain and sent toward its surface, thereby creating the higher surface measurements that were so misleading in our prior trials.

We had inadvertently caused poor brain flow distribution by our decisions about the anesthesia drugs, leading us now to realize that lowering the anesthesia dose was essential. Yet we *still* needed to keep the subject unconscious.[62]

So we sought a new answer — and found one in an available alternative drug. Adding Nembutal (a brain anesthetic) would induce brain coma (ensuring the pig did not awaken) — but did *not* lower blood pressure.

Another piece of the puzzle had been successfully added!

But we weren't done yet.

One Final Element

Brain swelling is a major problem following brain injury, as the brain resides within a rigid skull casing. It simply cannot expand, so that any water gain worsens damage. Dangerous brain swelling (from water) becomes accelerated if blood pressure is high during early reperfusion. Because of this, using a higher blood pressure can be dangerous. This introduced another challenging dilemma.

As I seek out research guidelines, nature is always my primary source. This stems from my recognition that problems arise whenever we make decisions that deviate from its rules. Conversely, following nature's proven patterns yields wonderful scientific remedies.

This principle holds true in designing medical care, as physicians often learn that "what they think is right" may be incorrect, because it differs from "what nature knows is right." That rule resurfaced as I reviewed the guidelines that have long been used to deliver blood flow to the brain. Conventionally, brain nourishment is delivered by a pump that provides a smooth flow without pulsations. This method is used universally, as nearly every heart-lung machine and blood delivery pump in the world will consistently deliver a smooth flow that is without waves.

Yet nature does not follow this rule. Instead, the body has pulsatile perfusion (as can be felt in our body's pulse), mirroring the pattern of the pulsations of ocean waves. Using this stimulus of mirroring nature, we developed an apparatus that furnished pulsatile blood flow. It worked. The pulsatile flow *improved* brain blood flow distribution, despite its delivering a lower average blood pressure! This is not a new concept. Its "ebb and flow" was elegantly described by ancient scholars like Galen in AD 180.

Time to Test

This step-by-step process to uncover what went wrong in our last studies set the stage for a new series of controlled reperfusion trials that would follow 30 minutes of no brain blood flow.

All our efforts were rewarded.

Excellent recovery of body and brain function was observed following our delivery of controlled reperfusion — and these findings were repeatedly achieved in other subjects![63]

We had done it.

The impossible became possible. *The unsolvable was solved.*

A feeling of fulfillment and glee came over everyone. We knew that this unique outcome might have enormous impact. Our excitement was overwhelming. We saw that so many patients could be helped. I believe we tapped into the infinite reward of research: envisioning its clinical application that will help the sick and buoy their families!

Our journey reminded me of a Winston Churchill quote: "Success is going from failure to failure without losing enthusiasm." A pathway we precisely followed.

Reflections on Success

This was a formidable experience of another type for us, because we, as cardiovascular surgeons, now entered a new arena: the untapped world of recovering the brain, rather than the heart. Our results pointed toward a potential sea change in the treatment of unwitnessed arrest and stroke victims worldwide.

Taking a moment to reflect on what we had done, I said to Brad, "You know, we couldn't have solved this 15 years ago. We didn't have the vast background of information, nor enough experience, to face such challenges." Brad agreed.

I wondered how many beginning researchers could have taken those steps, and could have used the data to work out the details? Our experience, coupled with unrelenting curiosity, made us better researchers. This knowledge fuels my dedication to the residents and research fellows who work with me for two-year periods. I am passing the torch, much as Julien Hoffman did with me from 1969 to 1970.

Yet, I couldn't help but wonder: if we didn't have that initial success with the first test subject to spur us on, would we have continued?

The answer is yes. We never embarked on a research project on which we gave up. An answer was always found, because the logic was sound. Some might suggest it was luck, but that is something I neither believe in nor rely upon. Instead, the "data is the data" and contains information that tells a story... though oftentimes one that needs to be uncovered. It is the world of science, requiring the sequential pursuit from observer to experimenter to observer, as mentor Claude Bernard taught us.

Please remember that our continued success in different aspects of research is not because "I am a man for all seasons." I never spread myself over multiple projects at once. Instead, for several years at a time, I devote enormous energies to a single project. The unwavering drive to find the solution of each study grew out of *knowing* an answer was attainable.

The Exciting New Future

I was particularly eager to continue exploring how our novel treatment might also transform the treatment of strokes — an enormous global issue.

I focused on this during one of my morning swims at 5:45 AM. Since 1997, I have been part of a UCLA club called the Bruin Masters. Early every morning, master swimmers meet and our coach runs us through different strokes, distances, and times. Besides being wonderful exercise, it is a place where I can also generate new ideas.

While swimming laps, I pondered how our results could lead toward a new protocol for strokes. I envisioned how cardiologists could immediately access a patient's blocked artery, then push a catheter beyond the obstruction to promptly deliver controlled reperfusion past the blockage — and protect the brain. Then the artery could be opened by angioplasty to restore normal circulation. The catheterization lab could function as "The Fast Response Treatment Wing."

All the necessary tools exist for this to occur, and hopefully the appreciation of our findings and their application might catalyze its development. But that can only happen if we safely extend the time frame *even further* without brain blood flow and get consistent recovery using controlled reperfusion.

Our next step!

Funding the Evolution of New Ideas

Friedhelm's report of his unique results, as well as our successful work at UCLA with Brad Allen, was published in major United States and European

Journals.[60–64] But this did not alter the strong resistance from cardiologists to having their catheterization labs used as a threshold for conducting such revolutionary approaches.

We were not deterred. We felt that as more studies were completed, there would be more and more compelling evidence of this lifesaving treatment's feasibility. As we had done many times in the past, we sent a grant request to NIH (National Institutes of Health) for financial support to continue the studies.

Novel ideas never find recognition because they *sound good*. Rather, they emerge into the spotlight after being tested. That might seem a natural progression to the public, but how does this really happen? As you have read in these pages, it is not as if some faucet opens so that truth flows freely from it. Instead, there must be sprouting of the seeds into ideas that create a new way of thinking, which must be transformed into innovative actions and results.

Such a venture needs a mechanism that permits the investigator to explore and overcome a broad number of unanticipated obstacles. This is where we enter the world of the laboratory research study. Yet there is an inherent dilemma to this approach: no funding entity wants to unquestioningly provide backing to unknown research.

Monies come from outside independent sources (they are virtually never supplied by the native institution, as none of my studies were funded by UCLA). The eternal challenge for the investigator is to convince others to financially support their research. This takes the form of a grant proposal.

The method behind this process is seldom discussed, as there's a Catch-22 to the procedure. This means to secure funding, you must first present a preliminary (pilot) study that verifies your capacity to achieve the stated goal.

The riddle is to figure out how one finances this vital exploratory study.

The usual practice is to use part of the funds from a prior grant to do the next pilot study. This does not abuse present available funds. There is no cheating, because the goals of the prior funded study were fully accomplished (as its pilot study was funded by the study that preceded it). This leap-frog approach to financing the groundwork for each subsequent study is simply a way of life in the world of research.

Again and again, I followed this route in my investigative work and its success paved the way for the evolution of each new idea during this 50-plus year career. It has allowed me success in a string of innovative pursuits thought unsolvable by traditional methods. This chapter on unwitnessed arrest falls into this category.

Startling Turn of Events

NIH was our primary funder, and we looked forward to using their support to pursue our next stage of discovery. Brad was made principal investigator and it was my thrill to help my former student succeed!

I was not prepared for the NIH response.

Following their evaluation of our grant application — which included submission of our video demonstrating the complete neurological recovery in test subjects following 30 minutes of total brain ischemia — Brad received a letter with their reply. Eagerly, we opened and read it.

Then we read it again.

The NIH reviewers indicated these dramatic brain recovery findings were not significant. This conclusion was reached despite the fact that such neurologic recovery had *never* yet been achieved anywhere else in the world. Despite our furnishing living evidence that these animals were able to walk and eat and drink after being dead for 30 minutes.

"Not significant?" Astonishing. I was stunned.

As said earlier, we are not entirely surprised when some of our innovations meet resistance by those completely invested in the past. But the NIH should be different, as it is in the business of facilitating new discoveries. We anticipated their excitement at this breakthrough. They recognized our track record, and were aware of their long history of funding our research. Most importantly, they received our video confirming complete recovery after 30 minutes of no brain blood flow. I could only guess they either did not look at it or did not believe it.

We made calls to appeal their decision, but to no avail. Our research is very expensive, and it could not move forward without new funding.

This rejection trampled our chances to explore applying controlled reperfusion after longer intervals of brain ischemia with unwitnessed arrest, and totally stymied our capacity to evolve new methods to treat stroke victims. The curtain suddenly fell on our efforts to change the devastation of brain damage, a now correctable problem.

I just sat at my desk, staring at their letter. I was frustrated, discouraged, and deeply sad for those patients who could not be helped. Yet this negativity was balanced by my knowing that we found the truth — the pinnacle of every scientific journey.

Turning Point

I knew the chances of continuing our study were now zero. No one else would fund this investigation.

It also meant that after 40 years of research, our laboratory must close. I made calls to find new places for my research fellows and lab technicians to work.

But for me personally, this was a momentous juncture.

On the surface, it seemed to nullify my lifelong excitement about developing and then testing an idea in the lab to see if it would ultimately work in patients. The lab is an astounding resource, for it is there that you plant the seeds of your thinking and allow them to bloom, as you grow exhilarated and gratified by the answers. Closing it stops this fruitful pattern.

This setback mirrors setbacks in research, in which failure in one area serves to raise the next question. What if I could do research without an experimental laboratory? I will reveal (in subsequent chapters) how my exploring the *unrecognized true nature of the heart's structure* and how it explains both normal and abnormal function — beautifully filled this void and led to unprecedented dynamic discoveries with far-reaching consequences.

The Uncertain Future

This memoir chapter on unwitnessed sudden death (and stroke) is the only one where my lifelong crossing from "bench to bedside" had not been completed. We had not compiled enough experimental data to justify its use in the treatment of patients.

Our intent to explore recovery after extending the periods without blood flow to 60 minutes, then to 90, then 120 had evaporated. Again, for me, the worst part of such abandoned pursuits is being unable to help the patients who would have benefited.

Our studies on sudden death showed we could solve witnessed arrest. That opened the door to helping people with unwitnessed arrest, which opened the door to treatment for strokes. Yet these portals have not remained opened, and rigidity reigns.

Innovation wasn't to be, at least not for now. But the truth always wins. Again, the only question is: when will it happen?

In the meantime, most recent statistics show approximately 795,000 people suffer a stroke every year. And that's just in the United States.

Something to think about....

CHAPTER 14

The Teacher's Highest Reward

Young surgeons are still students after graduating from medical school. They continue to learn by becoming residents and fellows. This educational path in cardiac surgery ends up creating its own version of a family — overseen by their physician mentor who guides them much as would a parent.

Those choosing to pursue scientific investigation will spend two years with a selected research team, whose leader develops an almost paternal role. During this period, the young surgeon's primary objective is to develop the skills that will shape their future.

They ask questions, learn how to use the lab's research tools and techniques to uncover answers, and sharpen written or oral presentation skills to help other physicians learn and use their work on their own patients.

Shoulders to Stand on

The educational path is never solitary. The writings of Claude Bernard taught me this. Our trek is only possible when we follow in the footsteps of giants. We must stand upon their shoulders and see what they did not. This starting place is crucial, since absence of such footing leaves us blind to envisioning tomorrow.

My own growth followed this formula. How fortunate I was to spend 18 months at the Cardiovascular Research Institute (CVRI) in San Francisco, overseen by Julius Comroe, and where I worked with Julien I.E. Hoffman.

Dr. Comroe was unique. He was so totally committed to education that he abandoned his career in pulmonary physiology to establish CVRI for young physicians, and create the solid cornerstone needed to start their professional lives. He is no longer with us (passing in 1984), but our abilities evolved from what he taught us. His students, including me, received the teacher's highest gift.

At CVRI, international fellows come together to acquire a wide range of medical training. They study the heart and the lungs, but also embryology, biochemistry, physiology, and the body's electrical activity.

Dr. Comroe established two primary educational avenues. First, he provided many prolific laboratories from which each fellow could select to obtain specialty training. Second, he created a series of courses for everyone, involving experimental design, biomedical statistics, mathematics (to design and analyze experiments, and determine meaning of data); plus, there were courses on how to read and edit a paper, present it orally, and how to listen and learn from talks given by others.

I vividly remember when we gave our talks, as he would assign specific chores to ten of the other participants. Each task focused on a different detail as we delivered the first 15 minutes of a presentation. Someone would watch how you used your hands, another observed your facial expressions, another looked at the quality and composition of your slides, another noted how you used your pointer, etc. He would videotape the talks, which you later watched on your own time. You were then armed with all these evaluations, ones that frequently described "how bad you were!"

This made you honestly face the weaknesses of your performance and make midcourse corrections. You then return later with a new five-minute presentation. Appreciating our limitations prodded us toward making an encore performance... to the same detractors who'd candidly pointed out our deficiencies before. Directly confronting our shortcomings made us better presenters.

Dr. Comroe knew the steps needed to fully develop our learning, *and* guided us into understanding how to use these newfound abilities toward educating others. He taught us that the data from our study's results was only the first stage. These raw facts set the framework to credibly communicate our findings. Yet he wanted our professional world to contain the *whole package*. This included not only discovery, but how to effectively share that data with others.

Dr. Comroe and Julien Hoffman were father figures whose influence became part of my worldview. I train my residents and research fellows the same way I was trained. *The legacy continues as the baton is passed.* This calls back to the immense value, satisfaction, and joy of giving that I learned as a child from my mother and grandmother that I describe in this book's introduction. For me, happiness is derived not only by helping patients, but also as a teacher, assisting those who in turn will give to others as well.

Launching Fellows at UCLA

When I first met with prospective and new research fellows in my office, I would ask: "Why do you want to study in my laboratory?"

There were three recurring answers.

First, "I want to learn to think differently. I have heard that is something you help your fellows to do." Indeed, that was my goal.

Secondly, "To hone my skills in writing papers for publication and learn how to make presentations at national conferences." Everybody knew my prior fellows published numerous papers.

Finally, each emphasized, "I hope to become well-recognized because of research and clinical studies I do with you."

I knew that nearly all incoming research fellows believed the measure of their success is "numerical" — they think *how many* publications they create is the benchmark to quantify the effectiveness of our collaboration.

My point of view was completely different.

As they each left my office, I asked them to look up the number of abstracts (summary of a scientific study) that a particular scientific laboratory had presented at the American Heart Association (AHA) meetings from 1973 to 1975, since in their minds, the number of presentations would "validate" the value of a prodigious single team.

They would come back to report, "I found about 140 abstracts were printed over this three-year period."

I then inquired if this yield of 140 abstracts provided a valuable indicator of the importance of this laboratory's productivity. The resounding answer was "Yes."

My final question was, "What new information did you learn from your review of this vast database?" The answer was always, "None."

This predictable response brings me back to Dr. Longmire's comment, who appraised these common criteria for academic success by stating that when the promotions committee evaluates the volume of written papers listed in your bibliography, "Sometimes they weigh them, sometimes they count them, but they never read them."

After the fellows gave their predictable responses, I would let them in on the *real goals* that I had in mind during their two years in my laboratory.

I would describe an illuminating experience, one that has happened with my prior fellows who uncovered new information: "It occurs while attending a national or international conference, where each participant wears a nametag for identification. When the meeting has a break between sessions, or while you go to the exhibit hall, or attend one of the cocktail parties... some physician walks over, sees your name tag, and asks, 'Are you the person who wrote the paper on such and such?' After you confirm that is you, this physician will say, 'Let me share something with you. On behalf of me and my patient, we are very grateful. Using what you wrote in that paper *saved a life*.' In that instant, you begin to understand the true importance of your work."

The power of this personal experience of being appreciated for one's contributions[65] reveals the correct goal of biomedical research. Reaching this height far surpasses the all-too-common ambition of presenting new work with limited merit. Finding a remedy for someone's illness — *improving or saving a life* — reflects the true harvest for your innovative efforts. Your work has meaning.

It's unfortunate that the belief in quantity (over quality) as a determiner of achievement prevails for many throughout the research community. In the university, this also translates into the "amount of physical space you are provided as the barometer of success" since everyone wants to have a big lab. But here too — it's not the size of the lab, but what you do in that lab. Yet this consideration is rarely heard as allocation of space remains the perceived touchstone for future accomplishment.

I remember when a senior surgeon, who had just come to UCLA, visited my basement office. He proudly informed me that he had 6,000 square feet of lab space. "That is wonderful," I replied, and then showed him my lab with 600 square feet of space (a 30 × 20 room). He expressed surprise. "Where is the rest of it?"

I smiled. "This is actually more than I need. The most crucial space required for research is only about eight inches." As he looked back quizzically, I slowly placed my forefingers on each side of my ears, conveying that the truly important work occurs in the area between them.

Bringing Up the Brood

It was some time after beginning to oversee residents that I was struck again by how patterns in life can be repetitive, as the training of cardiac surgery residents brings them into the fold much like your children. You give them input and guidance, and then observe their output. As with children, you teach students without any certainty of the end result. You don't know how they will turn out or what pursuits they will follow... and then all of a sudden you see it has paid off.

That can be a study they choose to conduct... or a way of *conducting themselves* that you didn't foresee. Again, this is much how it can be with your own offspring, as I was reminded some years ago.

The excitement and challenge of life as a cardiac surgeon and researcher carries a downside. You are up at five in the morning to perform morning rounds with patients and residents, and often don't return home until ten at night. When do you find time to spend with your children and your wife? You look for ways to make up for all the moments you missed.

Opportunities for one-on-one contact with my children arose during the bounty of international trips I took to conferences to describe my research and clinical work. Every year, I brought each of my daughters alone on a trip with me as I traveled to these different countries. Just the two of us.

One of my favorite destinations was Paris, where it also happened that my hero, Claude Bernard, wrote my bible, "An Introduction to the Study of Experimental Medicine." On such a trip, I took my oldest daughter, Nicole, when she was 20 years old. We were having a wonderful time, prancing playfully through the Parisian streets. But my lighthearted preoccupation came with a price tag. Small metal barriers lined the street, and *voila* — my shin hit one of these, causing a gash in my leg.

Even though I was the trained doctor, Nicole, at age 20, took charge. She called upon all her academically-learned French to search out a suitable physician in Saint-Germain-des-Prés. After we mounted a flight of stairs to his office, I received a couple of stitches and an antibiotic ointment. But my discomfort persisted, and before my eyes, Nicole suddenly became both doctor and nurse, comforting me and supervising my "recovery." Her generosity of spirit was delightful. She cared for me in the way I would nurture my students.

By the time of our trip, Nicole had already started college and was effectively out of our nest, leaving our world for a new one beyond. So it was especially pleasing to witness who she had become. Giving has always been one of my guiding principles. It was wonderful to see that my lovely daughter had taken on this trait.

I felt similarly gratified once my residents and fellows left my academic haven, as I often received a special "kudo" after having trained them for two years. Working in our lab took place in the midst of their overall education, after which they returned to their clinical residency at UCLA to treat patients. The other residents, without lab backgrounds, became curious about our graduates as they repeatedly asked, "How did you develop such a keen ability to sort out clinical diagnoses and treatments?"

The answer reflects the "teaching of thinking" concept that is used to problem-solve research dilemmas. The intense concentration and orderly sorting of facts gets directly transferred into resolving clinical puzzles.

As a result, they use this perspective in their selected fields away from the university. My hope is that these mentor's "seeds" will guide their future.

I delightedly witnessed a parallel as I watched my daughter Nicole develop her career. She works with computers (and still remains astounded by the snail pace of my understanding of her tasks). Several years ago, she informed me of a promotion that put her in charge of 17 coworkers. Pleased to learn of her advancement, I asked about her goals for this new position. She thought only a moment and answered, "To create an environment where they can learn and grow."

I was so proud of her, and happy that my attitude had made an impact. As a famous beer commercial once said, "It doesn't get any better than this."

Bearing Fruit

The area of study that each fellow pursues after graduating is selected by the student, not the mentor. The highest gift a teacher can receive is if that student becomes a teacher and uses knowledge gained in our laboratory as the jumping-off point for developing their own independent studies to help others.

An additional wish for me would be that someone who worked with me on ischemia / reperfusion injury of the heart might try to generate groundbreaking ideas for using this process of returning blood flow after there's been an absence of it also in other organs. As previously said, I believe our discovery reflects a biologic process (meaning it occurs in all organs). But until proven, this conclusion is only a personal opinion.

I also fully realized that budding researchers are taking a great risk by electing to address dilemmas in unexplored areas. Failure can damage their reputation and possibly curtail their career. There are no guarantees. Yet a successful pursuit of landmark objectives may favorably launch their future.

Friedhelm Beyersdorf did just this when he returned to Germany. He evaluated restarting blood flow to the leg after its arterial blood supply was blocked. Similarly, Bradley Allen in Chicago would study reflow after lung transplantation, as well as initiate studies on reperfusion damage after liver transplantation.

Every investigation was done completely by them. I had no involvement. But these studies were special for me, as my students were about to stand on the shoulders of their mentor — and travel to places that I had never visited.

Limb Ischemia

Some may have seen a movie where a physician — witnessing a patient with a cold, pale-looking leg and feeling no sensation other than pain — then states, "Dead leg. We must amputate immediately."

That realistic scene would play out in many hospitals, as sudden obstruction of blood supply to the limb causes the classic symptoms of pallor, paralysis, no feeling except for pain — along with contracture of the muscles (a kind of "charley horse" that is profoundly uncomfortable). This occurrence leads to one conclusion: remove the leg.

But is that the only conclusion?

We know that such leg contractures also occur *temporarily* in many athletes, sometimes from overexertion. Yet there will consistently be complete recovery from this severe and uncomfortable cramp! But when this same condition happens after an artery is blocked — suddenly this symptom is considered the "final negative marker" that has only one solution — amputation.

These situations are not identical, but they do share a commonality that relates to how the cell adjusts its internal calcium concentrations during stress. Knowing this, Friedhelm simply asked — *is contracture truly terminal for a leg without blood flow?*

It's What's on the Inside that Counts

Sudden closure of a leg vessel can happen for any of several reasons. A blood clot could form in its main (femoral) artery due to hardening of the artery and an irregular surface on its inner wall. Or a blood clot might form elsewhere, such as the heart, and travel through blood circulation (called an embolus) and end up in the leg. Or the artery may clot due to irritation by a catheter tube (inserted to help the impaired circulation) that remains in place for several days.

In the case of a clot, logical reasoning would suggest removing the clot, not amputating the leg. But logic doesn't always win.

That's because efforts decades earlier to reestablish blood flow by successfully removing a clot — had caused a devastating aftermath in these patients.

Resuming a new flow allowed toxic substances that had developed within the dead leg tissue to suddenly wash out into the general circulation. As a result, serious injury to the kidneys, heart, lungs, and brain — and massive leg swelling — would sometimes follow this treatment. In such cases, death rates rose to 20 to 30%, so attempts to restart blood flow were abandoned in favor of amputation. These drastic complications would not occur with leg amputation, as it only had a 1% mortality rate.

Friedhelm recognized the dismal prognosis of traditional treatment — and simultaneously appreciated how controlled reperfusion successfully treated the heart. This disparity (the heart recovering after controlled reflow and the leg dying after normal blood reflow) prompted him to explore using *controlled reflow* in the "dead" leg.

Could regular blood reflow be the culprit behind this damage after a leg has had no blood flow?

A logical conclusion. But this theory needed to be tested.

Before starting treatment on a patient, Friedhelm needed to confirm in the lab that no irreversible damage would follow six hours of no leg blood flow when controlled reperfusion was used. If successful, this observation would precisely parallel what happened when we studied the effects of six hours of heart ischemia at UCLA — and thus show that just as with the heart muscle, the leg was not dead either.

The team now under Friedhelm's guidance, first mimicked *conventional treatment* by returning normal blood in an animal subject. They found sudden and complete damage to a leg that looked normal before reflow. These dire sequences included massive leg swelling... abrupt blood potassium rise (due to toxic washout from the damaged leg) that significantly altered heart rhythm... and kidney failure due to the toxic proteins (myoglobin) released from the leg's damaged muscle.

Controlled reperfusion would now be used to test his novel concept for the extremity. He established laboratory guidelines for treating the leg by using the already established heart controlled reperfusion protocols.

So what happened?

It worked beautifully every time. No problem developed following its delivery, as the test animal's leg and the body completely recovered. None of the adverse and sometimes lethal events that followed regular blood reperfusion were observed.[66]

Friedhelm updated me by phone and I joined him in his elation!

We both knew what would come next.

Bench to Bedside

The role of the lab is to become a bridge to the patient, and Friedhelm would now use this innovative experimental knowledge to test how controlled reperfusion worked in 11 patients with "clinically dead" legs deemed to have "terminal contraction." Only then would he know if the success in the lab could be transferred to the sick patient.

The results were sensational. These included complete relief of leg contracture as normal function returned to the recovered muscles, while washout injury to other organs was absent![67]

With this discovery, a vision emerged for a new landscape of treatment by vascular surgeons, as they (not cardiac surgeons) are the ones who encounter this leg ischemia problem. They could now save jeopardized limbs and restore their function, while avoiding the untimely death or other adverse consequences that result from returning normal blood reflow!

Friedhelm called once more to tell me of these dramatic new findings. I was thrilled because one of my students had beautifully blazed a trail in a new arena of clinical care. Our excitement about the heart now rang equally true for the leg. This clinical confirmation allowed us to ponder an even broader future: *could controlled reperfusion help other organs as well?*

Friedhelm needed to report these remarkable findings. He sent me his draft for review and I realized that extensive editing was needed. It was my delight to pitch in and then return it to Germany. Friedhelm asked me to be coauthor. I disagreed, advising him that placing my name on this landmark work would be a mistake.

"A hallmark of innovation," I contended, "is recognition of the innovator. The readers may think this was my work if my name is on it, and it is not."

My decision was firm, but we agreed to make me a coauthor on some future report, for the leader here was Friedhelm, not his teacher. My extraordinary pleasure was in watching my student make a monumental accomplishment. Nothing more was needed.[68]

Further Proof

The next step for Friedhelm was to have colleagues at other centers use his treatment and see if their outcomes upheld his findings. A pair of German cardiac surgery centers joined this first clinical trial by using controlled leg reperfusion on 19 patients with extended limb ischemia, each having an average of *26 hours of no blood flow.* This challenge introduced a *striking test* of our concept.

Only three patients (each having severely damaged hearts — cardiogenic shock) died. Each of the other 16 patients completely regained normal limb function after controlled reperfusion. The corroboration of this concept by others was overwhelmingly positive.[69]

It was relatively easy for Friedhelm to convince other cardiac surgeons to test out controlled reperfusion in their patients who developed post-operative problems in their extremities. They could simply adjust the reperfusion setups that they routinely used during cardiac surgery.

However, getting vascular surgeons to consider this new approach was much more complicated.

I learned this firsthand when I was a visiting professor at the University of Illinois Hospital in Chicago, where Brad Allen was on their faculty. We were discussing Friedhelm's work at breakfast when Brad said, "We have a patient with a jeopardized limb where contracture is present. There was complete loss of blood flow to the leg, due to a clot forming around a catheter device in his femoral artery that was used to help his heart perform better."

I immediately suggested, "Let's go see him."

After visiting the patient, I proposed to the cardiac surgeon and the patient's consulting physician (who was a Professor of Vascular Surgery) that controlled reperfusion might reverse this apparently terminal leg injury.

"It will never work," countered the vascular surgeon.

"We have evidence that it can. Try it."

The vascular surgeon was certain an amputation was needed, but agreed to try the procedure. As the procedure was performed... he was astounded at the immediate and positive role that controlled reperfusion played in this patient's recovery.[70] The vascular surgeon watched the leg muscles that were rigid from contracture become remarkably malleable, along with an absence of the anticipated swelling and other complications.

Unfortunately, the road to acceptance of new knowledge is long and arduous, before the core of thinking changes to allow its general adoption. Toward that end, Friedhelm helped develop a *prospective randomized trial* by vascular surgeons in Germany and Austria to treat advanced leg ischemia. "Prospective randomized trial" means that some patients would receive normal blood while others would receive controlled reperfusion. The key requirement for validation is to use properly selected patients, and to precisely follow the established methods of controlled reperfusion.

There was great anticipation for validation of Friedhelm's breakthrough discovery. But the vascular surgeons did not adhere to the controlled reperfusion protocols... and no difference in results was found.

My credo is always, "If it does not work, either the idea is wrong, or the procedure was not done right." We knew that "the idea was not wrong," because truly "dead" contracted legs *had* recovered in previous studies. The failure here *was because the surgeons failed to do controlled reperfusion properly.* This conclusion is substantiated by the 24 patients who had just been summarized in Friedhelm's analysis. Their recovery proved the idea was correct.[69]

Unfortunately for patients, this poorly conducted trial buried any chance to recover doomed extremities. Yet, I know the opportunity will resurface again... because truth always wins.

Lung Transplantation

Finding that the controlled reperfusion approach worked equally well for the heart and leg, supported my fundamental belief that ischemia and reperfusion injury was a biologic process that could be applied to treating other organs.

One such area might be organ transplantation. The donation of healthy organs from an individual to replace diseased ones in another, when successful, can vastly extend the life of the recipient. Still, the process of removing an organ from a body introduces a period where it receives no blood flow, which lasts until the organ has been placed into the recipient. The only safeguards conventionally used to avoid injury are cooling of the donor organ (to lower its energy needs), which is then followed by return of normal blood flow after it is placed in the recipient.

But could this normal blood reperfusion lead to injury?

This became an area of interest for Brad Allen at the University of Illinois. Brad had studied using controlled heart reperfusion following acute heart attacks with us at UCLA from 1984 to 1986. Now in 1997, he noted that in preparation for lung transplantation, a lengthy period of time without blood flow (four to eight hours) was needed to transport the lung from a donor in one city to the recipient at his hospital in Chicago. He wondered if lung reperfusion injury occurred as a result, and if so, could it sometimes hamper success of the lung transplantation procedure? The question that naturally followed was: could controlled reperfusion avoid such a problem?

Of course, before he would try controlled reperfusion in lung transplant patients, Brad would test the effects of transplantation — with both normal and controlled reperfusion — in the lab.

The trauma of normal blood reperfusion was confirmed — by removing the lung of a piglet — exposing it to two hours of warm ischemia (no blood supply and no cooling) — and then replacing it into the same piglet (a procedure called "lung re-implantation"). Reflow of *normal* blood was given. Severe lung damage resulted, as lung vessels became constricted and thus raised their resistance to blood flow. They also became stiffer, swollen (from added water), and tiny capillaries near the breathing sacs (alveolar) filled with fluid.

Conversely, subsequent tests with using *controlled reperfusion* for 10 minutes — resulted in normal lung vessel resistance, no lung stiffness or swelling, and normal capillaries.

Brad took it a further step. In prior lung transplantation studies, Brad had found that adding a white blood cell filter would counteract toxic byproducts caused by white blood cells (WBC). So he added a WBC filter during controlled reperfusion, which produced even better results.[44]

Brad realized the next important step in the experiment would be to mimic the lung being kept cold, as it is transported to the recipient before transplantation. He simulated this process by again providing controlled reperfusion into the transplanted lung — *after* it had experienced 24 hours of cold storage (in an icebox). Amazingly, the positive results *following 24 hours of ischemia* precisely mirrored the findings when controlled reperfusion was delivered after two hours of ischemia at normal temperature conditions![71]

These excellent findings were critical to protecting the lung during its transplantation... *yet they also protected the other (normal) lung* in the recipient's body. That's important because *normal* blood reperfusion of a transplanted lung can cause a washout of toxic substances that circulate to injure the non-transplanted lung — similar to what happened following normal blood reflow when treating a dead leg, as was described in Friedhelm Beyersdorf's studies.

Protecting the normal lung is vital, since the patient must rely on it if the transplanted lung does not properly function. While its injury from conventional reperfusion would be on a lesser scale than that of the transplanted lung... this normal "back-up" lung would experience diminished reserve function as there would be heightened resistance to blood flow, increased stiffness and swelling, and small capillary damage.[72]

It was hoped that all of this could be prevented with controlled reperfusion — and indeed it was. Healthy lung function *was normal* after 24 hours of storage when controlled reperfusion was used.

Human Trials

These experiments established the findings necessary to allow controlled pulmonary reperfusion to begin to be used with patients undergoing lung transplantation.

That next critical step was done on patients at the University of Texas — and results were excellent.[73] Medical teams there were elated by the positive outcomes. Brad and I were particularly delighted and encouraged because everything that we had hoped for was proven true.

This approach has now subsequently been used at UCLA in over 100 patients.[74] Unfortunately, at UCLA, the recommended ten-minute duration of controlled reperfusion (using both the solution and white blood cell filter) was arbitrarily reduced by the transplant team, even though there had been no supplementary studies to support such a change. The results were still good overall, but further investigations are needed to evaluate the effectiveness of this shortened protocol, compared to what was originally recommended from the experimental studies.

This could be an important consideration, as the *long-term effects* of lung transplantations introduce another concern. We had always found that reperfusion damage is worse in the organ's inner shell, as was quite evident in the heart and brain. It is similarly true with the lung, as its inner cell lining of small breathing tubes may suffer long-term damage and cause a non-reversible condition called bronchiolitis obliterans. That results in inflammation and closure of the small breathing tubes. A tragedy unfolds in which lung transplantations that seem initially successful, may later lead to patients dying prematurely because of this lethal complication.

While the UCLA results thus far show a reduction in the development of bronchiolitis, it is too soon to fully tell the long-range consequences. There needs to be long-term testing of those patients that received normal blood — and those who received properly delivered controlled reperfusate — to determine if this lethal complication is also avoided by the new approach.

The Liver

This path toward proving the universal benefit of controlled reperfusion to various organs is an ongoing journey.

Though explorations with transplantation had so far only focused on the lungs, the trauma of ischemia (absent blood flow) is prominent in patients undergoing *any* kind of organ replacement. As with the lungs, the only conventional protection against this comes from cooling the removed organ... which is then followed by normal blood reperfusion after it is placed in the recipient's body.

As I've mentioned before, one of the thrills of working in a university is the interchange between practitioners of different disciplines. This was certainly true for organ transplantation, as UCLA has the largest liver transplant program in the United States. Its leader, Ron Busuttil, fully understood the enemy: the problems associated with ischemic reperfusion injury. Such injury led to awful consequences. The transplanted liver becomes congested, swells, and toxic enzymes wash out into the body. Extensive care is required, yet the liver may still fail completely and the patient succumbs.

Our ears were always open to hearing of new problems to solve in this area, since we believed our answer to the ischemic reperfusion process can benefit any organ. With this in mind, Brad Allen suggested we do a pilot study of controlled reperfusion after liver transplantation.

We first needed to determine if extensive injury indeed followed two hours of warm ischemia and normal blood reflow. This finding would become the yardstick by which we could measure the effectiveness of our approach. As it turned out, the challenge of such injury was a severe one. Both pigs undergoing warm ischemia and normal blood reperfusion died. Each exhibited the symptoms of severe liver damage before their death.

Now it came time to test our methods. Our experiences with the heart and leg and lungs rang true again. The two pigs receiving controlled reperfusion had *complete recovery.* And every indicator that might have pointed toward damage returned to normal within 24 hours.

Just as there is great significance to having others confirm positive results with patients (as Brad's success with patient lung transplants was duplicated by the Texas researchers), the same was true for documenting this extraordinary lab recovery. These positive experimental results were verified by one of Ron Busuttil's associates, who repeated our study in his lab. Our team had no part in that research, yet again — there was no reperfusion injury. A pattern became evident, as their liver findings mirrored the same return to normality that we had encountered in our studies of the heart, brain, limb, and lung, and in Brad's two pilot studies of the liver.[75]

This validation of Brad's results, which paralleled the successes of controlled reperfusion in other organs, led me to present my thoughts on this issue at a special conference at UCLA. The intent was to develop a Controlled Reperfusion Theme at our university. I provided an overview of the established benefits to this innovative approach for restoring blood supply after ischemia in different organs. Representatives from every department that did clinical transplantation attended, as each had experience with patients who had suffered ischemic reperfusion injury.

Everyone listened raptly, especially when Ron described his astonishment at observing mental normality in pigs who received controlled reperfusion after liver ischemia. He contrasted this to the metabolic chaos (and sometimes coma) that can typically follow normal blood reperfusion. Ron was taken aback, because the clinical appearance of mental normality meant that there was no washout of toxic substances from the liver. This included an absence of the generation of ammonia, a chemical that causes hepatic coma during the near terminal end-stage liver disease.

While the transition to using controlled reperfusion of the liver in patients has yet to happen at UCLA, its seeds have been sown into the mindsets of those in attendance. Again, from my perspective, it is not a matter of *if* it will happen... but *when* such truth will win.

It was gratifying to watch Friedhelm Beyersdorf and Brad Allen mount new steps on the scientific ladder. They used controlled reperfusion concepts to protect the diseased limb, the lung, and open the door to protecting the liver. Their capacity to identify, experimentally test, and then clinically implement a treatment that never before existed — provided the powerful foundation needed to allow controlled reperfusion to be tested in a spectrum of diseases — ones that had never before been solved in this manner.

It was everything a teacher could ever hope for.

Credit Where Credit is Due

The truest gauge for scientific accomplishment is how ideas become beacons to rethink problems, and lead to new solutions.

In all this, there is but one ultimate focus — the patient — who will benefit from the implementation of innovative changes. As I repeat to each incoming resident: personal acknowledgement is never the objective. The goal is *the creation of ideas that transform action.*

At UCLA's annual Longmire Surgical Society Dinner, residents and faculty that trained with Dr. Longmire during his 40 years gather together. We typically recount endless amusing stories that had occurred within our hallowed halls. Traditionally, graduating residents who had done outstanding work would receive awards during this event. On rare occasions, other people are recognized as well.

I was there with my wife, sitting with friends, when to my surprise, it was announced that I would receive the Longmire Legacy Award. Only two or three of these awards have ever been given in the 20 years since these dinners began, and I had no idea I would be receiving it.

What happened next was equally unforeseen.

One of my prior research fellows, a cardiac surgeon, was the president of the Longmire Club. When he introduced me, he said to the audience, "I want to tell you a story about Gerry Buckberg that I'm not sure anybody has ever heard. It's something that occurred when Gerry's breakthrough concept of blood cardioplegia was to be presented at the American Association of Thoracic Surgery in 1978."

At this point, I *really* had no idea what he was going to say.

He continued, "I happened to be present when Jim Maloney, the Division Chief of Cardiothoracic Surgery at UCLA, came to inform Gerry that he should present the paper. Maloney reasoned that it was Gerry's idea, and his presence would make a positive impact on the over 4,000 surgeons who would be in attendance, especially since it was to be the first paper on the program due to its merit."

My prior student smiled to himself a moment and resumed, "Gerry — being Gerry, then pointed to me and told Maloney, 'Our research fellow did the experimental and clinical analyses and should make the presentation.' Of course, Maloney being Maloney, persisted. 'No, you have to present it.'

"Finally, Gerry looked Maloney in the eye and said, 'Look, I won't do it. Either my research fellow makes the presentation, or I will advise the meeting's organizers that the paper will be withdrawn from presentation.' Obviously, Maloney finally agreed."

Several in the audience at the Longmire dinner laughed at this as they knew me quite well, thus fully appreciating my consistency in such decisions.

The dissemination of new medical information usually begins with a presentation at a major medical meeting, typically by the named leader of the study. Yet, everybody already knew it was my lab. Consequently, when the selected fellow demonstrates a superb effort, it elegantly reflects the leader's presence. Besides, each research fellow is just beginning their career, so that presenting an important paper may boost their launching.

Rewards for Awards

Satisfying recognition comes from first discovering the truth, and then from others using your concepts to replace less successful treatments. This desired progression originates with our research presentations given at major surgical society meetings, where the work of those who have met these requirements is sometimes acknowledged.

In 2000, The Society of Thoracic Surgery established the Earl Bakken Award. It is named for the man who designed the first wearable cardiac pacemaker and co-founded Medtronic, which manufactures it. The award is intended to honor those who have made exceptional scientific contributions that notably improved the practice of cardiothoracic surgery and the quality of life for patients.

I was privileged to receive their first Lifetime Achievement Award for my work on myocardial protection, and needed to make some remarks at the ceremony. As I contemplated what to say, I was struck that it seemed miraculous I was even there. I said that "the kids on Clarke Place in the Bronx, where I grew up, could not have conceived that the guy who played stickball in the street with them would be receiving this organization's first lifetime achievement award."

Of course, I also talked about having my work applied in clinical care and how its use touched people's lives, which was more gratifying than only publishing our findings in journals. I acknowledged the enormous contributions from my research fellows, and accepted the award with genuine gratitude. … Yet internally, I couldn't help but think of all the discoveries we had made that still needed to be accepted and implemented.

Then the perfect illustration of the phrase "Rewards for Awards" arose *after* I received the Bakken Prize. The convention still had a couple more days to go. As I walked into meetings and visited cocktail parties, I was approached by person after person after person. Somewhere between 100 to 200 surgeons from all over the globe thanked me. Expressing appreciation for my helping their practices become safer — and making their patients better.

This was the true honor for my work on myocardial protection. These individuals were often not affiliated with universities, or in positions to influence the widespread approval of new treatments. Rather, they were in private practice where cardiac surgeons focus on a singular pursuit: "How do I make my patient better?" Their generous acknowledgments confirmed the success of my principal goal — helping others through my work. I experienced each of these unique rewards in a private, one-on-one setting… yet each conveyed to me that the power of my discovery had far transcended its public recognition.

I offered a grateful smile to each of those coming up, and told them how enriching their comments were to me. No more needed to be said.

Inside, I knew it was a job well done. *My work had meaning.*

CHAPTER 15

Unanticipated Interlude

As with science, life flows in waves. Surging us past troughs of uncertainty between the crescendos of new discovery. Both in professional undertakings... and within oneself. Such a pattern occurred to me in 1996, originating from the most unexpected of circumstances.

I was with my family in Missoula, Montana to present at a conference attended by prominent surgeons from all around the world. After completion of the event, I was scheduled to return to Los Angeles and operate on a high-ranking official in the Indonesian government, who was traveling to UCLA for this procedure.

The conference went well, and on the final day of our presentations, there was a special evening barbecue along the river. Before dinner, many of us planned to ride horses through the area. But when I mounted Il Nigro, my aging steed, it took one look at me — a rather large rider — and decided "Not a chance."

He reared up... and bucked Uncle Bucky.

I landed hard on my arm and was in great pain. But mostly I remember thinking, "Damn it, I was supposed to operate on this important political leader and here I am flat on the ground." My elbow was broken. They took me to a tiny private hospital in the area to check me over... and discovered I had atrial fibrillation (abnormally fast and irregular heart rhythm).

While most people with atrial fibrillation experience a rapid heart rate, sense a "flub-dub" in their chest, and encounter fatigue without much exertion, I'd had none of these symptoms. Because I was an athlete, my heart rate remained low, between 45 and 55, and I wasn't tired. My condition only became evident when an electrocardiogram was taken prior to the expected brief surgical procedure to reset my bone. Yet once I knew I had atrial fibrillation, I could self-detect it by feeling my own pulse and sensing its irregularity.

The next morning, I returned to UCLA, where I saw a cardiologist who confirmed the diagnosis and reassured me it was not dangerous, and my elbow was fixed the next day. The subsequent treatment of my atrial fibrillation was straightforward. I was given a medical drug that would hopefully convert the rhythm back to normal (sinus) rhythm. In the meantime, I was placed on Coumadin, a blood-thinning drug used to prevent development of a clot on the surface of the heart's atrium. This complication may happen because fibrillation causes a quivering of the atrium, instead of allowing the muscle covering the atrium to contract normally. Consequently, the entire wall of this non-functioning thin muscle now acts like a flat lake, becoming the ideal flaccid area where a clot can form. The biggest danger from such a clot is that it can break off and become *an embolus* that enters the blood stream and travels someplace to obstruct blood flow. The greatest hazard is its going to the brain, causing a stroke. Concern about this fearsome complication is why the patient is always given an anticoagulant — a blood-thinning drug.

Fortunately, return of my natural heart rate occurred in about two months — literally on the same day I was scheduled to be admitted to UCLA for electrical defibrillation, thereby canceling the need for such a treatment (which is best avoided if possible, since it entails a number of steps, including an anesthesiologist putting you to sleep while you undergo brief electrical shocking of your heart with a defibrillator to return normal rhythm). Self-detecting the return of my normal heart rate was easy, since I was evaluating its consistency by checking my own pulse rate.

Even though I was having no other symptoms, the change to a normal rhythm was very welcome. I was quite eager to have my regular heartbeat restored so that I could get off the Coumadin medication. There is a significant concern about bleeding complications in the brain while on this drug, should you experience an unexpected event, like a bump on the head. Such an incident during treatment with a blood-thinning drug may result in a 30% death rate.

Because of such concerns, I stopped taking Coumadin as soon as I developed a normal pulse rate, whose continued regularity (which I would self-check) confirmed an absence of atrial fibrillation. My customary activities continued: research and teaching, performing cardiac operations, and a busy travel schedule to present at national and worldwide centers where I'd be invited to speak about our work on myocardial protection.

Forgotten Dreams

But my smooth routine soon became interrupted two months later in Tokyo, Japan, where I awakened one morning and found myself in my hotel bathtub. At first startled, I quickly deduced that the bruise on my cheek must have occurred from hitting a faucet on the tub, after having fallen in late at night when using the bathroom.

I checked my pulse — it was irregular. I thought I had gone into another bout of atrial fibrillation. That could vary my heart's output and lower blood pressure enough to diminish the oxygen supply to my brain and cause a fall. I could detect no other neurological symptoms or injuries. So I visited Sapporo the next day to give another series of lectures and help one of my former UCLA fellows operate upon a patient at his clinical center, all without incident. My normal heart rate (beats per minute) promptly returned after taking a brief dose of heart medication.

Yet all was not the same.

Following my return to Los Angeles, my secretary observed that I was repeatedly asking the same questions of her and others, something she'd never witnessed before during our 15 years together. I immediately went to a neurologist, whose testing showed that my short-term memory was impaired. There were no other neurological problems, but a magnetic resonance imaging (MRI) study of my brain was performed that day.

Results were not good. My brain artery vessels were normal, but I had sustained a stroke. There was a loss of two-and-a-half centimeters (about one inch) of tissue in the brain region responsible for recent memory. Called necrosis, this tissue was now dead, likely caused by an embolus (traveling blood clot) that came from my heart.

This event was shocking to me, especially since I had remained in a normal heart rhythm for two months following my conversion (return to normal rhythm) from atrial fibrillation. I contacted a cardiology colleague, who astounded me further with information of which I was completely unaware. He told me that after *an extended period* of atrial fibrillation like I had experienced, the atrium does not immediately recover, even after the successful treatment. It does not contract at all — even though there is restoration of a regular ventricular heartbeat, which can be confirmed by checking the wrist's pulse or with an electrocardiogram. The atrium chamber acts as if it was "stunned" — meaning it is like a motionless flaccid lake, despite allowing the return of uniform electrical ventricular impulses.

As I reflected on this new information, I realized it resembled what happens when the heart gets stunned as described previously in the chapter on heart attacks. Or the "daze" that a boxer or football player feels after a blow to the head causes a delayed neurological recovery.

This circumstance exposed a loophole in my knowledge. The consequence of this "stunning" after recovery from atrial fibrillation is that there continues to be a stagnant, non-contracting atrium — that provides a smooth non-moving surface that is perfect for clot formation. While I knew Coumadin was given to combat such clots, I thought this drug was discontinued as soon as atrial fibrillation was no longer present. I was not alone in this belief. Other surgical colleagues, including Jim Cox, a good friend and the surgical world's expert on treatment of atrial fibrillation, were equally unaware of this "stunning" complication.

How could that be?

As surgeons, we only deal with very short periods of atrial fibrillation. It occurs in about 30% of patients after open-heart surgery, but this fibrillation usually stops after a few days, and Coumadin is promptly and correctly discontinued when heart rhythm becomes normal again. But when atrial fibrillation has continued for a prolonged period of time, as it had in my case, the return to normality is not so simple or quick. Though my cardiologist had said nothing about this to me, I learned that when there has been a long period of atrial fibrillation, Coumadin should continue to be taken for another couple of months, even after a return to a normal heart rhythm. It is then stopped only after a contracting atrium is seen and confirmed by echocardiogram.

Thoroughly understanding what happens is crucial because the heart is a pump, not simply something carrying electricity like a television set without moving parts. Despite absence of atrial fibrillation, it was still not squeezing properly. The union of electrical impulses *and* contraction is essential for normality.

This dichotomy further emphasizes the importance of ensuring accurate communication between different medical specialties. Failure to do so has enormous impact upon people's lives, by causing complications that may otherwise be prevented. It was unfortunate that this baseline knowledge was not known in the surgical community... especially by me.

My goal in seeing a neurologist, aside from his confirming the diagnosis and impact of the stroke, was to better understand my condition. My first question was whether I could operate. Fortunately, while I was advised not to undertake any new procedures, I could carry on with things I had done previously. I listened to this advice and all went well, as there was no impairment of long-term memory.

However, my limitations of short-term memory became increasingly apparent, particularly while reading newspapers. I was not able to remember headlines describing a story's subject matter, and struggled to comprehend the articles as I could not recall the content of previous paragraphs. Wishing to counter these negative effects of my condition, I met with a cognitive therapist. She began by giving me a series of tests to challenge my capacities and judge my performance. The examinations turned out to be extremely perplexing and distressing, since she had me try a variety of things that I could not do. It candidly pointed out my present deficiencies, clarifying the depth of my brain damage that resulted from a stroke that impacted only a small region.

I was frightened once I recognized the extent of the injury. There were no physical impairments other than those to my brain, yet depriving this resource to an individual whose world revolves around intellectual pursuits — causes a psychological burden that overshadows everything else.

Harsh Reality

Unfortunately, the full gravity of my new existence became appallingly clear when I helped a resident do a reoperation procedure on a patient of mine.

As there had been a previous surgery on this heart, we would first have to deal with scar tissue, which was wrapped around much of the heart tissues and formed a kind of casing. In such circumstances, the surgeon needs to cut away some of the scar tissue to free and mobilize the heart again, like you would have with a normal heart. This would be necessary so we could then start the heart-lung machine and correct the underlying cardiac difficulty.

However, I did not sufficiently oversee the resident's technique, specifically in making certain that placement of a drainage tube within a blood vessel was not done in too aggressive a manner. The result was a major tear in the main upper vein (superior vena cava), which returns blood to the heart. Massive bleeding ensued. We quickly responded, but it was impossible to control the site of the hemorrhage because tissue on the surface of the vessel was pulled apart, as there was no elasticity in the scar tissue encasing the vessel. Bleeding was torrential. We promptly started the heart-lung machine to capture and return the blood. But this action was not effective.

I quickly summoned a senior surgical colleague to help us. We were able to control the situation and ultimately correct the underlying problem with the reoperation. But the heart was severely damaged during the process and the patient succumbed three weeks later.

The potential for such injuries is why risks are always greater with re-operations. Even though such problems are the reality of heart surgery, I could not stop blaming myself for my role in allowing the damage. I questioned my decision to assist the resident, though this approach of allowing residents to perform surgeries under supervision is how many were performed at the university, and the approach I had followed for 25 years. While I realized conceptually that these were tough procedures with very sick people — and like every cardiac surgeon, knew this hazard was a part of our world — I wasn't considering that.

I focused upon condemning myself for this tragedy.

The Depths

The end result of this internal self-recrimination was the development of a profound depression that totally altered my universe.

I immediately stopped operating, and could not provide educational help to my research fellows. I essentially became non-functional since I could not address any medical problems. The symptoms of this mental state took over my thinking, interfering with all aspects of my professional and social life. I withdrew from everything, becoming a shell of the person I had been. Inactivity replaced my productive lifestyle. The emptiness of this plunge into despair had no boundaries, without a foothold to rebound from or a ledge to grasp. It felt like a freefall.

While medical professionals provided me with psychiatric drugs, they had no positive effect. Though such medications are reported to help others, I realized the escape from my depression would require the generation of *a solution that came from within*. This disease imposes the greatest inward challenge anyone can confront, its resolution only evolving by guidance from the human spirit. In order to climb out of my abyss, I needed to find my own answer.

Light from Shadow

Despite how consumed and isolated I felt, I would discover I was not alone. I read a wonderful book on depression, *Darkness Visible*, by William Styron, which describes the way this illness engulfs one in despair. This brilliant author described the ravages of this disease upon his existence, and emphasized that creative individuals — those who devise and find their own way out of the despondency — have a better chance than those relying only on the advice and tasks defined by others. Knowing that I was creative by nature gave me hope.

My understanding also expanded after I read *Tuesdays with Morrie*, by Mitch Albom. Unlike my situation and the one described in Styron's book, where the mind was affected while the patient lives within a normal body... Morrie's body was shattered by Lou Gehrig's disease, while he remained mentally intact. Even as his physical condition continued to decline, Morrie's vibrant spirit never faltered. Though my situation appeared to have no solution, Morrie's story told the wonders of how the mind can overcome everything.

But could mine?

Sink or Swim

While Styron's book helped me to better grasp what was occurring and Morrie's tale encouraged striving forward, there still seemed so little to hold onto, to guide me, or even impel me forward.

Our ability to think is what uniquely defines each of us as individuals. Descartes described this by observing "I think, therefore I am." It's what drives us. Without that capacity, who are we?

I was an intellectual person who had always used that ability to perform those actions most important to me. But my brain had been taken away. My intellect was crushed. Everything had been taken from me. I lived in a sense of doom, because "if I cannot think; I am not."

Submerging

The time frame of this disease seemed endless. Days and weeks and many months passed without any reprieve from this mental morass. At the same time, I moved my UCLA office up to the 6th floor, after 27 years in a basement space that felt like living inside a submarine. I now had a wonderful office with a view... yet I simply sat at my desk, staring at empty shelves and my boxes of books in front of me. I didn't care even to take out one of my books. I sat there like a piece of deadwood... listening to the bells in an adjacent church, tolling hour after hour, the only progression in my stagnant world. I awaited arrival of the last clanging bell signaling the end of each successive day when I could leave this moribund existence... only to return again the next morning.

I realized that whatever I was already trying wasn't getting me better. I couldn't wait for — nor expect — nature to spontaneously shift it. I had to find some new way to recover myself. Yet I still did not know how to meet this challenge.

My desolation led me to take several steps that would change my world. I needed to purge all of my burdens — escape from the responsibilities that I could not meet. My ability to do the things I spent my life doing had simply evaporated.

First, my career as a clinical surgeon came to a halt. The skill that had been my life's work was thwarted. Second, I advised our major Journal of Thoracic and Cardiovascular Surgery that I could not continue my editorial responsibilities due to an unspecified medical problem. Third, I now needed to find places for my research fellows to work, since it was impossible to mentor them during our research program that I could not oversee. Fourth, this decision led me to also notify the National Institutes of Health (NIH) that my previously approved research grant had to be placed on hiatus, since a medical problem impeded our progression toward finding solutions to our funded project.

Finally, I would need to cancel 10 to 15 international lectures that I was scheduled to give, since I was not up to the task of presenting. I was basically getting rid of everything. My professional life was ending.

Moment of Truths

I remember being at home preparing to cancel my presentation lectures, starting with a conference in Argentina. Additionally, I was supposed to arrive there early for a pre-conference visit — to oversee Argentinean surgeons employing methods of heart protection that evolved from our studies.

My wife, Ingeborg, had gone to Europe to visit her family. I sat on my lawn alone… as I contemplated my fear of sharing with others my full cognitive limitations. Equally meaningful, I confronted the unbearable horror that the life I had so relished, could indeed be finished. I had already given up my lab, my researchers, my editing duties. Cancelling my Argentina visit and all that followed would be the final nail in the coffin. Everything would be over. But what choice was there?

I thought about how there is an intrinsic difference between how individuals confront these situations. One can either choose to hide their frailties, or confront them by taking the position that it is better to move forward, even if that means you may "fail" in a very profound and obvious manner. I recognized this second choice also describes the basic nature of the surgeon — whose *actions* define his credo — rather than searching for ways to escape any challenge. The surgeon's way is to *move forward* into things… particularly when the stakes are high.

I recalled how this had been so well-put by Claude Bernard, my conceptual hero from the moment I read his book, *Introduction to Experimental Medicine.* This legendary French physiologist described the world as being occupied by either observers or experimenters. The observers were like astronomers who watched the stars and recorded what they saw. But the experimenters saw the world with a belief of why certain things might be the way they are, and then did studies to understand the reasons behind what they perceived… perhaps uncovering solutions to a problem.

I sat straight up in my chair, realizing I had been living the life of the observer, watching what was happening to me, not testing circumstances to see if what I had experienced so far could be changed. I was behaving like a traditionalist, taking a position that bars progress.

I was planning to cancel the Argentina visit since I *expected* that I would fail. I didn't want to relive the sense of failure that followed the devastating operation that spawned my depth of despair. But then, despite my haze of depressed thoughts, I realized something elegantly straightforward: the only way that you *really* fail… *is to fail.* You cannot fail because *you think you are going to fail.* Actions, not fears, must be your credo.

I decided to visit Argentina as planned.

This bold decision followed the same natural path of experimental testing that guided my professional career. Escaping reality at home made me an observer of my own life, and I needed to take charge of it.

While I didn't know it at that moment, that choice and this trip would have a tremendous influence on the rest of my life.

Through Fire and Water

I would keep my commitment to present at the Argentinean conference in Mendoza — the first in a long while, ever since my condition had been so severe.

But I would stop beforehand in the medium-sized city of Cordoba, where a group of ten outstanding young surgeons, who would likely become their country's leaders in cardiac surgery, were gathered to try my technique of heart protection. The patient was to receive grafts to replace blocked vessels, and they wanted to use arteries for the grafts rather than veins because they lasted longer. Conventional methods of protecting the heart were often inadequate for the lengthier periods without blood supply that were needed to implant these arterial vessels. So they wanted to see if my protection method would be effective, while I oversaw its use. Everyone spoke English and I was asked to "scrub in" to participate in the operation, but I answered that I would rather observe. None of them realized the nature of my stroke and its role in generating my depression.

Ten young doctors in green gowns and I encircled the operating table as the surgeon performed the operation while using my techniques. Everything seemed to go well and they gave protection in exactly the way that I had described.

But as the surgeon took the patient off the heart-lung machine when he finished, the heart showed a markedly impaired capacity to contract. It would not beat effectively! Pharmacologic drugs to enhance the heart's contractile ability were immediately given, but these agents did not work. The patient was dying.

I determined that the damage was not related to myocardial protection. That had been administered perfectly. I believed the issue was that the graft connections were done incorrectly, and the heart was not receiving a sufficient supply of blood. The impaired performance of the front and side of the heart looked exactly like a region that had undergone a major heart attack — one getting insufficient blood supply due to vessel blockage.

I realized that they were not looking to me for an answer... but I had one.

"I know the cause. The protection isn't the problem — that was done well. There is a problem with the graft connections, so that the heart is not getting proper blood supply. This is a correctable problem, but it means restarting the heart-lung machine and revising some of the hook ups. This approach now requires using veins to replace the arterial conduits [the arteries they used for grafting] whose surgical connections are faulty."

Mine was a sole voice amid this group of potential leaders of heart surgery in Argentina. Following my battle plan would require the cardiac surgeon to stop the heart again, and then *impose an even longer period* of no blood supply to a heart that was now already damaged. Their alternative involved shoring up the failing heart by administering even higher doses of drugs, together with need to sometimes implant a mechanical device to support circulation if the high drug dose was ineffective — to tide the heart over in the hope it would improve after the procedure.

My proposal was based on my confidence that heart protection was excellent — so that the reasons for impaired heart performance must be mechanical (the operation itself). Their opposition was based on, "If you think the patient is dying, why would you want to take his blood supply away again?" — which dealt with the symptom of acute heart failure, not its cause.

So we were confronted by two diametrically opposed choices: simply accept there is heart failure after a procedure and support the heart with drugs or devices... or accept responsibility for having caused the heart failure by the operation itself and correct the cause.

The team of young surgeons observing the procedure was not convinced my answer was correct. However, decisions during surgical operations are not made by vote. Instead, final judgment belongs to the responsible surgeon. The gravity of this impaired cardiac performance required that something had to be done fast, and the surgeon performing the operation made his choice. "I'm going to listen to Gerry. We're following his approach."

The patient was immediately hooked up again to the heart-lung machine. Cardioplegia was given again. The surgery began again. The new surgical connections were carried out as I had suggested.

Answers to the choices we make during cardiac surgery are often quickly apparent, as the efficiency of the heart (or most importantly, its inefficiency) becomes evident as soon as the heart-lung machine is turned off. What would the answer be?

We passed this final test with flying colors. The performance of the heart was totally restored to normal function.

Reality Reboot

From Cordoba, I went forward to the conference in Mendoza, Argentina, where I would address an international gathering. As it would turn out, my worry about my depression causing me to fail during a presentation was unfounded. My lectures went very well. The buoying up that I experienced during the operation in Cordoba likely added to my self-assurance.

Yet even more deeply, I was reminded in Mendoza that the real beauty of traveling to teach is the opportunity to exchange ideas with other participants. Their broad range of experience provides a wonderful forum to share knowledge. My mind, which had been so terribly thwarted and dormant for the past 18 months, was energized as interchange among these colleagues would open the door to new possibilities... and new frontiers.

What kept recurring in my mind was the distressing theme of heart failure that would so often develop following a heart attack.

The most perplexing part is how this progression is hidden at first, as initial mortality is reduced from 20% to 5% by angioplasty. Instead, it only rears its ugly head many years later — as the region's scar from the heart attack never recovers, and the remote muscle (the still functioning muscle portion away from the damaged region) stretches more and more to compensate — until the heart is no longer able to adequately perform. The patient's life becomes increasingly diminished and ends prematurely.

I knew the common treatment for this is to place a graft with new blood supply to the impaired remote muscle, or repair leaky heart valves. But these interventions do not solve this worsening problem. The true enemy was evident — but only if we observed how the *heart's geometry* is markedly altered by the heart attack. It was a problem that deeply deserved a fresh and full examination. Recent figures show over 550,000 cases of congestive heart failure are added every year to the 5 million patients already with this disease — in the U.S. alone.

My new eagerness for understanding the role of geometry in heart failure was stirred by my now recalling the work of Vincent Dor, a French cardiac surgeon who I had previously visited in Monaco. He emphasized that *the scar was the culprit* that caused the heart's structure to change from a football shape to more like a basketball.

Yet Dor pointed out that failure happens following a heart attack in a heart that *deceptively looks good* on the surface... since returning normal blood flow by angioplasty makes the bulging heart no longer bulge. But this treatment *fails to* return contraction to the dead inner and middle layers of muscle of the heart attack region. His successful approach to countering this, involved performing a procedure to exclude the scar so that the rebuilt heart is returned to its more natural elliptical form... *but this is an operation no one else had done.*

My conference in Mendoza reignited my commitment toward determining if he was correct. Indeed, if his approach was effective, we would have a powerful new tool to confront congestive heart failure — *the major cause of death in the world.* One that would overcome the ineffectiveness of all traditional treatments.

The siren song of heart failure was now calling. To explore this world, I would need to pursue a series of persuasive and valid findings that explained why this disastrous event happened, and set the sails for many new investigations to further advance our thinking. This search would also draw others into this quest for a solution to our greatest health care challenge.

Percolating Passions

These were the seeds that permeated my thinking, and persisted throughout my visit to Mendoza, Argentina. The evolution of this new approach became the "secret ticket" out of my depression. I was flooded with ideas on how to develop this concept. I wanted to assemble a team of the world's top leaders in cardiac surgery. As this was a revolutionary idea among those experts that treated heart failure, I realized I would need to go and individually meet with each handpicked surgeon, wherever they practiced, to determine if they would become part of a newly formed group to challenge this immense global problem.

Once settled on this new plan, I decided to put on paper my concept of the journey we would all undertake together. The ideas flowed endlessly throughout my flight home from Argentina. While everyone else was seeking sleep during the 17-hour trip to Los Angeles, the little ceiling light above my seat stayed lit as I fervently wrote. Energy raced through me as I composed page after page after page, creating 70 consecutive handwritten pages of notes describing every ramification of this whole process of countering heart failure and all the studies that could be done and how to make best use of them. These pages would serve as the blueprint for our study, which I would take with me as I traveled the world to meet with each of these renowned surgeons. These meetings will be described in the second of these next two chapters on heart failure.

I completed my pages and leaned back in my seat. I was alive again. My capacity to think was returning as well, no doubt thanks to the remarkable capacity of the brain to form new neural pathways to compensate for damaged tissues. My internal voyage back to myself — had worked.

New Journey

Riding in the car toward my house after landing in Los Angeles, I took a moment to reflect on my ordeal. Styron had been right on target, since the deep depression that had consumed my world during the past year and a half... had simply evaporated within the seven days in Argentina that now launched me onto this new creative effort. His describing the depths of depression had an astounding impact, as my course remarkably paralleled his.

During my depression, I shared the power of his book, *Darkness Visible*, with my daughters, sending each a copy so they could better comprehend what was occurring with their father. My youngest daughter, Gia, happened to be getting her master's degree in social work at the University of Minnesota when she read it and was astonished by the remarkable parity of Styron's story and mine. With my consent, Gia wrote about my experience as part of her postgraduate studies and sent me a copy. I was moved that someone so close to me could so fully grasp my private trials.

Wishing to acknowledge Styron for his contribution to me, I located his address and forwarded him a note, describing myself and adding Gia's report. He promptly responded and defined our liaison by stating, "We have a brotherhood."

Styron's creativity was the road to his recovery, and the remainder of this memoir will define how I followed my own internal path in resuming my life and passions. For me, creativity means filling an empty room with new ideas, testing them, while making ongoing changes during learning. My return to normality was not through drugs. It was generated by the excitement of uncovering the new uncharted realms that would consume my spirit, energize my attitudes, and rekindle a new sense of myself.

My imaginative future was brimming, as initiation of this congestive heart failure project carried with it the chance to develop a means to help patients — the centerpiece of my universe. It would lay out the game plan for the next ten years of my life.

I had returned home. *I was me.*

CHAPTER 16

Congestive Heart Failure: Education to Enactment

After returning to Los Angeles from Argentina, I fully involved myself in trying to solve the immense, worldwide problem of congestive heart failure. I had found direction.

My secretary, who 18 months earlier had been the first to notice changes in my memory, now recognized a huge shift in my demeanor. She asked, "What happened to you?"

"Everything. I'll tell you about it later. We have work to do."

Her face lit up, her long-absent smile returning.

We set about getting my office in order. Books came out of boxes and onto shelves. Clutter was removed. I could suddenly appreciate the view out of my sixth-floor window... and envision what I was about to undertake.

I thought about how the medical community presently viewed congestive heart failure. Even though it was the largest problem in cardiac care, *almost nobody understood why it impaired heart efficiency, or had any idea how to fix it.* Treatment focused on creating better drugs to offset the symptoms. These may have helped patients live longer... but the quality of their lives still suffered terribly, ultimately ending in premature death. This was the best that the medical community could offer.

But I knew something they did not.

The Truth

A guiding principle is that you cannot treat what you do not understand. Too often it is assumed that what *we imagine* to be reality is the truth, and conclusions are drawn from that belief.

What I knew was this: heart failure developed because impaired heart muscle function caused inefficient performance. And I knew why.

Everything that most everyone believed about heart motion was wrong. To begin with, ask nearly anyone in medicine and they would describe heart action as *compression and dilation* — portrayed by making a clenched fist and then opening it. This type of function was first described by William Harvey, who famously discovered and wrote about the body's circulation in the 1600s.[76] His basic belief of how a heart functions has persisted ever since. In fact, the earliest two-dimensional imaging tools (injecting dye into a contracting heart and observing its image, or from an echocardiogram) supported that the heart acts almost like a piston — by compressing its volume to effectively drive out blood to meet our body's needs — and then drawing backward to refill for the next beat.

Harvey's conclusions replaced all earlier theories and became the standard for the next 400 years. His beliefs were taught in all medical schools.

It just happens that these beliefs aren't true.

How could that be? As is so often the case, people only see what they expect to see. This includes the world of medicine. For example, surgeons like myself, who watched the heart beat inside an open chest, thought it displayed the pumping action that Harvey described — because that's what we were taught to expect. We did not perceive the twisting motion that Galen, a prominent Greek physician, surgeon, and philosopher, had reported in AD 180. He was the physician to the gladiators... and witnessed this natural twisting motion after looking at the heart through the open chest wound of a fallen warrior.

Galen's observations have since been verified by today's *three-dimensional* measuring tools (like magnetic resonance imaging and speckle tracking echocardiograms), which now can document that the normal heart *twists* to eject blood, and then *uncoils* to fill.

Consequently, it is impossible for a hand to accurately mirror a normal heartbeat by clenching the fist, a motion that makes all the fingers simultaneously close and then open. Instead, a *sequential* clenching motion must be used — moving from little to ring to middle to index finger — to create a *dynamic whorl* as they close and compress.

Functionally, the biggest determinant of cardiac efficiency is the heart's twisting spiral motion, as these whorling movements reflect the same motion that exists within a hurricane or tornado. By contrast, the commonly believed compression or piston movements play only a minor role in the normal heart's effectiveness.

The Battle of the Bulge

Sitting in my office after returning from Argentina, I realized our first step toward solving the enduring riddle of heart failure would involve these functional differences between the normal spiral *twisting* heart — and the much less effective heart that occurs in cardiac failure, which *only squeezes* as its natural elliptical shape changes to a spherical dilated (stretched) form.

I recognized that heart failure has continued to be an awful problem in cardiac care precisely because its causes had not been clearly understood. What was known is that a heart attack causes death in a cardiac region where there had been an interrupted or insufficient blood flow, so that a scar replaces the normal muscle. Please understand that this term "scar" does not mean the narrow scar most people envision when they have a cut on their arm or leg. Instead it describes the dead and functionless muscle area in the heart that has lost its blood supply.

The result of this scar is that a *bulge* or aneurysm now develops, as this previously normal contracting region (when the heart's shape was elliptical or conical) will now stop squeezing, as it thins and billows with each heartbeat. (**Figure 1, left image**) The patient is kept alive because the heart continues beating thanks to the remaining live muscle that did not suffer a heart attack (as *its* blood supply had not been obstructed).

Yet all the patient knows is they feel chest pain, the tell-tale indicator of a heart attack.

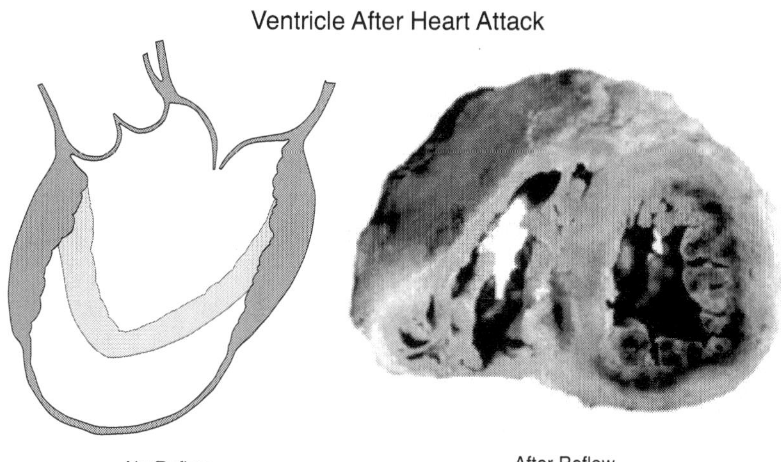

Figure 1: On left: cardiac shape when there is no blood reflow after a heart attack. Lighter gray is V-shape of normal heart, which becomes spherical (darker shading) after injured muscle thins and billows.

On right: cardiac shape after blood reflow showing extensive damage in darkened area of scar in inner shell and deeper muscle. The outer muscle shell is undamaged, but function does not recover, despite return of its shape toward normal.

As previously described in the chapter on heart attacks, the victim is rushed to the hospital, where a cardiologist performs an angioplasty to open the blockage in the artery (or uses drugs called thrombolytics that dissolve the clot). When the artery opens, symptoms rapidly improve: the chest pain lessens, and the blood pressure and the cardiac output come up, while the filling pressure in the lungs and the pulmonary artery pressure go down. *The bulge disappears.* The patient survives the heart attack and the angioplasty team takes pride in a job well done. The patient's life has been saved by thwarting the immediate risk of dying from the heart attack.

But the picture is not as clear as had been hoped. The formerly bulging dead muscle within the heart attack region has now shrunk to a smaller, thickened... *but still non-contracting* region. (**Figure 1, right image**) Clues to a more gloomy future may already be forming — for even if only 20% of this injured muscle is without function, the scenario of progressive heart failure will begin to rear its ugly head.[77]

Remote Compensation

However, this grim future isn't *immediately* evident. That's because the body is truly remarkable. It strives to stay alive, and the way it does this after there's a scar, is to have its *remote muscle* (the still-functioning muscle area away from the scarred tissue) compensate to keep the heart pumping.

Some of this was already known. In fact, cardiac surgeons can also become involved after an acute heart attack — to perform coronary artery bypass grafting to better restore blood flow to this remote muscle that is now so critical to the patient's survival (and also may repair or replace a leaking mitral valve when needed).

Unfortunately, despite being able to surgically improve the remote muscle's viability, surgeons are also helpless to stop adverse long-term outcomes — since congestive heart failure may develop, despite the presence of successful coronary artery bypass grafts. And the disease will finally prevail.

But why?

Not Making a Difference

This quandary deeply troubled me. I joined many other cardiac surgeon colleagues in realizing that many of our heart attack patients suffer a degradation of their health over time. This tragedy had played out in my own life, with my father's experience. It pained me greatly to watch this robust man growing short of breath after only minor exertions. His walking became difficult, normal activities became impossible, and finally, he became incapacitated and was stuck in bed at home much of the time. He had to go to the emergency room every two weeks and no longer enjoyed living. It was terrible. He was a cardiac cripple.

Yet in all the intervening years, I watched other patients suffer just as my father had, these same dire circumstances repeating themselves despite advances in medical treatment and new drugs. In fact, studies showed that these surgical procedures that restore blood flow to the remote muscle and /

or remedy a leaking valve after a heart attack — offered no better long-term results than patients who had no surgery.[78]

As a result, an astounding conclusion was reached. Cardiologists suggested we abandon these operations entirely, in favor of keeping these patients on drugs instead.[78] To me, this seemed like throwing the baby out with the bath water... instead of finding out *what* the problem was with the bath water.

I kept asking myself, "How can this be? I did everything correctly in these procedures. We improved flow though the coronary vessels, made leaky valves function properly, and prevented cardiac damage during the operation by using our heart protection methods. *Yet, despite these advantages, our surgical operation did not fulfill our expectation of having the patient experience a long and healthy life.*"

To me, this failure to have a long-term improvement *meant a fundamental cardiac problem had not yet been corrected.* The answer had to be that we did not get to the disease component that caused this heart failure. We all were frustrated by this dilemma. Worse, no one knew what to do to change it.

...Except someone had found the missing piece.

Monaco: Gaming Tables... or Operating Tables?

My work on controlled reperfusion had generated international interest, and years before my trip to Argentina, I was invited to Monaco, France to share my theories and knowledge.

Being a kid from the Bronx, my image of Monaco centered upon the grand gaming rooms and financial intrigue glamorized in Hollywood movies. But from a personal perspective, gambling had never been important, because those pursuits involve only educated guesses... and guesses were not my passion. Thus, the allure of the casino tables had no effect on me. Instead, my goal was to expose medical audiences to a sure-fire winner by demonstrating the benefits of controlled reperfusion in treatment of an acute heart attack.

Little did I know then that my visit to this fabled city would be the catalyst to my eventual search for the answer to heart failure.

Teacher Becomes Pupil

This quest was initiated when I visited my host, Vincent Dor, in Monaco. Dr. Dor had been Chief of Cardiothoracic Surgery at the University of Nice. As with so many of my trips, I went to teach — in this case, about using controlled reperfusion to prevent a scar from forming after a heart attack. Yet I came upon someone from whom I could learn.

It was at this time that Dr. Dor declared he had discovered something startling: *he knew why heart failure occurred... and had found a way to fix it.*

He had my full attention!

Dor confidently stated that it was "this *scar* — this dead tissue inside the heart after a heart attack — that was the cause of heart failure." It was the first time I had heard of this analysis.

Further, he claimed *the secret behind solving heart failure* — was to rebuild the ventricle into its natural elliptical shape.

I still remember my immediate reaction. The ventricle? *Nobody* had ever tried to deal with the ventricle to treat heart failure. Why would they? Once a patient received angioplasty or thrombosis drugs, the ventricle would again have a normal surface. The heart's bulge would have disappeared.

It was then that Dor looked at me and reiterated something I already knew: when the thin bulge disappears after angioplasty, that area of the heart becomes thickened — but it remains *akinetic* (does not move). He pointed out that confusion arises in the minds of the surgeons when they see that heart surface has no visible scar (bulge). They believe no incision should be made into this normal-looking region (even though a scar still exists within its inner shell). But he then emphatically pointed out: "If it doesn't squeeze, what difference is there if it doesn't squeeze because it is bulging, or if it doesn't squeeze because it contains a scar beneath its normal surface?"

That's when he reemphasized, "The essential problem is the scar that remains."

His observation astounded me. I knew it was a straightforward procedure for surgeons to treat the thin-walled aneurysm to eliminate this bulge. They simply remove the billowing portion to return the heart back to its normal shape. But performing this procedure had become a rare event, since most patients underwent angioplasty instead, so that the heart attack region became a smaller, thicker — though still functionless — muscle.

Yet nobody except Vincent Dor worried about how to surgically treat the scar *remaining* in the non-contracting muscle after angioplasty. Why would we? We knew the *remote muscle* (that region of live heart muscle *away* from the scar) would compensate to pump blood and keep the heart going.

So while a scar remained after a heart attack, there was not a broad understanding that it was related to heart failure.

Until now.

Dor again stressed that the irreversible scar caused by the heart attack *must be surgically excluded* from the working (or functioning) ventricular chamber, as its presence causes the abnormal changes in ventricle size — and that altered shape is the structural basis behind the progression toward heart failure.[79, 80]

The Shape of Things to Come

Dor's work showed that *the world was wrong.* The answers to heart failure were not a mystery! It had to do with geometry — and the twisting heart.

Though described previously in different ways, I will summarize this to further clarify its role in congestive heart failure:

A starting point for understanding this process is that the heart is *naturally elliptical* in shape, with a *helical* (spiral) structure that provides a powerful and efficient twisting motion to pump blood.

But when there is a heart attack, a scar (dead tissue) will form in the *entire section of the damaged muscle.* This involves 100% of the heart attack muscle's ventricle wall, leading to billowing or bulging of this non-contracting muscle mass.

The return of blood flow will make this bulge disappear — *but the scar remains,* now occupying 50 to 60% of the heart muscle's inner shell. The scar's extent changes (from whole muscle to just inner shell), but impaired performance within the scarred region does not. *There is no recovery of contraction... regardless of whether the scar occupied either 100% or 50% of the injured muscle.*

To keep the patient alive, the *remote muscle* (that portion without a heart attack) must beat more strongly to compensate for the injured area's lack of contraction. But the heart stretches as this is done, and as *the ventricle widens over time, this dilation* will wear down the remote muscle's ability to function.

Dor elaborated that this change in the heart's geometry causes the heart's normally *elliptical* or football shape to distort into a more *spherical* or basketball-like shape. (**Figure 2**) The result is its natural powerful twisting mechanism turns into a less efficient compressing piston (which ironically will *now* closely resemble the heart function that William Harvey described in the 1600s — mimicked by the clenched and opened fist.)

As this remote muscle continues to weaken, heart failure symptoms appear and progressively worsen, and finalize in death.

Until now, no one had ever talked about how the scar affects the ventricle or how it changes the heart's geometry. Yet as I listened to Dor... clouds of confusion gave way to the exciting light of clarity.

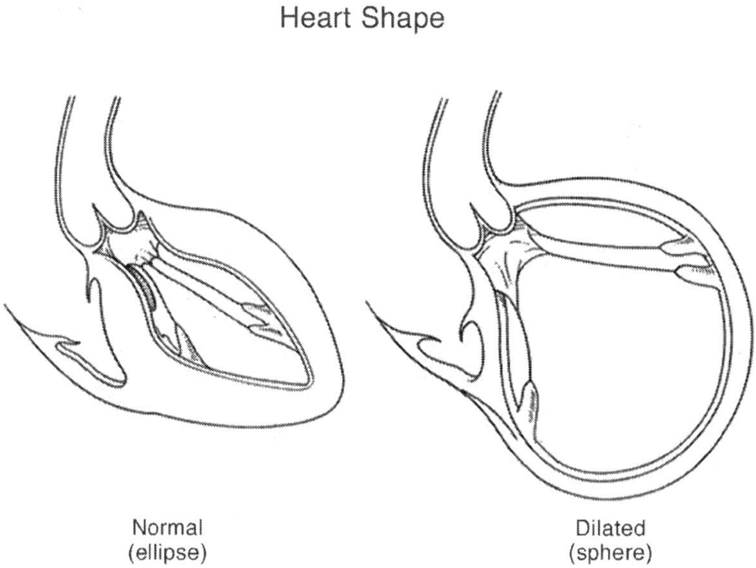

Heart Shape

Normal
(ellipse)

Dilated
(sphere)

Figure 2: Cardiac shape of normal heart (left) is conical.
Spherical configuration on right represents dilated heart in heart failure.

How apparent things can become if we stop to truly see, and are not simply obedient to what has always been believed.

I joined Dor's new thinking and exclaimed, "Finally, this makes perfect sense!"

The Grand Solution

It was by listening to Dor that I finally began to understand that the solution to this post-heart attack dilemma could not be accomplished solely by the delivery of medications, or by surgeons performing coronary bypass grafts or mitral valve corrections. These are incomplete remedies.[81, 82] The fundamental reason for poor outcomes arises from the medical world's failure to address the geometric change from the elliptical heart to the ill-fated spherical shape.

Part of the problem in understanding relates to an accepted medical objective called "muscle salvage." This refers to the goal of keeping the muscle alive. Prompt use of angioplasty results in only 50 to 60% of the heart attack muscle becoming scarred, instead of 100%. Yet when this happens, the term "salvaged muscle" (referring to the other 40 to 50% of outer muscle that's saved) creates a fundamental misconception. Despite the "saved muscle" now having a normal surface appearance — *the area beneath it is dead and scarred,* and the whole region does not function.[22] Yet surgeons consider the normal surface to be healthy, and deem it "off limits" from getting cut into.

It is essential to abandon this misconceived limitation, since the proper treatment of heart failure is *to surgically rebuild the scarred ventricle*. Dor's work showed the solution was straightforward: operate on the spherical heart to get rid of the scar, and then reconstruct the natural elliptical shape. Only one other surgeon, Adib Jatene from Brazil, had simultaneously come to this conclusion.[83]

Yet to me, *this was the potential game-changer.*

Though some of us were aware that these thickened muscles after angioplasty were not able to squeeze, we never acted upon this. We too thought they were inoperable.

But Dor had already performed these operations — with great success.

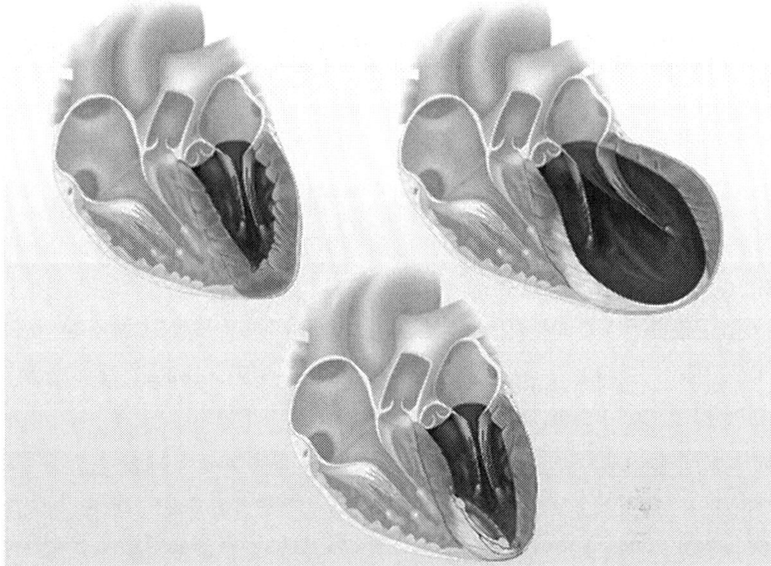

Figure 3: The geometric changes described by Dor are shown in this image.
Upper left is normal heart with conical shape. Upper right is dilated heart after a heart attack with the white area showing the scar, as the chamber dilates (expands) to compensate, and becomes spherical. Lower image shows ventricular restoration that excludes the scar and rebuilds the normal conical shape.

He recognized that the scar nearly always involved half of the ventricular septum (a muscle that forms the curtain between the left and right ventricles), and knew that stitches in such a squeezing muscle may not normally hold well. So he developed a new procedure called an *endoventricular circular patch plasty operation*. It beautifully sews in a patch of synthetic material to safely exclude the scar.[79] So to be clear, "excluding" the scar does not mean surgically removing it. Rather, we restructure the heart shape — so the area where the scar is located is *excluded (isolated)* from playing any role in the heart's function. (**Figure 3**) Dor showed me videos of several of his operations. Each outcome was nothing less than amazing.

I realized that while conventional surgical and medical protocols for heart failure focused on the "two Vs" — treating the blood *vessels* and the heart *valves* — we had ignored the third V — the *ventricle*. It was the *"triple V" — vessels, valve, and ventricle* — which together played the vital roles that needed to be dealt with simultaneously in treating congestive heart failure.

Confronting the Culprit

While I had learned all of this some years before my trip to Argentina, I had been fully occupied with my cardiac operations and research activities. Yet my interest in exploring this avenue blossomed at the end of my depression.

A number of years had passed since we showed that giving controlled reperfusion after a heart attack (described in Chapter 8) *prevents the culprit scar from ever occurring,* thus avoiding subsequent heart failure. Yet this approach to treating a heart attack had not yet been widely adopted, so I now turned my focus directly toward addressing the scar causing heart failure in these large dilated (stretched beyond normal size) hearts. In other words, I shifted my pursuits from trying to avoid the detrimental scar… to learning how to exclude it.

I knew that Dor's method of treating heart failure (by excluding the scar and making the ventricle look normal again) needed to be proven to the surgical cardiac community, if we were to galvanize a new approach to correct the ventricular cause of heart failure. To ignite such a fundamental change in thinking requires a major study to confirm that other surgical teams could match Dor's results. To achieve that goal, I intended to create a new international team.

Our primary objective would be to *prove that the cause of heart failure is the scar, and then correct it.* This concept would be tested by restoring the normal size and shape of the ventricle with the Dor procedure.

A totally new surgical solution for treating heart failure would emerge if this was successful.

Changing the Game

As noted, I needed to pursue this new ventricular approach to solving heart failure because until now, the use of controlled reperfusion after an acute heart attack (that would keep the culprit scar from forming, as discussed in

Chapter 8) was not generally accepted. Said most simply, the primary treatment goal needed to change from preventing the scar, to correcting the abnormal ventricular shape that is caused by the scar's presence.

Despite the inherent shortcomings of normal blood reperfusion after a heart attack, the enormous contributions of conventional angioplasty or drugs that dissolve the clot should not be disregarded. Each treatment achieves the powerful common goal of opening the closed artery, and such success yields a reduction in how often sudden death and / or early heart failure can develop. This treatment lowers the high mortality that would otherwise occur if the closed artery was not reopened. Angioplasty contributes a dramatic finding because it reduces initial mortality from 20% to 5%.

Yet despite these improvements, the culprit scar in the ventricle remains, and its presence causes the later development of heart failure. The timing of this ill-fated complication? That depends on when the remote muscle stretches enough to make the ventricle develop a spherical shape.

At Great Cost

The importance of finding answers becomes greater as we realize a dire truth: the frequency of heart failure has continued *undiminished*.

The incidence of cardiovascular disease fell 30% between 1995 and 2009[84] — *but the incidence of congestive heart failure remains unchanged*. There certainly has been progress in treating congestive heart failure through improvement in drug therapies, including agents that alter calcium metabolism and relax arterial blood vessels, and specialized diuretics that limit potassium loss. While we are grateful for these support medications that reduce symptoms and prolong life, we also note the challenge to cardiologists who continue their search for drugs to counter heart failure's many effects. This quest seems impossible when one considers the broad spectrum and sheer number of different body processes that are negatively affected. This also points to the ineffectiveness of trying a "one by one" approach to offset each of these numerous symptoms, which result from the body receiving profoundly inadequate nourishment due to a poorly functioning heart.

Aside from the physical and emotional costs, there are substantial financial costs associated with this as well. Present treatments for heart attacks and heart failure make up this nation's and the world's largest health care expenditure. It may reach $1 trillion per year by 2030 in the U.S. alone.[38]

The bottom line is we are not solving the problem. Instead, we are finding ways to make sick people live sicker longer, taking one expensive drug after another.

Who Will Get Heart Failure: *The Secret of Volume*

The debilitating symptoms and continuing high costs stemming from this terrible disease lead the patient or their family to ask a natural question: "Is there a way to predict who will get heart failure?" This is a thoughtful question, because not every heart attack results in heart failure.

There is an answer, and it again relates to the scar. Progression to heart failure begins if more than 20% of the heart muscle is dead, as this area forms the scar.[77] When that occurs, *an increase in the ventricle's volume* (the ventricle size, determined by the amount of blood in the ventricle at end of contraction) results as it dilates... with the heart sometimes progressing to become spherical in shape rather than elliptical.

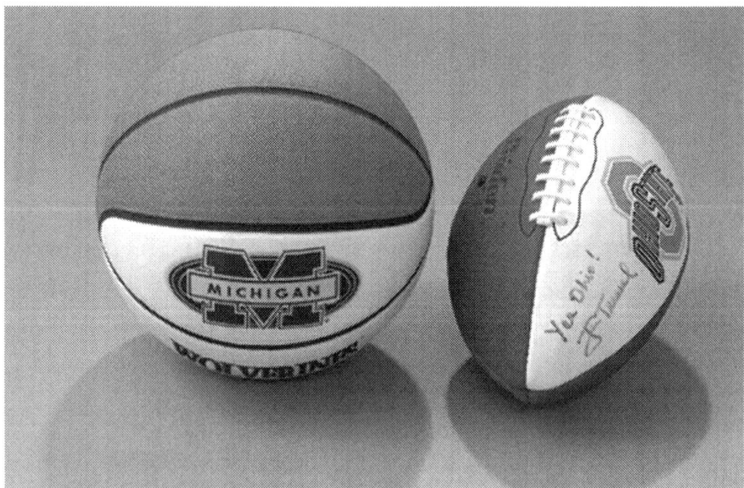

Figure 4: Athletic analogy, with spherical / basketball shape (left) and normal conical / football shape on right. I went to Ohio State, where the spherical Michigan shape represents our enemy.

Again, from a sports perspective, the elliptical heart is like a football (having a spiral twisting motion) and the failing abnormal one is more like a basketball (having a squeezing motion). (**Figure 4**)

I had never paid attention to — or measured — ventricular volume until Dor finally revealed this information to me in Monaco. But I learned there is a five-fold greater chance to develop heart failure when the size of the ventricle starts to more than double, from the normal 25 ml/m2... to 60 ml/m2.[85] Subsequently, *death* from congestive heart failure also correlates to these increasing volumes. The larger the volume, the more often and more quickly one succumbs. For instance, people with 150 ml/m2 will perish much faster than those with 70 ml/m2. (**Video 1**)

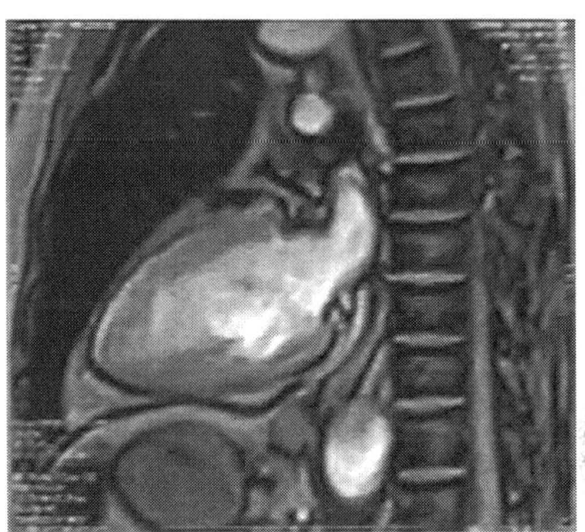

Video 1: The normal efficient ventricle with an elliptical shape is shown first, followed by a failing dilated heart with a spherical form, which also makes the mitral valve leak due to stretching of its parts.

www.vimeo.com/buckberg/failing-normal-heart

Nobody can predict exactly how long it will take in a particular person. This depends on how much the ventricle volume enlarged after the initial heart attack. But it has been shown that if the volume is more than 60 ml/m2 after the initial attack... heart failure and ultimately death rates can rise to 40% during the first year.[86] The reason is that larger ventricle volumes require the remote muscle to function in an increasingly abnormal way, wearing it out faster.

It should be noted that these dilated hearts that cannot contract efficiently — are the cause of heart failure in only about half of our patients. Congestive heart failure can *also* be due to another cause. The other 50% of patients develop this condition when ventricular size and geometry are normal, but the heart does not relax easily. This second issue will be addressed later in Chapter 22.

Size IS Everything

Given this perspective, there needs to be a reassessment of the importance of volume. The knowledge gained from its measurement is vast — since a spherical cardiac shape (from an enlarged ventricle) becomes the constant factor that explains the development of heart failure *from multiple causes.* (**Figure 5**)

Three such causes are described below (and in **Figure 5** on the following page) — with *shape* again being the consistent factor in each:

- First, as we've discussed, in *coronary artery disease,* a scar forms where there has been a heart attack, and the remote, viable muscle expands to compensate by contracting more forcefully. This stretch will cause a spherical heart shape.
- Second, a spherical shape also occurs from *valve disease* when either the aortic or mitral valve leaks. Ventricular volume increases as the heart must pump extra blood to the body to compensate for the leakage from an insufficient heart valve.
- Third, a similar spherical form develops in patients who have a *disease in the ventricular muscle* (from a virus, for example), despite their having normal coronary arteries and valves.

The ramifications from these examples are clear: the medical community needs to understand *why* enlarged ventricles are so detrimental to heart

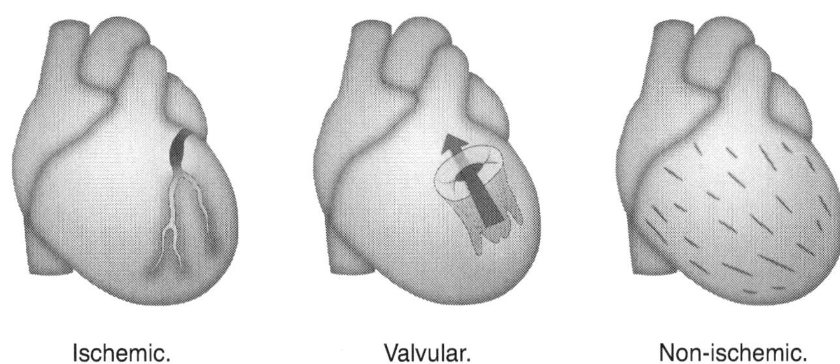

Figure 5: The three causes of a dilated heart include: on left, a heart attack due to a closed coronary artery; in center, a leaky aortic or mitral heart valve; and on right, direct damage of the heart muscle.

function, *and* that the solution is straightforward. They relate to the heart's architectural structure.

The Right Fiber = Good Health

This isn't about dietary fiber.

To truly understand why this spherical shape causes the heart to perform so much less efficiently, we need to visualize the heart not only from the outside, but also from *within the ventricle.* The external change to a sphere shape is obvious... but heart failure also changes *the muscle fiber orientation (the angles of these fiber pathways)* within the wall of the cardiac muscle. (**Figure 6**)

As you see from the illustration, the *slanted or sloping fiber pathways* (at 60°) that exist in a normal elliptical heart... become more horizontal (extending from side to side, rather than at angles) when the ventricular shape becomes circular. Why is this important? Because this accounts for the decrease in the heart's ability to function — as *the twisting ability disappears* — and is replaced by the inefficient, clenched fist version of pumping that also increases chances of a premature death.[37]

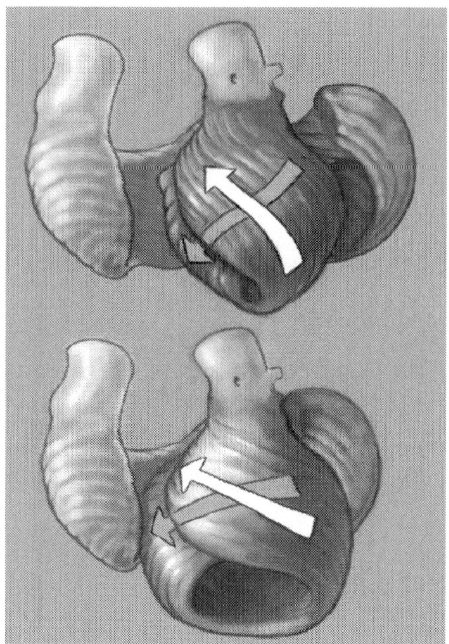

Figure 6: Anatomy and muscle fiber arrangement in normal heart (upper) and dilated heart in heart failure (lower). Note the fiber angles are at 60° in normal heart, and more horizontal fibers at approximately 30° angles in failing heart.

The dynamics of how the differences between the natural elliptical shape and the spherical contour account for the discrepancy in heart efficiency are shown in **Video 2,** taken in the operating room. It contrasts the performance of a normal heart with one that is dilated and failing.

Drugs cannot fix this geometric problem responsible for poor heart function, but correcting the abnormal spherical structure to restore the natural elliptical shape *will*.

Why was I so certain?

The rationale for my confidence wasn't limited only to what I had learned from Dor in Monaco. Or even my later discovering the additional vital contributions of Adib Jatene of Brazil, who had come up with a similar approach in 1984.[83] The reason I was so convinced was that before I had flown to Argentina, before I composed my 70 pages on the plane ride back...

I had performed this procedure in a patient with profound heart failure.

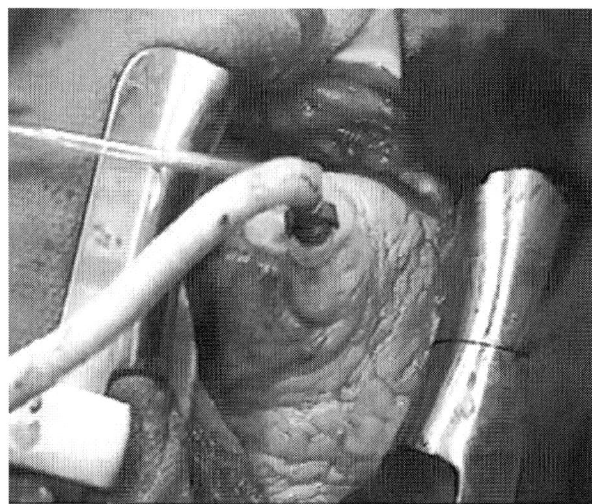

Video 2: In these two sequential videos, the first shows the natural twisting motion of the normal heart with a natural elliptical shape. The second video component shows the inefficient performance of a failing dilated heart.

www.vimco.com/buckberg/twisting-and-dilated-hearts

Hands-On Knowledge

The circumstances leading to my conducting this operation arose out of a UCLA/Asian link we had established. We visited Asian countries to demonstrate our techniques, and welcomed Asian teams to UCLA for learning. It was during a trip to Malaysia, not long after visiting Dor, when I told Yahya Awang, the Chief of Cardiac Surgery in Kuala Lumpur, about this new technique for heart failure that Dor had come up with — in which we change the geometry of the heart.

Soon after I returned home, I got a call from Yahya, who asked me to see a patient in severe heart failure following a heart attack. The patient had been treated with angioplasty and no longer had an aneurysm or bulging segment. But he was in very bad condition, the situation grim enough to justify the patient traveling to UCLA for treatment.

My thoughts immediately flashed on what I'd recently learned from Dor. This was my chance to see if his approach worked. But I had never performed this operation before... and needed to better understand how to do his procedure in this severely compromised patient. Dor had given me a videocassette showing his procedure, but it was not viewable at the hospital since it was recorded in the European PAL format. After many hurried phone calls throughout campus, I learned there was one PAL player in the Campus Library. Surprisingly, this was my first visit to Powell — the main college undergraduate library — and after some hunting, I found the machine and studied the tape.

Armed with the certainty that this was the right procedure, and supported by Dor's technical guidance, I embarked on my first treatment of heart failure by changing ventricular geometry in a patient.

When the patient arrived at UCLA from Malaysia, he was not in good shape. Yet he trusted that I would help him. We scheduled the procedure.

In the operating room, I informed the team, "We're going to conduct an innovative kind of approach today, unlike anything we've ever done before. We will open the chest and shall find a ventricle that has a smooth, ordinary-looking surface, yet it camouflages the deeper internal scar that develops from the heart attack. The scar is why the ventricle dilates [enlarges] and causes poor function. We will exclude it and return the ventricle to its natural shape."

Everyone in the room was silent. No one had heard of such a procedure.

One of the team asked, "Who else does something like this?"

"A surgeon in France named Dor. It is a new procedure, something others have not done. But I think the potential answer to heart failure may be changing the heart's geometry. It is also likely, at the moment, this patient's only chance."

We began.

The team was understandably wary. Surgeons are always afraid to cut into a ventricle if it looks normal on the surface, because the stitches don't hold well when you try to put it back together — since you are trying to make stitches in a muscle that's squeezing.

But as we went forward, I explained that Dor's solution to eliminate the tension from that area was by using a patch in the ventricle, to prevent the ventricle from tearing apart due to its torsion and twisting. It is similar to patching a tear in a rubber raft. If you were to try to fix the damage by scrunching up the rubber on either side of the tear and joining them together, it wouldn't hold very well. But if you put a patch over the incision site, this takes all the tension off the tissues that remain in their normal position. Patches were not new to cardiac surgeons and were already used in a variety of operations, though never one like this.

The team fully engaged and followed every step. All went well with my inaugural procedure, and we restored the normal heart shape. (**Figure 3**)

The resulting heart motion told the functional story — as we observed the recovery of the twisting movement! There was immediate, remarkable relief from heart failure after the spherical ventricular chamber was returned to its more natural elliptical shape. Everyone around the table was mesmerized. I was ecstatic, and envisioned the tremendous potential for this procedure.

The memory of this success never fades, as I recall this initial operation each day in my office. At his three-month follow-up, the patient returned and gratefully presented me with a beautiful Royal Selangor Pewter Clock from Malaysia. It sits on the wall above the entry door to my office.

This gift's intrinsic beauty of harmony and form wonderfully matched the new aura of self-assuredness that characterized the patient after my first case of ventricular restoration. Before surgery, the man was a shell of who he had once been. He felt like he was living on borrowed time. He was filled with anxiety and had little hope. After the procedure, he was a different person. His long-absent confidence, steadiness, and power had returned. He wasn't dying. He wasn't wallowing. He was a proud human being.

He continued to visit me periodically, always recalling the devastating experience during his bout with heart failure. He then described the bounty of symptom-free living that has followed our rebuilding of his ventricle. Remarkably, this reality is instantly observable when he enters my examining room, as his vitality and joy of living flow from him. This great gift made me appreciate the magnitude and beauty of Dor's contribution to the world of congestive heart failure.

This patient's operation would be the only such procedure I would do at this time. Nobody at UCLA sent me any cases like this, as no one understood what was occurring with heart failure, nor its association with ventricular volume. That is why I knew I had to build a team made up of the world's top cardiac surgeons. Together, we could bring this to the world's attention.

It was an adventure waiting for the right time. *That time had arrived.*

The Game Plan

In my office, I reviewed my 70 pages of ideas and strategies designed to document and validate this new game plan. I was pleased to see my thoughts were just as compelling now as they were during my impassioned airborne writing session.

It was clear that guidelines needed to be established for treating a region that was not typically approached by surgeons. Dor had shown that incising into such a normal-looking cardiac surface to exclude the underlying scar is a straightforward operation with proven benefit. My role now was to help accumulate data to make surgeons aware of this remarkable procedure.

Thus, the need for our study.

Replace… or Restore

Significantly, our study would finally present an alternative to the only other present surgical approaches for treating irreversible heart failure: heart transplants or insertion of mechanical devices. Rather than resolve a severely failing heart by subjecting the patient to a transplant from a donor, or having it taken over mechanically… why not use a far less aggressive procedure that fixes the heart that is already there by restoring its natural ventricular shape?

This alternative restoration would avoid the problems with transplantation (whose drugs can cause hardening of the arteries, kidney problems and cancer), or inserting heart assist devices (that can be accompanied by bleeding and clotting problems). I reasoned that bringing the heart's function back to a more natural state was a better choice.

Opening Minds

Beyond educating surgeons about this approach, I knew another hurdle would be the role of cardiologists — as they are the gatekeepers who determine the course of treatment for patients. Cardiac surgeons won't be sent patients whose ventricle they can restore, unless they are directed our way by cardiologists. For that to happen, we would need to show cardiologists why they should expand their focus beyond correcting the bulge (aneurysm) after a heart attack.

Yet at this point, no one except for Dor and Jatene (and once myself) had done this kind of surgery. In fact, just as this memoir reveals how new ideas frequently encounter resistance, Dor had already joined our endless cadre of innovators who experienced surgical opposition. His initial papers were rejected from publication in the *American Association of Thoracic Surgery Journal* (the leading publication in cardiac surgery). The journal's reviewers could not conceive of cutting into a ventricle that had a normal, non-scarred surface. It was ridiculous from their point of view.

Their response reminded me of how Spanish leadership had tried to bar Christopher Columbus from his journey to the Americas, believing he would fall off the edge of a flat world. While the globe was actually spherical, these stalwarts of yesterday failed to explore for tomorrow.

Dor told me of this dilemma when I met with him, adding that abstracts for his presentations had also not been accepted for presentation at our annual AATS meeting. But I was so impressed by what he taught me, and with my own success in treating a heart failure patient, that I offered to help him rewrite his manuscript. I took on this task after speaking with our journal editor, John Waldhausen, who asked me to simultaneously write an editorial to accompany the Dor submission. They published Dor's revised paper and my editorial together in the same issue.[79] In my editorial, I suggested calling this rebuilding technique the "Dor Procedure" to honor his enormous contributions, and this is how it came to be known.[87]

But this early publication did not sway the medical community. Nor did I expect it would. It was just a first step toward changing the world's perceptions of heart failure.

We Who Climb Do Not Climb Alone

As I was preparing the next stage for creating a new worldwide study toward solving heart failure, I recalled Julius Comroe at the CVRI in San Francisco, many years earlier, coming into our class of postdoctoral scholars one day while holding a drawing of a mountain. The image showed no evidence of a trail up its surface, yet a surgeon was conspicuously perched upon its peak after doing a heart transplantation.

Comroe began by saying, "I know you all want to be excellent — standouts in your field." He then had us survey his picture as he asked us to describe why was it possible for this surgeon to stand so proudly on the mountaintop after doing a heart transplant. Had he performed some Olympian leap from the ground due to superhuman prowess?

"How did he get there?"

As we pondered what Comroe's point might be, he turned the picture around to show us the back of the hill, strewn with boulders. "He did it by climbing upon the boulders carved by so many before him — whose numerous contributions made this possible through X-rays, EKGs, antibiotics, blood transfusions, anti-rejection drugs, etc."

"Nobody leaps to the top of the mountain," Comroe continued. "You get there because you can step on these boulders that have been created for you, one after another, on your journey toward new ideas. What's more, there will be times that someone else will be on the top of the mountain — helped by the boulders you provided for their ascent."

His message was that it was never "me, me, me." It was about the concept of the TEAM.

It was just such a team that I was about to form.

CHAPTER 17

Congestive Heart Failure: Enactment

Establishing a new clinical treatment for congestive heart failure by changing ventricular size and shape required that we establish a small team of outstanding international centers from the United States, Europe, Asia, and South America. Their collective task would be to see if they could repeat Dor's results and improve the prognosis of heart failure patients using his method.

The "Magnificent Eleven"

I set out on a worldwide romp to meet with each of these handpicked physicians. I used my 70-page document to explain my plan to test this geometric concept in heart failure, and asked if they would participate. Contacting each beforehand, all I told them was, "I want four hours of your time to consider a whole new way of looking at heart failure." I also emphasized that this trip was entirely at my own expense. I didn't want any travel, hotel, or meal expenses provided. I just wanted their attention during this four-hour period.

Suitably intrigued, no one turned me down.

Each meeting took place in a different locale. I felt somewhat like the lead character in the original film of *The Magnificent Seven,* where Yul Brynner's character travels to wherever he must to recruit the best people for his team. I met Francis Fontan, the leading surgeon in Europe, at the Hermitage Hotel in Monaco, in an empty ballroom far from everyone so we could concentrate. In Milan, I was picked up at a small airport by Lorenzo Menicanti and went to his home, where we drank Cuban rum and talked about the future of this treatment. Hisa Suma and I conferred in a luxurious Tokyo office building. I was with Sergio de Oliviera at his penthouse in Sao Paulo, Brazil. I ate with Fred Loop, the CEO of the Cleveland Clinic, in his elegant office, where my presentation would not be interrupted by anyone except for the private waiter who served us lunch. I also visited Nick Kouchoukos in St. Louis, Irv Kron at University of Virginia, Eric Rose at Columbia University, Connie Athanasuleas at University of Alabama, Friedhelm Beyersdorf from Germany, and of course, Vincent Dor of Monaco.

Engaging Discussion

I began each presentation by focusing on the fact that the heart attack region contained dead muscle. It did not contract when it bulged, nor when it shrank following angioplasty. The essential fact was that a scar formed after a heart attack, was treated by reperfusion, and was now hidden beneath the normal muscle on the cardiac surface. Yet the effect on the heart was not limited only to the scar that had replaced previously contracting muscle. It will also impact the "live remote muscle" that is now completely responsible for the heart function. This area stretches or dilates as it compensates, and this progressively impairs its performance.

Following this explanation, I introduced Dor's novel surgical approach that excludes the dead scar and rebuilds the natural elliptical heart form, which will improve function of the remote muscle, and restore the heart's ability to contract properly by twisting.

I knew I was presenting a unique challenge, because a surgeon would now have to take the unprecedented step of incising *a normal heart surface* to gain access to and exclude the underlying scar — and then do a new procedure that returned the heart's shape to normal. Surgeons would be faced with an operation that none of them had ever performed before (except Menicanti, who was Dor's student) — nor had ever heard of.

Yet these participants were undeterred because they had forward-thinking minds. Each was captivated by the possibility. They were not daunted by the task of incising the normal ventricular surface in order to reach the scar that lurked beneath. All of them knew there were ways to confirm that a scar was indeed present before cutting into the heart: by looking at the EKG to confirm the heart attack, viewing a ventriculogram to confirm the heart's inability to contract, and by using commonly accessible isotope tests to verify the existence of a scar.

The use of these tests prevents the mistake of incising a normal heart surface, only to then find no underlying scar. Such an error could easily happen if one relies *only* on a heart's inability to properly contract as an indicator, since limited or no contraction can *also* occur in non-scarred hearts if the blood supply is inadequate. You can imagine a surgeon's anguish if they were to incise a ventricle in a critically ill heart failure patient — only to find there was no scar! Fortunately, these readily available safeguards prevent this mishap.

The joy of interacting with these very smart colleagues was dazzling, as each posed new questions and / or made innovative suggestions that expanded my knowledge. Though everyone was excited about what I presented, each also exercised their freedom to introduce divergent views. Part of why I'd selected these leaders was that I knew they would honestly tell me if they thought I was heading in a wrong direction — and why. I did not orchestrate these meetings to sell an idea, but rather to discuss and to discover, as well as to teach.

I certainly threw down a new gauntlet for our potential team, as these renowned leaders of cardiac surgery would not participate if this approach did not make sense to them. Yet the power of this new idea was infectious, as was their clear vision for the immense impact it might have.

Every one of them said yes!

Now numbering 11, our team was formed. Each agreed to a group meeting during the next American Association of Thoracic Surgery (AATS) conference in Boston.

The Path Forward

An open mind was the number one requirement I had for members of the team. This requirement transcended any stipulation that they be part of an academic university. Many of these distinguished colleagues had left the university system and established successful programs outside its walls. The *spirit of inquisitiveness* drove their never-ending pursuit to grow, and set the stage for creating better heart care.

I also hoped our initial work together might provide the underlying basis for developing an even grander future exploration. Success in reproducing Dor's findings could motivate the National Institutes of Health (NIH) to sponsor a prospective randomized trial to study heart failure. Cardiologists and cardiac surgeons would work together toward a common goal. That is important, since cardiologists must accept that while their medications may help heart failure patients live longer, these drugs fail to alter the basic geometric reasons for impaired ventricular performance. This recognition opens the door to a new intervention of changing ventricular shape that will blend nicely with their drugs — to finally counter heart failure.

If successful, this joint effort could lead to a new treatment that would help an enormous pool of patients.

I made one additional request of team members. I realized that their prominence meant their status did not need further enhancement, so I suggested they each select a younger colleague to join us, whose career and reputation could blossom if this project was successful. I now could see a grand package evolving. A new idea, the development of an inclusive global view... *and a baton being passed to a new generation of respected surgeons.*

Vincent Dor of Monaco had recommended his outstanding student and colleague, Lorenzo Menicanti from Milan, whose fresh ideas became a breath of spring. I selected Connie Athanasuleas from Birmingham, Alabama, who had collaborated with me previously, was technically superb, had great capacity to make discoveries, and possessed an incredible aptitude for gathering insight by distilling knowledge from his comprehensive view of the medical literature.

A Change of Heart (Protection)

As it happened, visits to my future team members were not the only trips I took during this time.

My belief in "traveling to learn" proved invaluable once more, following a visit to Randas Batista in South America. I saw him perform rebuilding procedures on *a beating heart* (cardioplegia was *not* used)! He was operating on big, dilated hearts caused by an infectious disease (there was no scar from a heart attack). But superb heart performance immediately followed his repairing these terminal ventricles, exceeding what I would expect from my blood cardioplegia approach.

I took a step back and thought, "This is really amazing!"

The flame of my curiosity beamed brightly, and I had to find out for myself if this approach would work. I went back to UCLA to test Batista's heart protection approach in animal test subjects and had outstanding results. A unique turn of events, as I was now in a position of contradicting myself! Wow, my position had been to tell the whole world about blood cardioplegia, but now I would advocate for another technique — while heart shape is being rebuilt.

I have always been a seeker of truth, so my next step was to use this beating method during ventricular rebuilding in a patient with heart failure. Connie and I performed ventricular restoration procedures on a small number of extremely ill patients in Birmingham, Alabama, with Connie as the principal surgeon. The heart protection was excellent using this new technique, and each procedure was successful. My willingness to change thinking became based upon the evidence, and guided my adopting a new approach to protection.

First Collaborative Meeting

In anticipation of the upcoming gathering of our group in Boston, I had T-shirts made up to commemorate our first meeting. They displayed drawings I created that compared a dilated unhappy heart to a conical healthy one, (**Figure 1**) with the name of what I thought our group might be called emblazoned across the top.

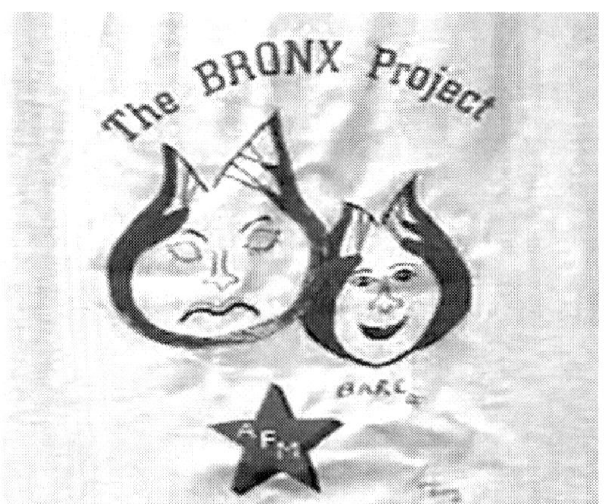

Figure 1: Bronx Project T-shirt, showing sick dilated heart on left and restored heart on right. The description is on accompanying video.

Video 1 of Bronx Project: Narration describes reasons for its name.

www.vimeo.com/buckberg/the-bronx-project

My vantage point of history guided me. I was from New York City, and knew that "The Manhattan Project" team developed the atom bomb to kill people to end World War II. Our job was to save people, so I called our group "The Bronx Project" after the borough where I was born, to celebrate our anticipated triumph in successfully overturning heart failure. (**see Video 1**)

Shirts in hand, all was set for our conference. I was also delighted that John Kirklin from Alabama would join our meeting to help us plan, and give his thoughts about the potential for our effort. He had been a mentor to me, and his presence added to the curiosity and scholarship needed for this new undertaking.

All international team members were there, including representatives from our U.S. centers: the Cleveland Clinic, University of Virginia, Columbia University, Methodist Hospital in St. Louis, Carraway Hospital in Birmingham, and UCLA. The brightest of the bright sparkled, with Kirklin and Fontan being the most famous surgeons in the United States and Europe, respectively.

Each cardiac surgeon was joined by a cardiologist, a pairing crucial to our mission of collaboration between surgeons and cardiologists. We had a busy room of 40 people, and the dialogue of the full-day event was superb.

My recommendation to change our methods of protection from cardioplegia (in which we stop the heart) to a method of operating on the beating heart (Batista's approach) was a surprise to the group. Indeed, it challenged a tradition that I had helped create, but I also knew it was the best technique in these circumstances.

Everyone looked at me, stunned. "You are the guru of cardioplegia and you're saying *to let the heart beat*?"

"That's exactly what I am suggesting. Especially since the area being operated on is dead and never moves."

I thought my decision would become a motivator for everyone to maintain such an open mind. My belief is the educational book never closes, and growth is not possible unless we are free to modify established methods.

Yet there is never a smooth pathway when climbing the hill to a new peak. My suggestion to change myocardial protection methods was viewed as a dramatic turnaround. Francis Fontan was astounded and loudly objected, and John Kirklin declared that our entire ventricular rebuilding collaborative effort had no future!

The first test of this team emerged. Such divergence of opinion was *exactly* the reason for my forming this group.

Stagnation comes from being surrounded by people who only agree with you. Plus, while Fontan and Kirklin were my heroes, they were also human. Their reactions did not properly reflect their wisdom, but matched reactions I have encountered throughout my career. I was undaunted, because decisions are based on truth, not upon opinions. Unfortunately, the conflicting tenor of this interchange prevented me from distributing the T-shirts... and the naming of our effort was postponed.

Subsequently, Francis Fontan tried the method of performing surgery on *a beating heart*, recognized its usefulness, and declared, "Bravo." He listened, thought, and acted. I also visited him in Bordeaux, France and he was thrilled to receive the Bronx Project T-shirt. John Kirklin would later be delighted to learn of the superb results of our group's effort, and became a supporter.

This is one of the virtues of splendid collaboration, as changes evolve when open-minded participants with opposing viewpoints... will subsequently use *evidence* as the basis for shifting their positions. Truth wins, not reactions. This differs vastly from the unbending views that characterize those with rigid thinking.

I was thrilled, because the actions of my heroes demonstrated exactly what champions are about.

Grand Adventure Begins

After our meeting in Boston, we agreed to meet again five months later in Brussels. In the meantime, surgeons in our group began performing these ventricular restoration procedures. To get this going, I visited U.S. centers to "scrub in" and assist them during their first case of ventricular restoration. Each operation was performed upon on a patient with a scar in a ventricle that had a normal (unscarred) heart surface. Interestingly, although our prior outcomes had achieved repeated success... the new surgical teams routinely anticipated a difficult post-operative recovery for these high-risk patients.

For instance, upon entering the operating room in one prominent East Coast center, I noticed they had a left ventricular assist device ready for use, as well as a bottle of nitric oxide. The senior surgeon explained these were typical precautions used in extremely sick patients, as the assist device will support a failing heart and the drug infusion can open narrowed lung arteries. This patient was very sick and they expected he would still be very sick after we finished.

But I countered, "No, I expect he is going to do well, as the procedure is really straightforward." I supported this contention by suggesting that "I help *the resident* perform the operation," and this is what we did.

Surgeons are often known to have a certain "panache," or preconception that colors our actions. For example, as the resident was performing the operation, the senior surgeon interjected that we should use a *continuous suture* to allow the procedure to move more rapidly — even though he had never performed this surgery. I politely said, "I've done a number of these procedures and *interrupted sutures* seem to work better, so let's try this one that way." We agreed and the case went smoothly, with excellent heart performance.

I needed to return to Los Angeles in the early morning, and when the flight had a stop in Dallas, I called the office of the senior surgeon to get a follow-up. I learned all was well with the patient, and the surgeon was in the operating room. His assistant transferred my call to the OR... and I asked the nurse to tell "Dr. Continuous" that "Dr. Interruptus" was on the phone.

A roar of laughter was transmitted from their East Coast operating room to Dallas. Everything was good.

No Tussles in Brussels

Five months after our Boston gathering, we had our next group meeting in Brussels. By this time, about 200 operations had been performed by members of the group. The protocols created for the Dor procedure had been followed, and some surgeons had performed their operations on a beating heart.

The overall results were outstanding, and matched the outcomes we had expected! Based on these triumphs, everyone agreed to expand the numbers of patients treated.

I decided to use this meeting to bring up my idea for what to call our group. While I loved "The Bronx Project," it was not met with widespread approval. Seemed like an incompatible mixing of my humor with their bleak view of heart failure. Alas, another name would need to be found.

We agreed to gather together again at the next American Association of Thoracic Surgery conference. As it turned out, these collaborative meetings would continue annually for the next ten years.

By Any Other Name

Our group still needed a title. While visiting Connie in Birmingham, he and I brainstormed ideas that included "Cardiac Renaissance" and "Rebirth." None of them seemed quite right.

Then Chris Athanasuleas, Connie's wife, suggested, "Why don't you simply call it the "RESTORE Group?"

Connie and I looked at each other. RESTORE was a much better choice!

Aside from "restore" meaning "bring back to normal," we believed our name should also describe our approach. Connie and I, and our cardiology colleague, Al Stanley, found RESTORE to be the pertinent medical word; it stood for Reconstructive Endoventricular (inside ventricle) Surgery, that returns Torsion (ability to twist), Original Radius (size), and Elliptical (shape of the left ventricle). It was adopted and has remained the name ever since.

Remarkable Results

As members of the RESTORE team began doing more and more of these successful procedures, we accumulated data showing the benefits of ventricular reconstruction — which we now called *surgical ventricular restoration*, or SVR. However, processing data from our participating centers became a major task, as our team was not functioning within a university, where statistical departments are readily available.

Fortunately, Connie found our answer in Birmingham. The eminent statistician, Dr. William Siler, agreed to participate. Bill had previously run the statistics program at the University of Alabama, and worked brilliantly and tirelessly toward analyzing the data collected from our national and international centers. Vigor was his modus operandi, and our extraordinary 82-year-old colleague remained active by continuing to scuba dive. Aside from being thrilled by his learned contributions, Connie and I were astounded that his energetic existence seemed to be linked to chain-smoking cigarettes and a continuous consumption of Coca-Cola.

Bill's work analyzed the collected data from *1,198* consecutive patients that underwent ventricular restoration by our team members. Other parts of the "triple V" — coronary bypass grafting and mitral valve repair — were also performed as we changed the size and shape of the ventricle in these dilated hearts.

Results were impressive.

Traditional patients with advanced symptoms of congestive heart failure typically experience a 50 to 75% three-year mortality rate[86, 88] — a disastrous outcome that rivals or exceeds death rates from cancers.

Yet a very different picture emerged from the data analyzing outcomes in the 1,198 RESTORE patients. Operative mortality (death while in hospital) was 6% in these high risk patients, and their five-year *survival rate* was 70%.[89] This was a new and dramatic finding of high long-term survival following treatment for advanced heart failure, and opened the door toward making even longer-term observations.

Yet longevity may not be the best final evaluation criteria in congestive heart failure, as quality of life is perhaps more important. Remember my dad who visited the emergency room every two weeks and lost his vitality due to incapacitating symptoms. Such an awful outcome is transformed by ventricular restoration, as the RESTORE analysis showed only 22% of patients needed to be re-hospitalized for heart failure during this five-year period.[90]

To help non-medical readers further appreciate the magnitude of this improvement, I provide here the worldwide benchmarks for symptoms of heart failure, as set out in the New York Heart Association Functional Classification. These are used to gauge how patients are doing:

- Class I — no symptoms
- Class II — symptoms occurring with mild exercise
- Class III — symptoms during walking on flat surface
- Class IV — breathless at rest and housebound

The cardiac cripple exists in classes III and IV, which is called advanced heart failure. This was my dad's fate at the end of his progression.

Most of our patients were *already* class III and IV when the RESTORE Group took them on for ventricular restoration. Yet following ventricular rebuilding, 85% of them achieved class I or II category status, demonstrating

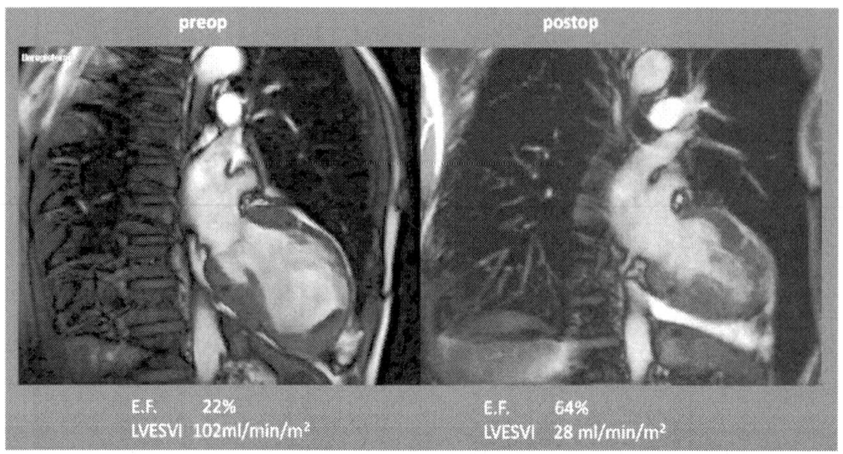

Video 2 of ventricular restoration: Spherical heart on left, with reduced function. After restoration (right), function returns to normal. (E.F is ejection fraction and LVESVI is left ventricular end systolic volume index) From the studies of Vincent Dor.

www.vimeo.com/buckberg/surgical-heart-restoration

the procedure's benefits: providing a fuller, more functional life over a longer survival period. The reason for such contrast is evident in the linked video (**video 2**) of how the heart performs before and after SVR (surgical ventricular restoration) — as the dramatic return to normal performance becomes apparent.

Exploring statistics further, we find that 50 to 70% of those class III and IV patients who *do not* undergo ventricular restoration will succumb to heart failure or sudden death (arrhythmias) within the first two years. However, sudden death is particularly rare in RESTORE patients — likely because this lethal complication is avoided by shrinking the ventricular volume (the ventricle chamber's size). A stretched ventricle chamber is the primary cause of the abnormal heart rhythms that cause sudden death.[91]

Surprisingly, discussions on the origin of heart failure arrhythmias written by electrophysiologists (cardiologists that treat rhythm disturbances) have consistently *neglected to mention "stretch"* as the principal condition that leads to sudden death.[92] The reason for this exclusion is that their looking at the electrocardiogram to determine the cause is quite different from looking at the abnormal rhythm's source: the dilated heart.

Hopefully, a new recognition of ventricle stretch as the primary cause will motivate others to address the dilated heart that produces these dangerous rhythms.

Ventricular restoration accomplishes this task.

NIH to Forward the Revolution

The RESTORE team formally reported its initial three-year results: 86% survival, avoidance of sudden death, and functional quality of life markedly improved over that from conventional treatments.[93] (These early findings preceded the five-year results that were just discussed.)

As I'd hoped, these positive outcomes stimulated the National Institutes of Health (NIH) to develop and fund a prospectively randomized Surgical Treatment of Ischemic Congestive Heart Failure (STICH) trial. A "prospectively randomized trial" means it will compare results of patients having *ventricular restoration* and coronary artery bypass grafting — against patients getting coronary bypass grafting alone.

The launch of this STICH Trial was itself memorable. The NIH invited our surgical luminaries to visit Bethesda, Maryland and meet with their director, Claude Lenfant (who would retire soon after), to offer us insight on how to submit a proposal for their financial support to test this new approach to heart failure.

The participants included Vincent Dor, the father of this method to rebuild the heart... Francis Fontan, the most prominent heart surgeon in Europe... Lorenzo Menicanti, Dor's student who had extensive experience... along with myself and a surgeon from Duke University.

The meeting took place in an NIH conference room. It was a unique experience, as Lenfant had never met Dor or Fontan before, and their animated conversations in French made me think of the U.N. conferring at the beginning of a new meaningful endeavor. Menicanti was gracious and presented me with a Montblanc pen, with a card that read, "To the maestro, for organizing this powerful new assault on our common enemy."

We were all thrilled that NIH was creating a trial to further legitimize our results. This would help bring such treatment into the mainstream. For their part, NIH felt the outcomes we had already achieved were highly notable. They ultimately allocated $45 million for the study.

The Show Must Go On

Meanwhile, SVR procedures continued to be performed independently from the NIH study, by our team and by other surgeons worldwide who were encouraged by our findings. In fact, by the time the STICH trial would be started (about two years after our NIH meeting), similar ventricular rebuilding results were recorded in *over 5,000 additional patients globally*,[94] documenting high survival rates despite advanced heart failure.

Randomization was not done in those cases (that is, none of these 5,000 patients were treated without ventricular restoration for comparison), but the drama of these remarkable findings was inescapable. Predictably, their excellent results matched our initial RESTORE outcomes, and *all* outcomes remained vastly superior to those following drug treatment alone, or those having coronary bypass grafting (done both with and without mitral repair) — but without ventricular rebuilding.[81, 82]

Some might question if there even needed to be a STICH trial, since we had over 6,000 patients (the RESTORE Group's 1,198 plus the additional 5,000) that proved our procedure worked. But the medical community generally believes that a prospective randomized study (as the STICH trial was designed to be), when conducted correctly, is the best type of study to provide credibility.

Thus, we happily expected the STICH trial to further advance this procedure into the mainstream. Naturally, we assumed they would duplicate our findings by following the established patient selection and restoration procedure guidelines.

Never. Assume. Anything!

Setting the Foundation

My initial involvement with STICH was to lead the Surgical Therapy Committee, whose designated role was to ensure that the SVR (surgical ventricular restoration) procedure was properly performed, and that only patients who met the guidelines for why they had developed heart failure would enter this study. These "entry criteria" were determined by international experts who had ventricular restoration procedure background.

Patient selection was straightforward. To be eligible for the study, they had to fulfill three criteria. First, be a heart attack patient with limited ejection fraction (emptying less than 35% of the blood in the ventricle with each heartbeat). Second, have increased ventricular volumes (ventricle enlarged to over 60 ml/m2). Third, their ventricle must contain a non-contractile (not contracting) area with a scar that occupied at least 35% of its perimeter. These criteria typically occur in heart attack patients that develop heart failure.

Surgeons also needed to qualify to participate, by having previously performed the procedure in five patients, and showing (four months post-operatively) that their operation reduced ventricular volume by at least 30%... increased ejection fraction by 10%... and had less than 10% mortality.

Fifty centers — both national and international — were selected to participate, and Duke University became the principal investigator that oversaw this study.

All should have gone well.

Off the Rails

Unfortunately, it was not long before it became apparent that this trial was heading in the wrong direction. ...*A very wrong direction.*

First, the team of participants was changed, expanding to 127 centers — instead of only the 50 originally chosen. This meant that many surgeons and cardiologists *who'd never performed surgical restoration* joined the bandwagon. The STICH leadership disregarded the criteria requiring that participating surgeons must demonstrate they can perform a safe procedure to qualify.

Moreover, *they changed the critical entry requirements* established by the Surgical Therapy Committee. These guidelines determined which patients could qualify to enter the trial.

Essentially, all fail-safe mechanisms were ignored. These decisions were made by surgeons and cardiologists without experience in surgical ventricular restoration. These "leaders" were focused more upon easing the criteria for patient recruitment — than upon complying with the agreed-upon selection and procedure guidelines.

Expanding the quantity of participating centers was done to overcome their difficulty in getting sufficient numbers of patients to meet the entry guidelines. It is possible that these criteria were changed in order to retain government funding of this study. Of course, if such a financial maneuver occurred, it took place at the expense of discarding the established and successful standards set by experienced surgeons.

We objected. But our voices were not heard.

Separate from this, another issue developed. Before the trial, Connie Athanasuleas and I designed an alternative patch that could be used to rebuild the ventricle. It was not publicly available, had not been used by the RESTORE team, and was not being recommended for use by others. The trial leaders stated the patch would be fine, as long the STICH trial received all income from it.

Cumulative disagreements ultimately led to our resigning from the STICH Trial.

This was disappointing for us. Yet leaving STICH did not diminish our interest in Surgical Ventricular Restoration, which grew as the RESTORE Group's activities continued. More and more successful ventricular reduction procedures were done.

However, the supervision of the STICH study, and its outcomes — only worsened after our departure.

Devastating Blow

The STICH results became highly flawed because of all the changes made by their leadership. Yet little could I predict how severely its parade of faulty and misleading data would negatively impact heart failure patients worldwide.

The STICH trial "statistics" showed that coronary grafting with ventricular restoration (501 patients) *was no better* than doing only coronary artery grafting alone (499 patients), judged by the patients' after-treatment tolerance to exercise, re-hospitalizations for cardiac causes, and death rates.[95]

The implication was enormous — as these findings were now used *to impede* the worldwide use of ventricular restoration to treat congestive heart failure.

But how could its failure to work in the 500 STICH patients, overturn the highly successful ventricular restoration findings in the RESTORE Group's 1,198 patients, and another 5,000 patients around the globe?

A powerful question. The answer is that everyone believed the STICH results — because this trial was funded by the esteemed NIH, and then reported in the well-respected *New England Journal of Medicine* in April of 2009. The world thus bestowed upon the STICH Trial a level of credibility that completely misrepresented the quality of the study — and its outcomes became accepted because of these sources. Yet no matter how prestigious the source of funding or reporting, accurate results are needed to make a legitimate conclusion. Without this, misguided conclusions are made — and patients with heart failure are deprived of an operation that can vastly improve their health and lengthen their lives.

Broken System, Battered Patients

The truth is, it is not at all difficult to recognize the flaws in the STICH study if one is willing to look. The purpose of my reporting them here is to make the reader aware that even a leading organization like the NIH, and highly regarded publications like the *New England Journal of Medicine*, are not perfect. Their status carries weight, but it is science that defines the truth. Evidence always wins.

For the trial to have validity, it first needs to have a proper selection of patients with the necessary medical condition, so that each surgeon can properly perform a procedure that will lower ventricular volume by more than 30%. (Achieving this reduction in ventricle size is what leads to patient improvement.) These guidelines were followed in the RESTORE Group's 1,198 surgical ventricle restoration patients, and in the additional 5,000 patients worldwide whose outcomes matched the RESTORE results.[89]

But the STICH trial changed the qualifying criteria for both patients — and for participating surgeons — and so could not reproduce these positive findings. They then concluded that the previous 6,198 worldwide SVR outcomes *were incorrect*... by using their own STICH data.

The key question is: how credible is their data?

I will now show that the STICH trial execution *failed* to provide "credible data" by enrolling improper patients... by failing to achieve the required technical outcomes established by STICH's own Surgical Therapy Committee... and by utilizing surgeons without experience in ventricular rebuilding.

These faults are not vague or subtle. They are *glaring*.

Selecting Improper Patients

Patients had to fit a series of entry criteria to be admitted to the trial — to match typical heart attack patients who then develop heart failure. So let's see how those were met:

- They needed hearts with a limited ejection fraction of less than 35%... yet *a fifth* of patients (19%) had an ejection fraction *above* that amount.[96]

  They should have been excluded from the trial.
- Ventricular volume had to be over 60 ml/m2 (and be measured again four months after SVR)... but *nearly half* of the patients (44%) *never even had a volume measurement taken* before and after the procedure.[97]

  They should have been excluded.
- A scar had to be present, and occupy 35% of ventricular perimeter... but *nearly three-quarters* of patients (73%) had *no scar measurements taken* before the procedure.[78]

  They should have been excluded.

(This meant 73% of patients *entered the trial without it known if they even possessed a ventricular scar.* Imagine the torment of a surgeon cutting open the ventricle in a sick patient — only to find normal heart muscle instead of a scar! Yet such unneeded ventricular incisions were made into the non-scarred hearts of at least 19% of the patients. And *their data was still included* in the surgical ventricular restoration study!)

- Of the only 27% of patients (267 of 1,000) that *were* checked for a scar — 46 had no scar — but were *still kept* in the study.[78]

  They should have been excluded.
- SVR is done for a scar after a heart attack — yet 13% of patients *never had a heart attack.*[95]

  They should have been excluded.
- 9% of patients *did not even undergo ventricular restoration* — yet were *still analyzed* with this group.[95]

  They should have been excluded.

How could such gross irregularities occur?

These problems stem from a failure to ensure that their own Surgical Therapy Committee standards were met, based on decisions made by the appointed STICH leaders (who, again, did not have any experience in ventricular restoration).

Remarkably, they issued new rules indicating that just looking at the external visual appearance of a poorly contracting heart provided enough evidence to do ventricular restoration — rather than documenting that an internal scar existed. This decision was completely incorrect, since the same outward appearance of poor contraction can simply be due to inadequate blood flow — and the ventricle should *never* be opened because of lack of satisfactory blood flow.

Improper Outcomes

The second major flawed area was in the assessment of the trial results, which had to meet certain conditions to be included in the evaluation. They are:

- Ventricular volume (the ventricle size, determined by the amount of blood in the ventricle at end of contraction) needed to be measured to determine if the goal to shrink volume was achieved. But such volumes *were not even measured* in 44% of patients before and after the procedure.

  Thus, how did they determine if the required amount of shrinkage was accomplished?
- When ventricular volumes *were* measured, there was only a 19% reduction in their SVR group — significantly *less than the 30% required* to be part of the reporting data.

  Those smaller volume patients should have been excluded.

Figure 2 compares the STICH finding of 19% volume reduction in 161 patient results — to the more than 40% average volume reduction in over 1,500 patients from the ten international centers that performed safe SVR procedures.[94] STICH's failure to achieve an adequate decrease in volume (more than 30%) demonstrates that the ventricular restoration procedure was inadequately performed.

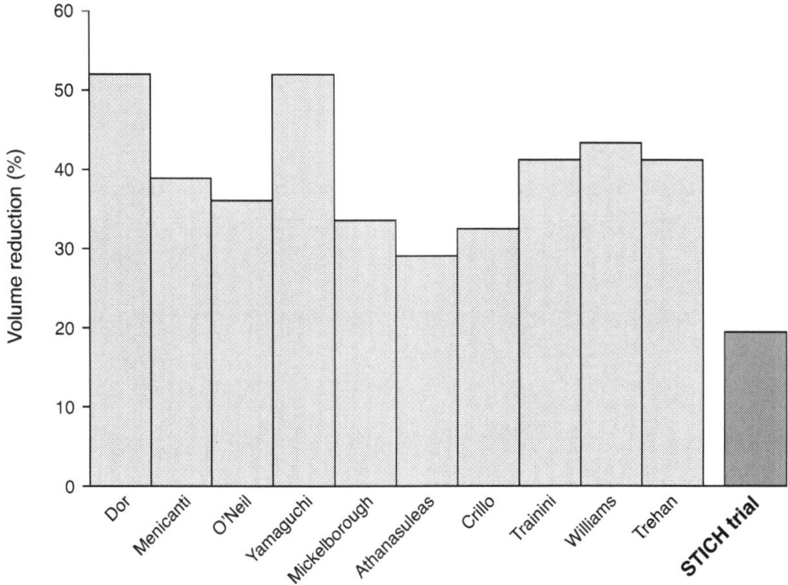

Figure 2: Percent (%) reduction in ventricular volume in ten worldwide centers when surgical ventricular restoration is done properly, with an average 40% reduction shown in ten columns on left. Right column shows only 19% volume reduction in the STICH trial, a dramatic contrast.

Selecting Unqualified Surgeons

Given the poor surgical results just described, one must ask: *how could this happen*? That answer is easy: as cited earlier, the study utilized surgeons without experience in rebuilding ventricles. The basis for this decision likely springs from STICH expanding the trials to take place in 127 worldwide centers from the initially selected 50 centers — in order to increase availability of test sites to acquire sufficient numbers of patients (and in doing so, ensure that the study would receive the financial support to continue).

But surgeons in these centers *were not trained* in this procedure. When our RESTORE Group began their trials, I went to different centers that would be performing the procedure and helped them learn how to do surgical ventricular restoration. With the STICH trial, the Surgical Therapy Committee had planned to do the same thing in the 50 centers originally chosen — but none of this was done after our departure from the study.

So there was no assurance that surgeons participating in the study had met the requirements of having already done this procedure on at least five patients — to demonstrate they could successfully reduce ventricular volume by at least 30%, increase ejection fraction by 10%, and have less than 10% mortality.

Consequently, operations were performed by surgeons who had *never* done this procedure before. Plus, given that 127 centers now participated, there would only be an average of four SVR cases conducted at each center. ...A *very* steep learning curve for a surgeon to effectively learn a new treatment.

Ultimately — recruitment, rather than competence — won the day. The study became a gigantic charade.

Consequences for the Heart Failure Patient

Unfortunately, the consequences of this flawed data and its analysis were used by the cardiology and surgical communities to substantiate their belief that ventricular restoration had no advantages over present methods (coronary bypass grafting and mitral repair only).

The statisticians summarizing STICH trial results made conclusions from the data they were given, but that data was not valid.

Regrettably, this data is still considered sacrosanct because it emanates from distinguished sources (NIH, *New England Journal of Medicine*). It guides clinical decisions in the vast population of heart failure patients, and unfortunately, prevents them from receiving the ventricular restoration procedure that will help them.

Attempts to Bring the Light of Truth… Go Dark

In an attempt to counter the study's misleading results, we asked the *New England Journal of Medicine* if we could write an editorial to formally respond to the published STICH report. But they would only allow us to write a brief letter to the editor.[98] We also placed reports in other major journals, but nobody listened, and thinking has not changed.[99]

Randomized Trials

People would sometimes argue that our RESTORE Group results were not part of a prospective randomized trial. Everyone believes that credibility can *only* come from a randomized study.

Yet history is a wonderful teacher, as many stories repeat themselves.

A prospective randomized trial *only has validity* if the selection criteria are met and all procedures are done properly. This lesson was notoriously played out in the 1980s, when the role of coronary artery bypass grafting was first being defined. The VA Hospitals did a prospective randomized trial in 13 centers, and found that coronary bypass grafting was no better than other medical treatment. They reported an approximate 6% mortality and found that many grafts had closed, and concluded that coronary grafting was unnecessary.[100] This is in line with the way the STICH trial concluded that SVR was not helpful.

It turned out that these poor results following coronary bypass grafting occurred because the surgeons at participating centers had performed an inadequate technical procedure. This flaw became evident when Fred Loop at the Cleveland Clinic posed a powerful counterargument.[101] He summarized results from 1,000 consecutive patients at his center and showed mortality was approximately 1% and graft closure was rare. The contrasts were astounding, as this rebuttal became globally accepted and the world of coronary bypass grafting exploded. It became the standard method of treatment for coronary artery occlusion (blockage). The lesson was blatantly clear: a prospective randomized trial does not work if you do not do the operation right.

To me, a natural parallel exists between these two studies. In one, if an open vessel is closed... open it. In the other, if the natural elliptical shape becomes a sphere... bring back the ellipse.

The Impact and its Meaning

The hardship of this failed STICH study does not fall on me or on members in the RESTORE Group, but upon the thwarted opportunity of the medical community to counter the world's most debilitating illness and on the patients it could have helped. The STICH trial's faulty results was like "placing nails into the coffin" — one used to bury a revolutionary treatment for this devastating disease.

This experience made my thoughts drift back to when I applied to medical school and talked about my favorite book, the story of Philippe Ignaz Semmelweis, who had said, "Wash your hands to prevent the spread of childbed fever." This truth was ignored. Certainly, "returning the dilated heart to its natural elliptical shape" aims at a similarly powerful objective.

When the STICH trial was being planned, a famous cardiologist met with me to say, "Gerry, if this treatment works, it will place a crowning plume upon your accomplishments." My response was that my prize is, "If no one else experiences my dad's debilitation when he died from the ravages of end-stage heart failure, nothing else is needed."

For that reason, I will keep trying to hasten its arrival.

The Matter of Time

One step in the right direction came when the limitations of the STICH trial became apparent in Europe.[102]

According to their 2010 Task Force, guidelines from the European Society for Cardiology (ESC) and European Association for Cardiothoracic Surgery (EACTS) contradicted the STICH conclusions — and recommended the consideration of using SVR in centers with high levels of experience — following proper measurement of ventricular volume and the culprit scar in potential patients.

Aside from these welcome scientific comments coming from Europe, the STICH trial continues to represent a huge tragedy in how health care procedures are delivered. Because of its flawed data, the report remains an enormous obstacle to the proper treatment of the international population of heart failure patients. These misguided findings have essentially stopped cardiologists from considering having the spherical, failing chamber rebuilt back to its natural elliptical, healthy functioning form.

Truth will eventually win, but the huge number of sick patients with failing hearts will unfortunately bear the brunt of the STICH report's marred data. They will continue suffering the devastating symptoms and unchanged death rates from heart failure until *this calamity* is overturned.

This distressing chain of events was properly summarized by Mark Twain: "A lie can travel halfway around the world while the truth is putting on its shoes."

It is time for the truth to be heard — and acted upon.

CHAPTER 18

Paco: Exploring the New Horizon

Some discoveries reverberate throughout the scientific community. Revelations by Albert Einstein and Sir Isaac Newton have altered thinking forever. The key to their power is simplicity. We will now learn of a third such revelation.

Each of our prior chapters has described a research adventure in which I was fortunate to chase after breakthroughs in critical areas of cardiac care, ranging from heart-protecting cardioplegia, to countering heart attacks, to healing heart failure. Each undertaking focused primarily on finding an innovative treatment for a particular condition.

This chapter's exploratory voyage is one *that would change everything.*

Many things we had learned before would now come into question. We were sailing onto an ocean that had never been crossed, with no buoys to guide us. Now that can be frightening. But I was not tentative because my curiosity *compels me* to find answers.

It is an exciting way to travel through life, and reflects how I have always lived mine.

This chapter is about navigating waters that would alter the future of the entire cardiovascular field... by unraveling a truth that has escaped detection throughout the ages.

Riddle of the Heart

Everything in nature has a reason for being as it is. From the massive spiral formations of our galaxies to the crystalline configurations of a snowflake, there is a governing pattern. This is also true for the heart.

Our heart is nothing less than miraculous. Consider that it beats more than 100,000 times a day, over 35 million beats a year, pumping blood (with help from squeezing arteries and veins) through blood vessels *over 60,000 miles* long.

Though the heart's accomplishments are clear, *opinions about how it achieves them differ*, even with all of today's technology that might explain it. This impasse continues due to a lack of agreement on how its movement during each heartbeat can be explained by its structure. It's a basic question — a puzzle you might expect to have been solved long ago.

Interestingly, it was.

And then *it wasn't.*

Today, debate continues in the medical community about how the heart's form and structure can account for its function. Yet the prevailing belief — endorsed by most in the medical field and taught in medical schools — is wrong.

Knowing the truth of how heart structure and function are intertwined is crucial for reasons that extend far beyond intellectual understanding. *Incorrect knowledge creates the major limitation to developing successful treatments of diseases caused by the disruption of normality.* Simply, we must understand how the heart works — in order to deal with problems that arise when it is not working correctly.

That achievement cannot come without a solid knowledge of structure — because *form defines function.* This is why physicians and researchers have struggled throughout history for answers to how structure and performance are linked. Without this foundation, treatments will relieve symptoms, but sadly, will fail to correct the underlying disease.

Current approaches to treating heart failure provide the cardinal example of this predicament, as heart failure continues to be the world's leading cause of death. The heart failure death rate essentially *remains unchanged* over the last 20 years, despite all our advances in medications and technology.

My prior chapters addressed heart failure caused by the poor contraction in a heart that stretches after a heart attack — but this dilemma happens in only 50% of heart failure patients. The other 50% develop failure because while their ventricles have good contraction, they cannot relax properly between beats. *Yet in both cases* — the vital factor is a disturbance in the normal structure / function relationship. Finding a way to correct the mechanical causes for both these conditions requires a powerful understanding of this interconnection between structure and function.

But this is only the beginning, as gaining such knowledge can lead to a series of groundbreaking approaches for a wide range of major heart problems. A gargantuan leap may then take place, as our treatments will extend far beyond just alleviating symptoms — *they will solve a series of diseases* — that presently have no remedy.

Contemporary Cardiac Conflict

Unfortunately, even though knowledge and technology have advanced, confusion about the interdependence of structure and function still exists, as it is based upon different *deductions* made by two medical disciplines.

The first field of study involves anatomists and pathologists. They examine hearts in an autopsy room, essentially looking at dead tissue, and then infer what happens in live tissue: the functioning living heart. In other words, they *observe form (structure)... but deduce function.*

By contrast, the second group, the imaging community, uses MRI and echocardiograms to *observe motion... and deduce the structure* that made the heart move.

In both, deductive reasoning is used in place of knowledge. Yet the answer is to *know* structure so it can explain function. Without this certainty, they may argue forever, as each holds onto their own bias. This mirrors the dilemma I have encountered throughout my professional life: the introduction of new ideas being rejected due to rigid adherence to conventional thinking.

Now, the starting point of having a bias is a good thing. It introduces a theory that must be tested by an experiment. That is how research is done. But once that experiment begins, the answer *is what nature tells you*, not what you think — or want — to happen. Fiercely grasping onto what you previously believed is where the dilemma surfaces, and such rigidity has repeated itself again and again in history.

For example, Ludwig Rehn encountered just such an obstacle in Frankfurt, Germany in 1896, when he performed the first successful cardiac operation by closing a stab wound by directly suturing (sewing) the heart. Before this point, the traditional belief was that cardiac surgery would be forever prohibited by nature, as everyone thought operating directly on a heart was taboo. Any surgeon who dared to do so was certain to lose the acceptance of his colleagues. Yet Rehn successfully showed that operating on the heart *was* feasible, and he became known as the father of cardiac surgery.

Some Things Don't Change (But Should)

Today, operating directly on the heart has been widely adopted. Cardiac surgery is routine. Truth won, not traditional thinking.

Yet divergent beliefs continue about how the heart works, and these beliefs have lengthy historical roots. The endurance of these disagreements on heart structure and function demonstrate the obstinate holding onto such bias... as *deductions* about heart movement — *made from examinations of dead hearts in the 1600s* — continue to be considered valid today.

Back then, as now, the heart was thought to be highly complex: a *cardiac Gordian knot,* containing muscles that appear to go in all directions. Its structure was believed far too complicated to ever be understood.

Today, the imaging community retains these same beliefs, despite their improved abilities to observe cardiac movements. Admittedly, only two-dimensional diagnostic tools were initially available, such as observing dye injected into the ventricle to show how the heart wall contracts, or using the echocardiogram to watch the heart wall thicken and relax during each heartbeat. Those imaging tests reinforced the long-accepted four heart actions of: narrowing, shortening, lengthening, and widening. But the current introduction of modern three-dimensional imaging showed two more motions: *twisting and uncoiling*. These last two of the six motions form the core of the working heart's movements.

Such truth is known, yet this knowledge has not yet seeded new thinking, as mainstream physicians, nurses, medical students, and the general public continue to describe heart function using the conventional four cardiac motions previously mentioned. For them, contraction for emptying is traditionally portrayed as the making of a fist, followed by opening the closed hand for filling.

Yet truth is what nature prescribes, not how man interprets it. Cardiac motion in humans has not changed for over 100,000 years... and *twisting remains the most important motion.*

Hallowed History

My long quest to understand the heart has been enthralling. It was along this pursuit that I recognized that today's conventional description of heart movement precisely matches what William Harvey stated in 1628, in his classic book, *The Anatomical Exercises, De Motu Cordis De Circulatione Sanguinis* (often simply called *De Mortu Cordis*).[76] It detailed the body's circulation system and was a monumental contribution. The title "Father of Circulation" bestowed upon Harvey was well-earned.

Intriguingly, my efforts to learn more of Harvey's enormous discovery on the circulatory system had led me to the rare book room in the UCLA library... where they kept one of the only twenty original copies worldwide of Harvey's text. How magical to enter this inspiring chamber resembling a cathedral and have the unique opportunity to hold a treasure, one we all regarded as part of the Holy Grail.

But the real significance of this landmark experience became my realization that humanity's imperfections existed even within such noble history. Mixed with the brilliance of Harvey's contribution toward understanding the circulation were his mistaken deductions about cardiac function. Harvey admits his limited comprehension by stating, "I believe that the motion of the heart was to be understood by God alone" as he watched the heart move.[76]

Claude Bernard's edict of letting nature define what is truth, rather than only using deduction, was relevant again. It is not that Harvey was entirely wrong about the heart's mechanism. The heart does have the compressive motion as he portrayed. But Harvey's explanation is incomplete. *Missing are the twisting and uncoiling movements* described in this chapter, which are key to the normal heart motions of ejecting and filling during each heartbeat. The intent of this chapter is to uncover the muscles that cause this fundamental twisting motion. Harvey's failing to observe this motion does not diminish his majesty. Instead, it simply points to the beauty of the endless trail to learn, discover, and grow.

We know this now, as today's 3D imaging display of the heart's twisting and uncoiling movements confirm these fundamental basic motions. ...But do we need such sophisticated new tools to tell us the truth about heart motion?

We do not, as the following look into the past will surprisingly reveal.

Hidden History

During the 1600s when Harvey lived, Giovanni Borelli, an Italian physiologist, physicist, and mathematician, proclaimed that the heart twisted — resembling the wringing of a towel in a wine press — to eject blood through the body.[103] Even before him, Leonardo da Vinci described watching a knife *rotate* during each heartbeat after being inserted into the heart of a pig about to be slaughtered.

But even these were not the first times such descriptions appeared. Walking *further back* in history reveals that at around 280 BC, Erasistratus, the recognized father of physiology, described this twisting. His observations were later reinforced in AD 180 by Galen, the physician to the gladiators mentioned earlier in this book, who observed the heart uncoil each time as blood is forcefully sucked into it.

Nature's tale is consistently revealed through its movements. But this truth is only apparent to the curious eye.

Turning Point

Acceptance of the twisting theory plummeted when William Harvey submitted his report on the circulatory system. The leaders of medicine in the 1600s embraced his conclusions, and armed with this perceived truth, stated that Galen's theories were inadequate and inaccurate. They were equally convinced that Harvey had also refuted Vesalius, the Flemish founder of modern anatomy, who totally supported Galen's concept that the pulse reflected nature, as evident in the "ebb and flow" of ocean waves and currents.

Harvey believed that the heart exerted a bellows action upon the circulation, mimicking exactly what happens at a fireplace when a bellows is compressed to add more oxygen to the flames. He insisted that pressure was the guiding force for moving blood from a high to a lower pressure area within the heart, simulating a piston pump.

Seeing is Believing… Or is It?

Harvey was wonderful, but not perfect. His conclusions about the heart's constricting and dilating motions were true — but they are only a minor part of its action. Yet his concepts blotted out all prior descriptions of cardiac coiling and uncoiling actions… and astoundingly have persisted despite current 3D imaging that firmly demonstrates twisting in normal hearts.

Most cardiac surgeons still live within the world of looking without seeing. We have clung to the imagery of compression represented by the clenched fist that we learned as medical students. It even carries through into the operating room where the twist happens… but we only observe what we long believed was true. Our focus upon the four motions Harvey described — shortening, lengthening, narrowing, and widening — makes us miss the vital twisting and uncoiling movements, because we fail to understand the structure that makes this happen. Yet as you can see, the twisting heart is evident in the operating room. (**Video 1 twisting**)

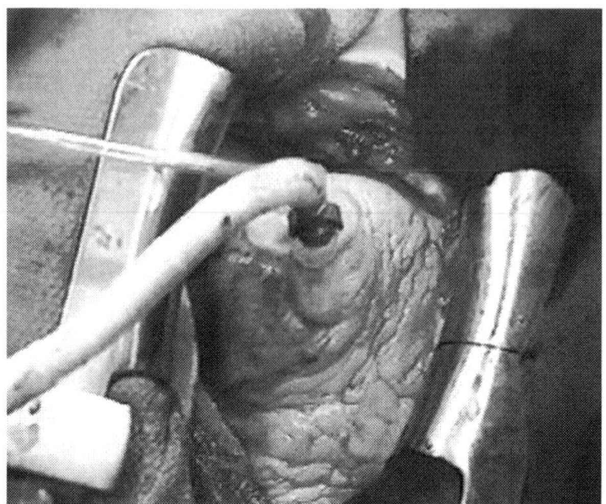

Video 1: The cardiac twisting motion in a patient undergoing cardiac surgery, as seen in the operating room.

www.vimeo.com/buckberg/normal-heart-twisting

Up to this point, this chapter has given you an overview of yesterday. Now I will unveil *my voyage into tomorrow*. It is linked to my becoming aware of the heart's *true structure*, and the ways in which this incredible knowledge will explain the mechanical forces that make the heart twist and uncoil. This is essential, because without this information, it is not possible to understand why the heart moves in such a way.

Hidden in Plain Sight: The Helix

It turns out the persistent belief that the heart is a complex rather than a simple structure has impeded acceptance of a different theory — one that involves a helix (spiral) configuration. Yet the reciprocal spiral coils of the helix are common in nature (as will be described in the next chapter).

As we'll learn, this helical heart architecture — and its surrounding wrap — defines the structure that accounts *for each of the six cardiac actions.*[104–108] This geometry was actually observed in the 1600s by English physiologist Lower and again in the 1700s by French anatomist Senec — but there has yet to be wide recognition of its impact on cardiac performance.

Heart structure never changes, but our perception of it does. In fact, this helical configuration was confirmed by a broad spectrum of the world's most prominent anatomists in the 1940s.[107] But they were perplexed by how the heart's muscle's configuration could create the geometric structure they were seeing. Moreover, this limitation prevented them from understanding how the heart's design could mechanically explain every cardiac motion — yet all agreed that the helix and surrounding wrap were the centerpieces of the heart's architectural form.

We just needed someone to provide these explanations.

Amazingly, such a person existed.

The next steps to my astounding adventure were about to begin.

Unraveling the Gordian Knot

En route to Murcia, Spain in 1998 to speak at the Spanish Cardiovascular Surgeons meeting, I had a stopover in Barcelona. While there, I visited surgeons at the University Clinics in Barcelona to describe how to use Dor's procedure to treat heart failure. We then did two operations.

After completing these procedures, Jose Pomar, the chief of Cardiovascular Surgery, asked, "Do you fully understood ventricular structure?" When I admitted my knowledge was limited, he told me of a retired cardiologist named Francisco Torrent-Guasp, who had made a remarkable discovery about the internal cardiac structure. "Would you like to meet him?" I readily agreed.

After the conference in Murcia, we traveled to Alicante, Spain, where Torrent-Guasp was to present his work before a group of cardiac surgeons that had attended the Murcia meeting. While I didn't know it then, this unplanned trip would open grand new doors to my understanding… and set the framework for my research and clinical efforts for the next 20 years, right up to today.

Paco, the Bearer of Answers

Arriving in Alicante, I was excited that my room was a suite on the top floor of a fabulous hotel overlooking the Mediterranean Sea. But rather than sitting to relish the view, I went immediately downstairs to see "Paco" Torrent-Guasp. (Paco is short for Francisco.) (**Figure 1**)

It was a memorable first meeting. We talked briefly before his presentation and I showed him some images of heart structure. Paco looked directly at me and said, "You do not understand cardiac anatomy."

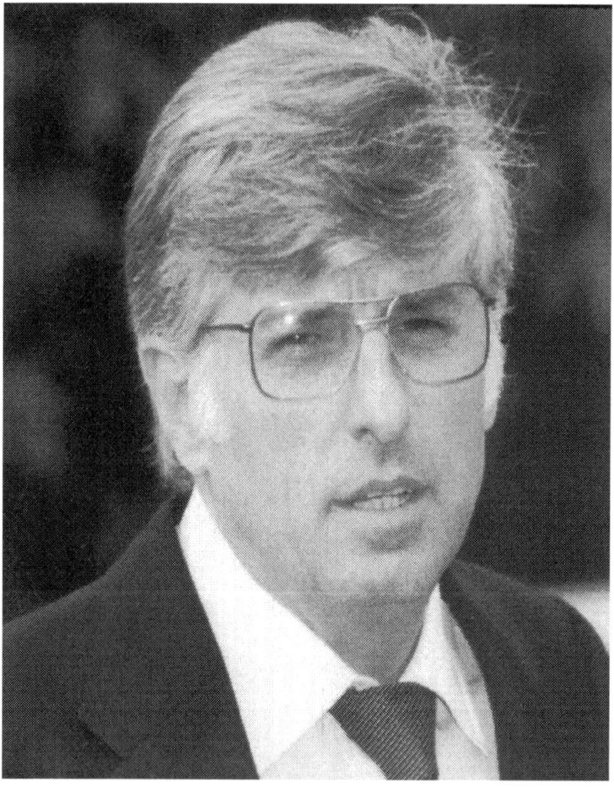

Figure 1: Francisco "Paco" Torrent-Guasp

I couldn't believe he'd say this to someone who'd been practicing heart surgery for nearly 30 years. Yet a primary objective to my travel is to gather new knowledge, so I awaited his presentation to learn about the differences in our views.

Paco proceeded to show us how he had "unraveled the heart" — figuratively and *literally*. I was captivated as he displayed how the heart's muscles would completely *unfold* to look like a string or an unrolled rope.

This architecture had a simple form *containing a coiled helix* (with obliquely angled or slanted fibers) that was *surrounded by a wrap* around its circumference (of transverse/horizontal muscle fibers)! Equally stunning was when he refolded the model, as it reformed the heart. This revelation is shown in an astonishing video of Paco "dissecting" the helical heart by using only his fingers to reveal its folding and unfolding characteristics, as described by its narrator. (**Video 2**)

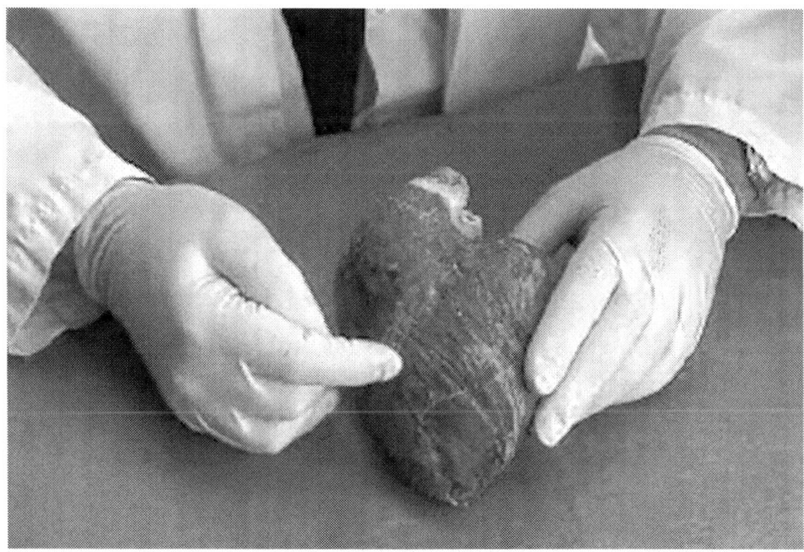

Video 2: Paco Torrent-Guasp unwraps the heart.

www.vimeo.com/buckberg/unwrapping-heart-1

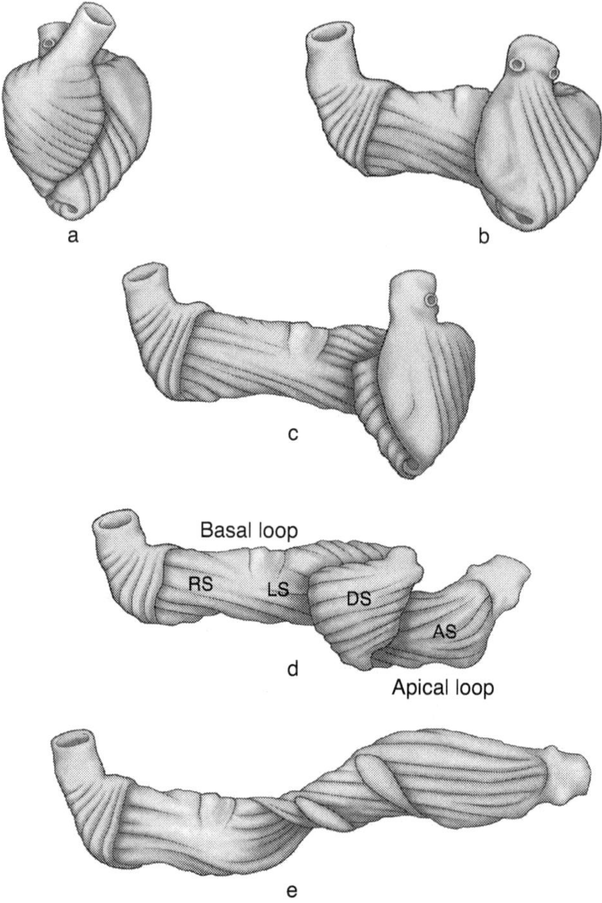

Figure 2: Unfolding of Torrent-Guasp's heart model. a) the intact heart. In b) the circumferential wrap of the base is unfolded as it covers the right ventricle. In c) the base wraps around the left ventricle and the helix is shown. In d) the helix of the apical loop is unfolded (on the right side) and its two parts of the inner coil (called descending segment or DS) and outer coil (called ascending segment, or AS) are shown. The left side shows the unfolding of the wrap or basal loop to display its right side or RS, and left side or LS. In e) the heart becomes an unfolded rope.

This unraveling reveals the different areas of the heart, as are indicated in **Figure 2**.

At this point, Paco declared, "Nature is simple, but scientists are complicated." This elegant observation reflects the clarity of his thinking.

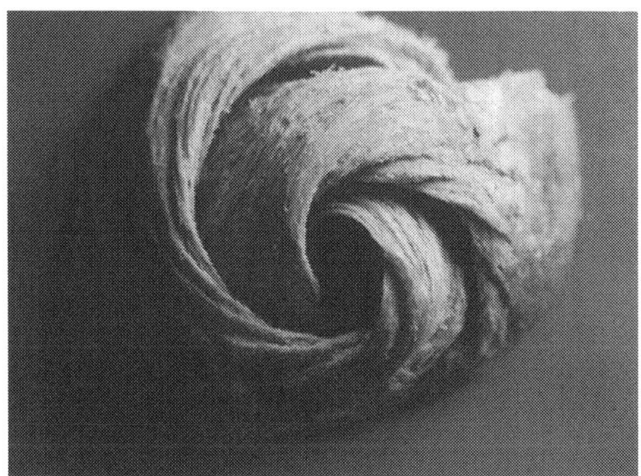

Figure 3: A view of the Torrent-Guasp dissection, showing the spirals that form the heart's tip or apex.

Paco further demonstrated that this helix has a *vortex* at its tip, meaning the heart muscle goes downward at a 60° angle, then makes a loop to *coil around* this tip, to finally move back upward at the same 60° angle — evolving a pattern that has a wondrous spiral-like arrangement that was best observed from the heart's tip: its apex. (**Figure 3**)

Paco's excitement about how this elegant structure could transform into movement was palpable. He called the working heart's motion… the Cardiac Dance.

His observations also had historical precedent, since his external cardiac structure mirrored what English physiologist Richard Lower had noted in the 1600s. Yet Paco took the *colossal next step*: uncovering the architecture's muscle pathways and solving the three-dimensional structure of the heart!

Paco called this heart configuration the *helical ventricular myocardial band* (HVMB), and named the helical muscles that go down to form the apex (tip) and then curl around to go back up… *the apical loop.* This apical loop can *shorten and lengthen*. He called the surrounding transverse/horizontal muscle (wrap)… *the basal loop,* which can *narrow (compress) and widen* the helix.

What Paco presented was nothing less than astonishing! It erased misunderstanding — and introduced a new and *uncomplicated* understanding of the heart's structure!

Its sheer straightforwardness made me revisit my favorite phrase, "Elegance is simplicity, confusion is complexity." Just as Einstein formulated $E=mc^2$, and Newton defined F=ma, Paco's documentation of a helix and wrap puts his contribution within the tiny number of *monumental discoveries* that shall change thinking forever.

If I was right, his contributions should place him within the legendary status of William Harvey, who defined circulation. Paco's road map of heart design will create a legion of new breakthroughs in cardiac diagnosis and practice.

Curiosity Catalyzed

I talked with Paco for four hours during dinner after his presentation. As we finished and were about to go our separate ways, I posed a new question.

"Paco, where do you live?"

"About 100 kilometers from here," he answered. "Why?"

"I would like go with you and learn further. Could we do that?"

Paco smiled and said, "Of course." I hurried back to my beautiful suite overlooking the ocean and checked out, having never even opened my bags. I drove with Paco and Teresa, his lovely wife, to his hometown of Dénia, arriving at 2 AM.

My first chore the next morning was to change my plane reservations and reschedule my plans (I was going next to Lausanne, Switzerland to lecture), so I could arrive two days later. Paco and I spoke for 18 hours that day. I learned that Paco had begun uncovering this knowledge about heart structure almost 40 years earlier by performing dissections as a medical student in Salamanca, Spain. But his data and work had remained consistently unknown to medical, physiological, anatomic, and surgical societies.

Paco showed me a fabulous teaching tool that he developed: a silicon rubber heart model that permitted easy unwrapping, and then re-wrapping, of the heart's apical and basal loops in only ten seconds. Its detailed markings mimicked the angles of the muscle fibers that existed in a dissected heart. It also displayed the *cleavage planes* — where the adjacent muscle tissue bundles could be separated to simplify the process of unwrapping the heart into a simple rope form, and then easily become rewrapped back to normality — just as it would in the dissection room.

I found this extraordinary. A secret that had been hidden for 2,200 years (280 BC to AD 1998) could now be revealed and displayed within ten seconds.

To further validate his model for me, he performed identical "dissections" on beef hearts obtained from a local butcher.

His demonstration of easily unwrapping the apical (helical) and basal (wrap) loops of the HVMB into an unfolded rope-like configuration needs to be seen to be believed. (**Video 3**)

Paco had unraveled the Gordian knot of anatomy.

We continued talking, and before I left the next day, I asked four additional questions: about embryologic development (the heart's formation and early

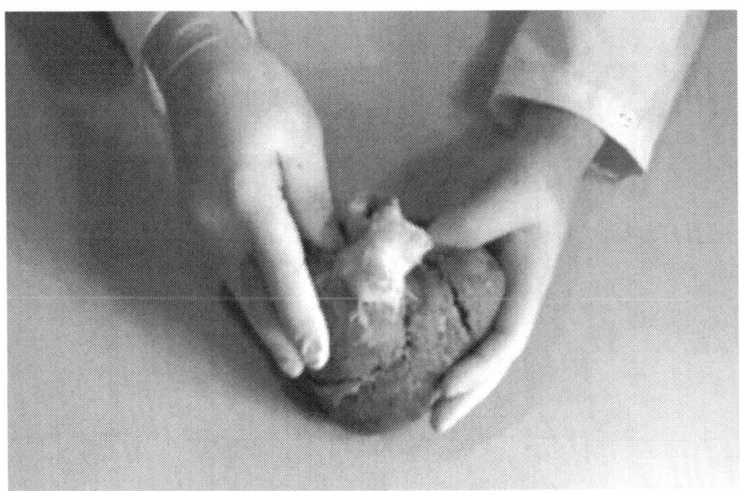

Video 3: Paco Torrent-Guasp unwraps the heart.
Note that he begins by unfolding the circumferential wrap to show the helix. Then he unfolds the helix to demonstrate that the heart looks like a rope after being unwrapped.

www.vimeo.com/buckberg/unwrapping-heart-2

growth)... the heart's electrical system... why his dissection differed from what was known about where the papillary muscles had their origin (that connect to valves at the junction between the atrium and ventricle)... and finally, how the right ventricle worked.

Paco did not have the answers, even though his knowledge of anatomy was astounding. Yet, I needed to have these initial questions solved if I were to fully support and advocate his approach.

I was galvanized because the far-reaching impact of this work was already apparent to me. This newfound potential to *correlate structure with function* could fundamentally explain the mechanical reasons behind many cardiac problems — by shedding new light on normality and how it is disrupted by disease — thereby guiding the evolution of novel treatment options. I centered

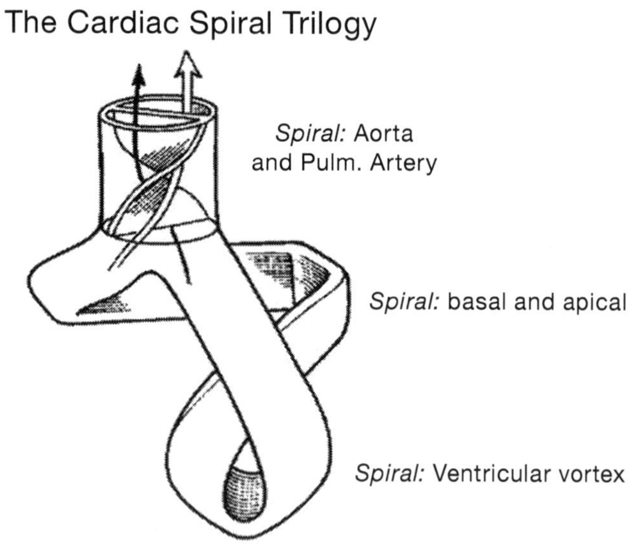

Figure 4: The heart configuration involves three spirals. The first (lower part of image) is at the ventricular vortex (at the apex). The second (middle of image) is where the circumferential wrap folds downward toward the apex to create the helix... that ends upward at the aorta (blood vessel that carries out blood from the left ventricle). The third (top of image) is where the two arteries leaving the heart — one going to the lungs (pulmonary) and the other to the body (aorta) — cross each other at 60° angles.

all of my research efforts on this objective. If successful, *a revolution in worldwide thinking would be created.*

Nature's Beauty... Unveiled Again

Paco's discovery was gratifying for another reason. Forms within nature have always been fascinating to me, in particular, the spiral structure found in everything from DNA to galaxies. The heart described by Paco introduced yet another spiral, as its three spiral patterns create a wondrous cardiac configuration. **Figure 4** illustrates this triple spiral design. First, the basal loop folds to become the helix, then it turns at the vortex (where the reciprocal spiral muscles form it) at the heart's tip, and then its outflow arteries (aorta and pulmonary artery) cross each other.

How simple, graceful, and if correct... staggering.

Will This "New" Anatomy Match Function?

Fortified with what I now knew, it was time to find out if we could answer the definitive question that had enchanted and exasperated researchers for centuries: "*Could this structure explain how the heart functions?*"

This pursuit hurled me into my grandest journey.

Resolving this age-old mystery required creation of a new kind of battle plan. Fresh tools were at our disposal, since we had Paco's model of the helical ventricular myocardial band. It helped us select specific sites to explore in a beating heart muscle. This allowed us to make motion recordings from within the helix that contained slanted (oblique) fibers, or in the wrap comprised of horizontal (transverse) fibers. The outcomes from this testing would allow us to confirm — or reject — Paco's helical ventricular myocardial band theory. I knew that if these findings were positive, we could at long last reveal how the heart performs its wonderfully dynamic symphony of motions... during every single heartbeat!

Many would think the key to such discovery would be sophisticated and expensive investigative equipment. But we did not have access to fancy MRI or Echo machines that cost $500,000 or more. Instead, we only had some inexpensive crystals to place in the heart. They acted like probes, recording an impulse that tabulated how the heart moves as it contracts. We used a device costing just $10,000 to record these findings. But that was all we needed.

Still, we knew we were facing a formidable challenge: how do we determine the probes' placement? We were essentially looking at a working heart without "signposts," as if trying to establish tactical positions within an unmarked battlefield. Doubt was inescapable.

While such uncertainty is always a part of research, I also realized we were armed with the unique architectural road map provided by Paco's model. *But only if its guidance was correct.*

To the Lab

Imagine the anticipation in our laboratory.

We started by mounting Paco's silicon model adjacent to our operating table, where it displayed the wrap and underlying helix muscles. With this precise replica of the heart directing us, we could position the recording (sono-micrometry) crystals in a living heart in the exact regions that Paco identified as the underlying helix and the wrap.

If Paco's model was right, and the crystal markers were correctly placed — the data inscribed from these recordings during each heartbeat would confirm that the three muscles (the two arms of the helix and the wrap) accounted *for all of the heart's movements.*

But if not, we must join the other frustrated investigators who had failed to find mechanical reasons for cardiac movement.

It was a daunting challenge to take on!

Our strategy was simple. Pairs of tiny crystals would be inserted (one cm apart) either into the horizontal fibers of the wrap, or along the diagonally angled helical bands on the outside and inside of the ventricle. The contraction movement of these muscle fibers would then be recorded in thousandths of a second to rapidly follow their motion.

Everything was in place. Nothing like this had ever been done before.

Needle in the Haystack?

Fortunately, we were not looking for a needle in a haystack, since we had Paco's helical heart model as the guidepost. Our search for the "holy grail" — understanding why the heart moved — began with our Spanish research fellow, Manuel Castella, doing these studies. I spoke with Paco and he was proud that another Spaniard would play such a key role, half a world away.

The study began. Tracking results were recorded. Our first answers came back.

We did not find success. This was clear as soon as Manuel walked into my office from the lab after our first experiment. His face was not hard to read.

"What happened?" I asked.

"We have a problem. The crystals are revealing abnormal and irregular contractions in an area of the heart. Actually, in three areas. I'm sorry, Dr. B., but it's not working as expected. The heart simply doesn't function the way Paco said it would."

I could see that Manuel was personally frustrated, as well as concerned about my reaction. But I wasn't looking for only "my" answers. I was seeking truth. Manuel's training needed to include this lesson. As Claude Bernard stated, if results are incorrect, it means either your idea is wrong, or your procedure is not being done properly. Exploring these barriers would become an essential part of our search, because Paco's model *can only be considered valid if it passes all tests.* A dazzling hunt was about to begin to understand every roadblock — to see if each reflected permanent obstacles, or could be explained and resolved.

I smiled reassuringly at Manuel. "Nature is telling us something. Let's find out what."

We returned to the lab.

The first issue related to the *absence of a clear contraction* from recordings of a pair of crystals in the deeper tissues on the lower side of the heart. Could this mean that the fiber arrangements in this region were different than what we had expected from the helix and wrap?

Manuel and I agreed on the next step. "Do an autopsy to find exactly where the crystals were positioned — a key factor — before we draw any conclusion."

We were on target, as the autopsy examination showed the recording crystals, inserted through the heart muscle, touched a papillary muscle on its inner surface. This small muscle contains *longitudinal* fibers that interact with heart valve structures. Paco's model was validated, because this tiny site has no helical or transverse fibers.

The second goal was to understand why there were persistently poor recordings at the heart's tip. This tip (called the apex) is formed by the vortex of the heart's inner and outer helix (as shown in Paco's model). I thought about this and told Manuel, "The heart's form and function simulates nature. For example, when it twists, the motion resembles the whorl of a hurricane or a tornado."

So I asked, "What happens in the eye of each of those storms?"

Manuel's face lit up. "Nothing. It's the area of calm."

"What if that was the same for the heart?" I posed. "The apex at the tip of the ventricle is very thin and located just beyond the twist of the vortex. Could this be an area that does not move?"

Exhilarated, we tested and confirmed this. The motionless cardiac tip *does* reflect the calm eye of a storm. Most importantly, nature demonstrated something, and we used that lesson to understand something else. This was proven from the *normal* shortening function that we recorded when crystals were placed *adjacent* to the apical vortex (but not on the tip of the vortex itself).

Finally, we faced the third roadblock. Recordings from the right ventricular wall showed these fibers contracting *as if* they were oblique (diagonal) — like those helical fibers in the left ventricle. It contradicted our belief they should be transverse (horizontal). How could this be?

Manuel feared this might be a crushing blow to the helical heart concept. Yet, just as one does when his car is lost on a trip, we needed to consult our road map.

I said, "Let's take another look at Paco's model."

So we opened the model, peered closer, and there it was.

"Look at that!"

Paco's model showed that this part of the right ventricular wall *did* contain deeper oblique fibers — similar to those on the surface of the left ventricle. An unforeseen finding, since we had deduced (but incorrectly) that this part of the wrap *only* contained transverse fibers.

The crystals simply told us what was there, not what we expected. They worked perfectly, and by doing so, they confirmed the accuracy of the fiber orientations within Paco's model! It was a stunning finding. We now had overcome all of the apparent roadblocks.

It was an amazing experience, because every time we came across responses we didn't anticipate, we were able to figure out why — using Paco's model for guidance. His myocardial band model could explain every logjam we encountered, and in doing so, solidified our confidence about the gigantic importance of Paco's discovery.

All of this took place over several exhilarating months, with new findings emerging during every step of the journey. Paco's helical model truly became the Rand McNally map that led to a unique and spellbinding understanding of how the heart mechanically works.

(Sequential) Timing is Everything

Our initial venture into decoding normal structure and function led us to an unanticipated prize. Manuel called, as he had found something, but did not disclose it. Instead, he urged me to come down to the lab.

"Dr. B., I know the general consensus is that the heart muscles all contract simultaneously to pump blood, like a closing fist. But look at these tracings."

He handed me recordings of crystal movements as the heart contracted.

"I hadn't noted it before," he continued, "but the crystals in each of the three muscle regions we tested do *not* all move at once [simultaneously] during a heartbeat. They moved sequentially."

Examining the data, I grinned. "This is fantastic! You're right — it shows the muscles are contracting sequentially — one after the other after the other. These direct muscle recordings confirm that the conventional belief of synchronous action [all moving together] like closing fingers all at once to make a fist *is absolutely wrong*. Instead, they follow each other, *like a whorl of a contraction*. Great work!"

The power of our understanding of form and function blossomed. The magnificence of Paco's insight explained all six motions of function by a cardiac structure of *just three primary muscles* in the heart (the two helix layers and the wrap)! Its beauty lay in its straightforward nature: the wrap *narrows* the ventricle and subsequently *widens* it... while the helix *shortens* the chamber and subsequently *lengthens* it... and *twisting* is caused by the *differential rotation of the helical muscle* (one portion going clockwise and the other counterclockwise), which subsequently *uncoils* to return the ventricle to its starting point.

How thrilling and elegant.

Controlled Power

Our explorations also led us to recognize another aspect of heart structure — one that helps explain the heart's incredible strength.

The heart's powerful spiral muscles that produce the twisting helix would essentially "explode" during its ejection of blood to circulate throughout the body — if not for the *wrap* that contains it. That is, as the helix squeezes forcefully, the sides of these inner spiraling muscles would naturally splay outward. But they are held together by this surrounding wrap. (**Figure 5**)

My previous analogy between the twisting action of a heart and the whorl of a hurricane was only partially correct. There is no wrap around a hurricane, so the hurricane spreads out far and wide (25 to 150 miles or more) because

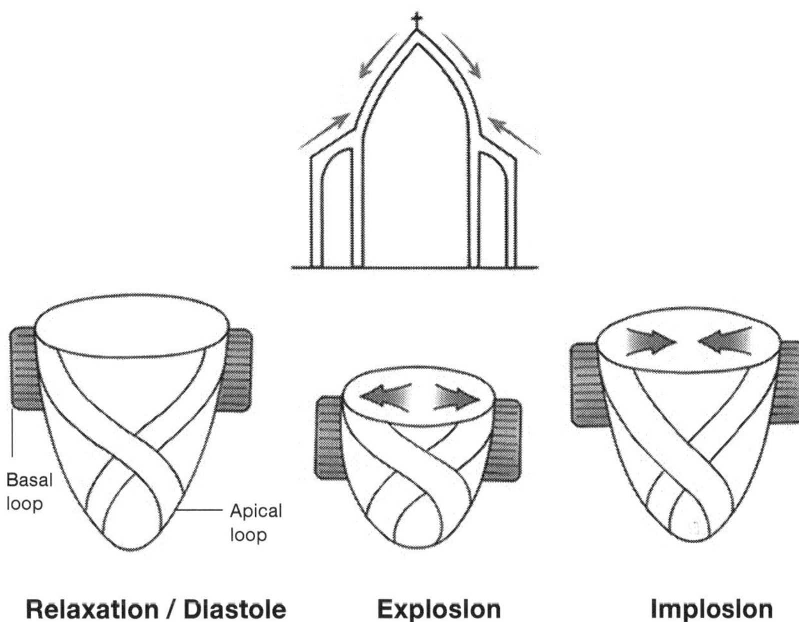

Figure 5: The bottom three figures show the relationship of the circumferential wrap (horizontal lines) and the figure 8 helix, with relaxation (diastole) on left, and ejection and suction in center and right. The wrap surrounds the helix and prevents its arms from exploding during ejection and imploding during suction.

Upper image shows how heart design is same as cathedral's gothic dome and surrounding buttresses.

it has no confinement. Conversely, the heart is more efficient because a wrap is part of its design, and this containment maximizes power to perform its majestic functions. *No energy is wasted.* The wrap also imposes a similar benefit when the heart develops suction. It prevents ventricular *implosion* — offsetting the ventricle's tendency to collapse — as the wrap holds the chamber open to avoid this consequence.

This inner conical shape and outside wrap made me realize that the heart's structure resembles a church's gothic dome. Think of the way this style of architecture contains buttresses that keep the dome from pushing outward and then toppling down. (**Figure 5**) This unique commonality led me during lectures to playfully ask my medical audience, "Which came first — the heart or church?"

A New Future

Our team was ecstatic as each of our preliminary experiments confirmed Paco's prediction of these major muscle fiber bundles — *and* explained the reasons behind heart movement. Paco had indeed solved the ancient enigma of myocardial architecture! We were so grateful for his discovery, which gave us the chance to help uncover this vast new universe.

The next question I asked myself was, Did I wish to spend many ensuing years studying this cardiac structure in order to understand the mechanics behind *normal* and *abnormal* heart motion?

My response was a resounding yes, especially since a broad spectrum of new imaging technology was forthcoming. These tools could be used to further verify Paco's architectural findings. And they did. New evaluations by magnetic resonance imaging, velocity vector imaging, and 3D speckle tracking echocardiography — all revealed an even clearer picture of the interaction between the helical and transverse muscle fibers.[104–106] For the first time, we'd solved the ongoing divide between *what* you see — and *understanding why* you see it. We could use Paco's concept of the heart's architecture to account for the results that the imagers found every time. *Bravo for Paco!* His theories became further validated as each newly available technology confirmed our measurements.

Of course, the real winner is not Paco... but the patient.

Paco's discoveries — and our affirmation of them — offered a *monumental shift* in our understanding of the heart. But how would the medical community react to this groundbreaking knowledge?

As we would find out, history tells a repetitive tale, one populated by the fierce stalwarts of tradition who are resistant to new thinking. They will hold onto old beliefs, despite a wealth of fresh data that confirms the helical ventricular myocardial band architecture can explain structural reasons for every cardiac motion.

Alternatively, a very different and pragmatic response is made by those who want to consider this new concept. They ask: "What does this discovery mean, and is it useful?"

That fundamental question addresses why the connection between structure and function is so powerfully important. Possessing this innovative knowledge yields a remarkable treasure, as it unearths a bevy of answers to problems that, until now, have frustrated the medical community. As we'll see, an eruption of fresh insights will evolve into successful solutions for a wide range of common heart conditions, whose treatments so far have only addressed symptoms.

I will explore these uncharted waters in the upcoming chapters, using this new knowledge as a guide to understanding — and treating — these previously *unsolvable* cardiac issues:

- heart failure in dilated hearts
- heart failure in normal hearts that cannot relax
- disorders in the ventricular septum and right ventricle
- heart pacemaker shortcomings

Creativity — Important to All My Journeys

Beyond continuing to play a key role in my developing novel solutions to these and other heart problems, my *creative energies* have always fueled the artistic portions of my life. Creativity is adventure, and blends both art and science.

A glimpse into my artistic endeavors will be presented in a sequence of chapters (bracketed between each of the remaining scientific chapters) to reveal how my curiosity energizes a convergence of art and science in my life. They will disclose:

- how the helix and heart interrelates with the human being
- a video presentation of the helix and heart that won an international prize
- heart function as reflected in a ballet called "The Cardiac Dance, Spirals of Life"
- the heart and Stonehenge — surprisingly similar constructions
- and finally, how *my art and my science* link with my lifestyle.

Paco's work took us a giant step forward, because it raised the curtain on a deeper understanding of heart structure and its function. Our feet would have remained fixed without this insight, leading us to only stand on today. But with it, the beauty of tomorrow unfolds before us.

It is a future filled with unprecedented breakthroughs that come by having *vision* — not from simply looking.

CHAPTER 19

Art and Science: Nature's Grand Design

One of the most wonderful things about a new scientific idea is its capacity to open a gateway to the next exploration.

Paco's discovery of the helical heart's architecture answered many unresolved questions, while simultaneously raising new ones. Each of these questions needed to be answered, for their solution will ensure the validity of his new helical heart model. The first query involved explaining the relationship between the helical heart's structure and how its electrical connections can stimulate its rhythmical motions.

Little could I have predicted that this medical pursuit would reveal connections between the heart, nature, and the human being.

Starting Point

The heart's electrical system was outside my area of expertise, so my initial step was to find a suitable scholar with an open mind who could listen, learn, and ask questions that might more fully uncover the helical heart's structure / function relationships. I selected Jim Cox, a renowned cardiac surgeon and the master electro-physiologist who had designed a groundbreaking surgical procedure to treat atrial fibrillation.

Paco (Dr. Francisco Torrent-Guasp) had unmasked the heart's hidden geometric form. For this reason, I asked him to fly in from Spain to join us at Georgetown University in Washington DC, where his revelations of cardiac anatomy could be shared with Jim Cox.

It was a momentous meeting. Jim was fascinated by how this concept simplified understanding the heart's form while explaining its function. He was further impressed by the beauty of Paco's silicon model. It allowed rapid unfolding of the heart into a rope-like configuration, and then refolded to reproduce normal structure. This phenomenal teaching tool allowed anyone to see the straightforward elegance of the heart's construction.

The Lecture

Neither Jim nor I realized the full ramifications of this concept of ventricular architecture. Yet we both recognized the enormity of its potential. At the end of our discussion, Jim asked me to consider giving the Basic Science Lecture at the American Association of Thoracic and Cardiac Surgery (AATS) conference in 2001. He knew our colleagues would consider Paco's work an exciting breakthrough.

The "Basic Science Lecture" is a high point of the association's annual meeting — the world's foremost gathering about heart surgery that is attended by 3,000 to 4,000 cardiac surgeons from all over the globe. As its president, Jim was free to select that year's speaker. Having me present was a bold stroke, as the purpose of the lecture is to have a lasting impact that addresses subjects that go beyond surgery. It is not just about discussing new approaches to performing an operation. In fact, only one other surgeon had ever given this talk. Instead, Nobel Laureates, renowned physicists, genetic engineers, and other prominent individuals had been chosen. But Jim recognized that the implications of what I would present could be vast. It would lay out a novel approach that may finally link cardiac form and function. (**Figure 1**)

Jim saw this as a way to spring open the previously closed doors to new ways of thinking (an enticing goal, as it also lined up with my teaching mantra). I gladly accepted.

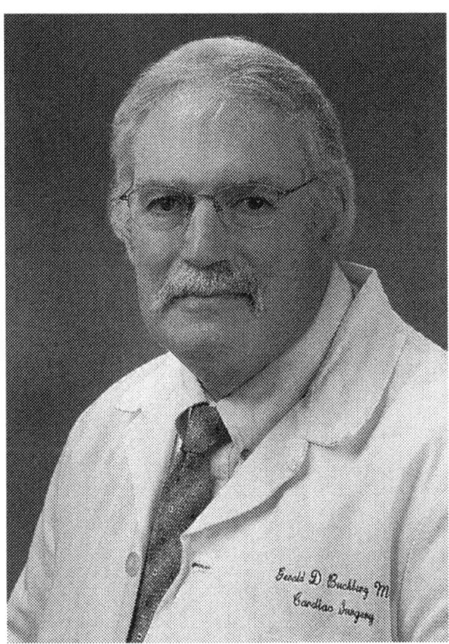

Figure 1: Gerald Buckberg M.D. at Basic Science Lecture at AATS in 2001.

The Challenge Ahead

It was quite an honor to deliver this lecture, and much thought would go into creating it. This would be far different from all of my previous presentations, each of which had focused on specific scientific cardiac topics. While I knew my subject would center on Paco's discovery, I also realized that if I was to introduce a new way of thinking, the talk needed to go beyond simply a discussion of the heart.

I needed to reveal that the structure of the heart is part of something much larger, a prelude to my exposing a concept that may give insight into the nature of life itself.

The lecture would blend art and science, and be entitled, "Basic Science Review: The Helix and the Heart." Later, I will provide a link to a video of the lecture. This chapter will detail how the presentation evolved, and the incredible discoveries along the way.

Let me now describe the education of me, the educator.

Journey's Beginning: The Student's Mind

As I would be exploring new territory, I wanted to embrace a learning strategy similar to one that I often used with my two daughters when they were growing up.

My workweek was always very busy, so I treasured the special time I could be with my daughters during weekends. One of the things I did was to take them on a walk down a canyon near our house... where we played the game of "discovery." Though we walked along corridors that we had traveled many times before, we'd look for different things each time. We talked about the concept of discovery, where you must be willing to see things freshly, and try to understand why they are there. It is the difference between "having vision," rather than only "looking."

I knew I wanted to touch on this process as I began my talk, as my lecture would be presented to a very accomplished and established collection of surgeons. Describing this discovery process would set the tone and hopefully help them open to a radically new way of looking at the heart and more. I'd cite the academic adage that "Students are often wrong, but always in doubt... whereas professors are sometimes wrong, but never in doubt."

I'd ask them to join me on this fresh "walk," as together we maintain this student-like attitude, one that has energized my quest for new possibilities during my over 50 years of finding ways to create interaction between research and clinical practice.

Pilgrimage to Discovery Began Long Ago

While beginning my research into organizing this lecture, I quickly realized my presentation must cast a wide net, so that I needed to create new correlations between the heart, nature, and the human being.

Yet I was uncertain how to justify connecting these three subjects. But Albert Einstein, my hero, reassured me. "All our science, measured against reality, is primitive and childlike, and yet is the most precious thing we have," he once said. His advice encouraged me to search for Nature's yet-unrecognized grander picture.

The heart was a fine starting point, but I quickly realized that Paco and I were not the only ones to enter this educational trail involving the helical heart design. In fact, we were not at all the first.

I found that the English physician and physiologist, Richard Lower, had described *helical fibers* back in 1669, when looking at the vortex at the apex tip on the bottom of the heart. He noted that the helical arms were like a figure-eight, with reciprocal arms that cross each other in a clockwise and counterclockwise pattern. (**Figure 2**) Then later, in 1748, the French anatomist Senec inspected the inside of the heart and noted a *similar* reciprocal pattern of helical clockwise and counterclockwise formations of spiral muscle fibers (he also confirmed this inner helix was surrounded by a wrap of horizontal fibers that could compress or constrict the ventricle).

The prevalence of interest in this helical design surprised me. I found that in the 1400s, Leonardo da Vinci, another hero of mine, focused upon the heart's apex, which he thought to be the motor of the ventricle. Leonardo was

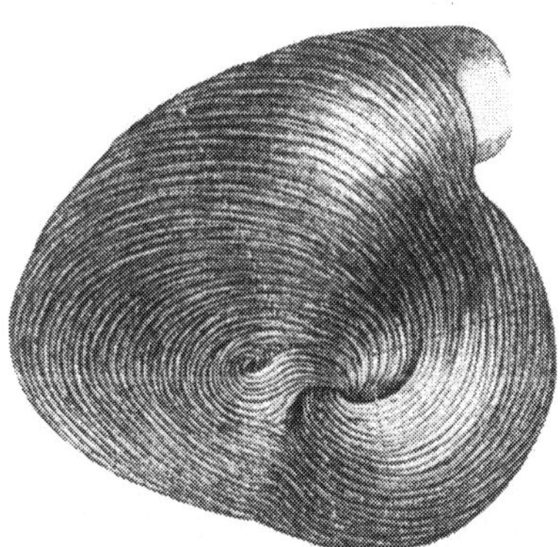

Figure 2: Lower's illustration in the 1600s showing a helix with clockwise and counterclockwise spiral formations of ventricular muscle. The vortex at the apex, shows the outside spiral arm turns in and the inside spiral arm turns out.

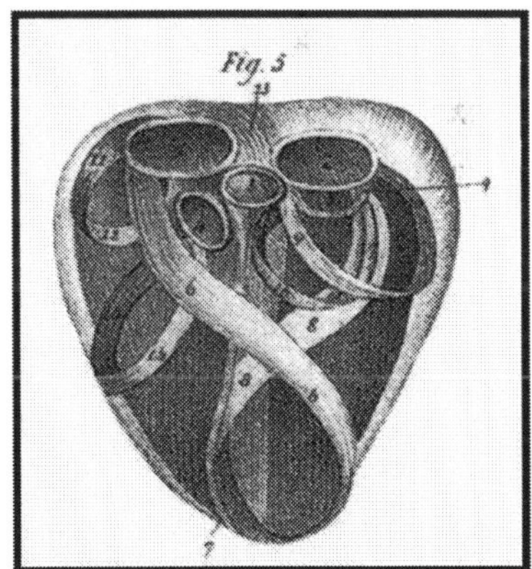

Senec's illustration in 1700s France showing the helical arrangement of ventricular muscle fibers create the cardiac architectural design.

intrigued by the reciprocal spirals in the blood flow patterns that developed as blood was ejected into the aorta.

I wondered what conclusions Leonardo might have drawn if he had been able to study (with the advanced imaging technology we possess today) the zebra fish, which developed 400 million years ago. I learned it also exhibits clockwise and counterclockwise spirals after heart blood is ejected into its aorta. This is especially thought-provoking as this fish's anatomy is *tiny* — its aorta blood vessel microstructure being only one-third the size of a human hair! (**Video 1**) Yet the configuration of its aorta is the same as that of the human, as are the spiral whorls of blood flow observed after each heartbeat.

Would Leonardo have considered the same idea that I was considering? Namely, that we humans are not unique, but simply play a part, just like the zebra fish, in nature's larger scheme?

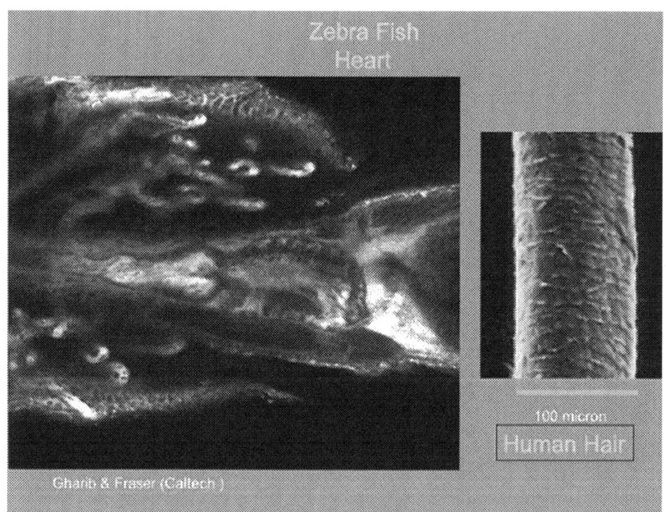

Video 1: On left is elliptical working heart of zebra fish, whose aorta and heart shape mirror the human's as commonality exists but the size differs: the five-cell thick zebra fish heart ejects blood into an aorta that is one-third the size of a single human hair (on right).

www.vimeo.com/buckberg/zebra-fish-heart

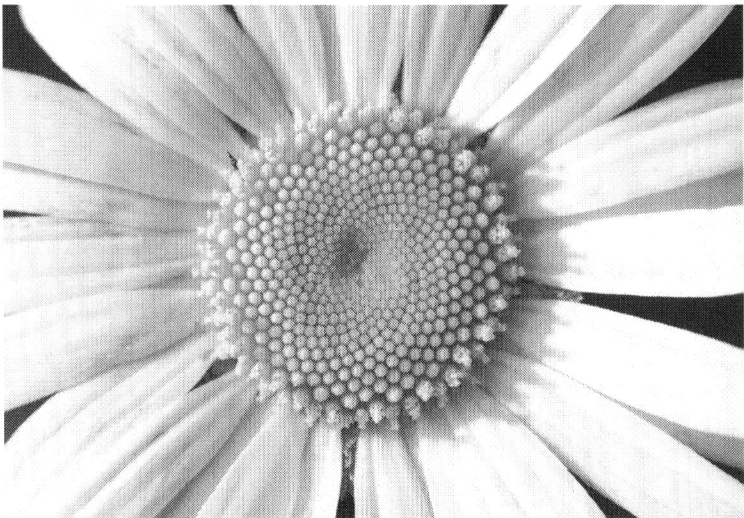

Figure 3: Reciprocal spirals in daisy, nature's design.

World Beyond the Heart

An even more enthralling observation was still ahead of me, as I would find that the heart was not unique in its clockwise and counterclockwise architectural configuration. This natural pattern exists across a vast scope of life, and reveals magnificence and harmony throughout nature.

Keen observation uncovers new understanding. For example, in botany, flower buds display this same reciprocal spiral arrangement. (**Figure 3**) Moreover, the tiny circles in the center "floral disc" expand as you go from center toward its outer rim. This marvelous growth design is called the "botanical logarithmic spiral theory of phyllotaxis." *The magical joining of science, mathematics, and life.*

I quickly realized that spirals were not limited to the heart or a flower's bud. You can see the same pattern in the growth of a pinecone. Even the nautilus shell contains a spiral. Moreover, I was astounded that a helix shape — similar to that of the heart, (**Figure 4**) becomes apparent if you view the narrowed (vortex) end of seashell when it is upright.

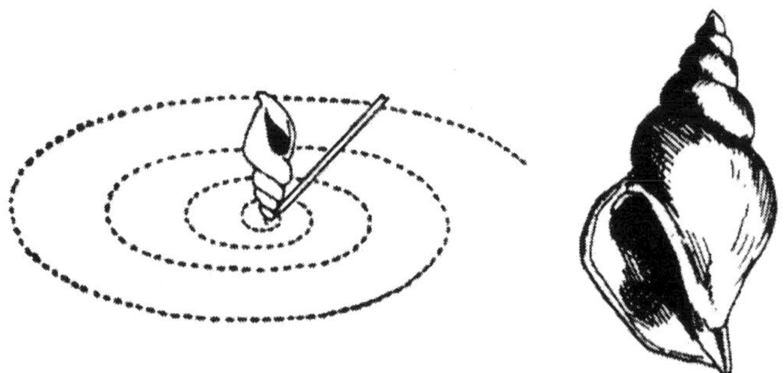

Figure 4: Demonstration of how the conical helix is formed from the flat spiral.

Ecstatic, I began looking further, and found helical patterns common to many animals with horns, such as the ram or eland. But again, this isn't a matter of visual aesthetics. It's a matter of function. These horns do not break during combat. Why? Because nature has provided a very sturdy structure by creating additional spirals *inside* the horns — again, the interweaving of spirals within spirals is exposed as one of nature's tricks.

My pursuit widened as I wondered: how prevalent might the spiral be in nature?

I found more and more examples. Looking to better understand this fundamental harmony drew me back even further in history to 600 BC, when the Greek mathematician Pythagoras defined the concept of the *golden section.* This relationship emerges from a simple rectangular figure. A line placed within it will create two proportional dimensions, as the ratio of the smaller component to the larger component... mirrors how the larger component compares to the whole. (**Figure 5**)

The numerical characteristics of this interaction were later discovered in AD 1250 by Fibonacci, who mathematically described a logarithmic spiral that identified a harmony between parts. He defined these proportions as 0.618.... (a number without end, infinite like that of π or pi). Placing these rectangular parts together (as in the diagram) creates a spiral. (**Figure 5, bottom**) It again shows the beauty of harmony *and* variance — yet another instance of spirals that maintain core similarities even while appearing in different forms.

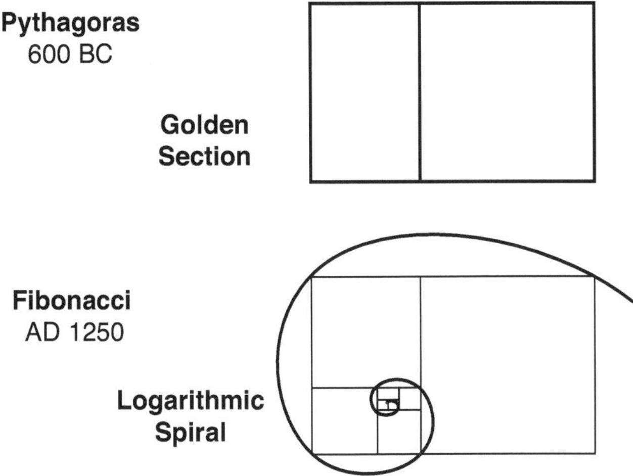

Figure 5: The golden proportion of Pythagoras (above) in 600 BC where the small is to the large, as the large is to the whole. Bottom is how interweaving the golden proportions will form a spiral, as described by Fibonacci in AD 1250.

Gargantuan Relatives

Enchanted by my findings, I again turned my attention to nature's smallest components. Leaping forward in time to 1953 and more contemporary revelations made through microscopic surveys, scientists were finally able to unveil the structure of DNA, the recipe for the master plan of life. And what did they find?

That DNA has *a double helix (spiral) structure.*

The scope of correlations seemed infinite, for I found other examples in microbiology as well as in the heart. Substances that ignite the proteins that cause the heart's muscle contractions (such as myosin, actin, and tropomyosin)[108] all display the double helix structure. The same spiral arrangement within calcium ions can be observed by using scanning electron microscopy to look deeply into a cell.

I was uncovering an entire symphony of interrelated double helix forms — each reflecting spiral configurations that are the "keys to the natural kingdom." This unity stretches across a spectrum from microscopic ionic images to the macrostructure of the galaxy of spiral whorls in the heavens above us! (**Figure 6**)

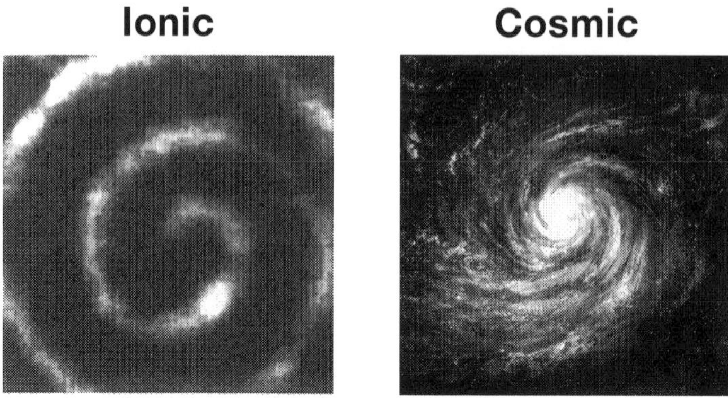

Figure 6: Gargantuan relatives, as the spiral exists in an ion of calcium, in the same way it appears in the cosmos.

We see many of the same patterns wherever we look, confirming an inevitable conclusion: *the heart is part of a greater design that exists within nature.*

Einstein believed in such possibilities, and, in fact, resisted the assumption of the innate randomness in the universe that was proposed by quantum mechanics. He famously said, "God does not play dice with the universe." In other words, God is not arbitrary in deciding how things will be. There is a grand plan, and I had found that the spiral and helix are fundamental to it.

As Close as Your Fingertips

Bringing it back to Earth and toward something relatable to us as humans, we can witness nature's spirals by looking at our own hands — our fingerprints. While all of us possess relatively similar-looking fingerprints, there are slight variations such that no two are alike. Amazingly, these overlapping clockwise and counterclockwise fingerprint spirals — resemble those at the vortex of our heart's apex! Could our "heart fingerprints" be another *unique human signature* and means of identification?

Even more stunning, while all fingerprint spirals are not the same, they all conform to the Fibonacci number, adhering to same 0.618.... ratio. Again, this elegance of agreement (innate similarity) and variance (with differences) prevails.

Impressionist Makes Lasting Impression

It was only after creating my lecture that I would realize my pathway into the "world of spirals" and *similarities with differences* probably began much earlier — starting with my fascination for a series of paintings by one of my favorite artists, Claude Monet, a French Impressionist. Long before meeting Paco, I was drawn to Monet's series of paintings from the late 1800s of haystacks near his home and of the cathedral in Rouen. In both cases, he painted the same objects numerous times under varying light conditions. I was captivated by how within each set of the haystacks and of the churches, he had identified commonality... while at the same time revealing variations. Each fresh vista differed due to the changing natural light. (**Figure** 7)

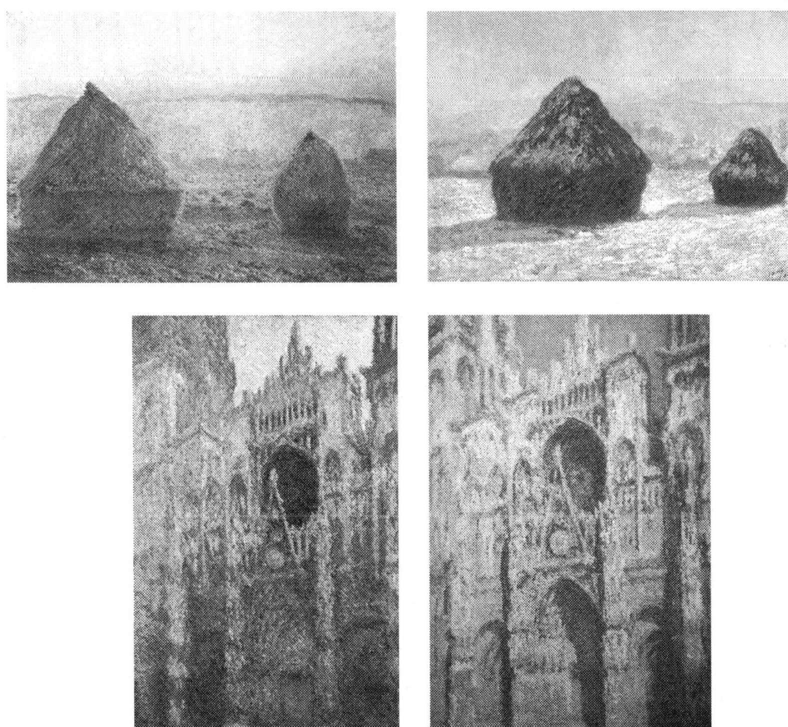

Figure 7: Variations within the same form by Monet.
Haystacks are above and Cathedral at Rouen below.

Though not conscious of it when formulating my lecture, I believe the impact of Monet's work predisposed my mind to search for the similarities and variances of the spiral. It was an unexpected alliance between great art and science.

Heart Architecture = Classic Architecture

The centerpiece of my presentation was always to be the heart, with the most powerful component to be my portrayal of Paco's contribution. I would demonstrate how he started with an intact heart, then unfolded it to initially show the circumferential wrap, and then separated the helical spiral arms in order to display the rope-like or "worm-like" structure of the unfolded heart. The majesty of its beauty heightens as Paco then refolds the splayed out form to perfectly rebuild the intact structure. (**Video 2**, a "replay" of the last chapter's video) I knew the audience would gasp at Paco's remarkable innovation, especially when followed by MRI images that verified these reciprocal spirals... and radioisotope studies that confirmed how this structure explains mechanical heart function. These tests established the vital bond between form and function — the essential groundwork of cardiac surgery knowledge.

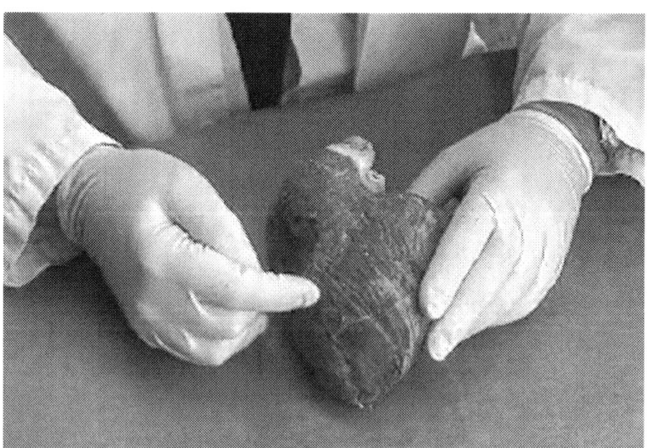

Video 2: Paco Torrent-Guasp unwraps the heart.

www.vimeo.com/buckberg/unwrapping-heart-1

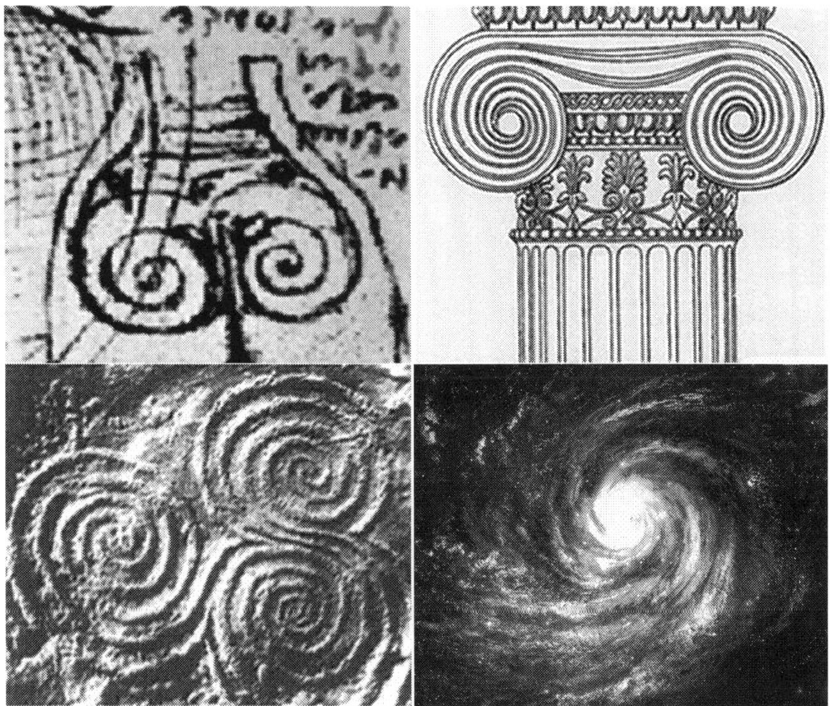

Figure 8: Similarity of spirals. Leonardo da Vinci shows heart flow into aorta (upper left), Greek columns (upper right), prehistoric graves (lower left), and in galaxies (lower right).

Yet beyond its presence in our own human form, we can also witness spirals in *what we build and create.* In fact, one might wonder (as I did), if it was simply those aortic reciprocal spirals in the heart that so impressed Leonardo… or whether it was the commonality they shared with the clockwise and counterclockwise spirals that existed at the top of Greek columns built in 500 BC… or the spiral images placed on graves by prehistoric people in 5000 BC… or the galaxy. (**Figure 8**)

Continuing to develop my presentation, I recognized further ways that man-made structures reflect our heart structure. The most obvious were comparisons of similarities between the heart's configuration and classical architectural design.

The Greeks built temples with columns to support its framework. These pillars needed to be placed close together in order to provide sufficient strength to support the upper horizontal beams and prevent them from collapsing. Yet this configuration only permitted a few people at a time to walk between the pillars for entry or exit. The next development was made by the Romans, who introduced a semicircle configuration, in which stresses were offset by a centerpiece at an upper central focal point. This was the point of greatest compression by arch forces. With greater space between pillars, more people could now walk through these semicircular forms, but there were still limitations. There was instability when higher and wider archways were used to facilitate traffic. This explains why the Roman Coliseum has three levels. A new design was needed.

An apex-like structure (having a singular, highest focal point) emerged, its form evident even in the simple huts and tents created by Celtics or Native Americans. These structures differed as their stress forces proceeded downward — and were counteracted by a buttress construction on (and within) the ground that maintained the integrity of the cone. (**Figure 9a**)

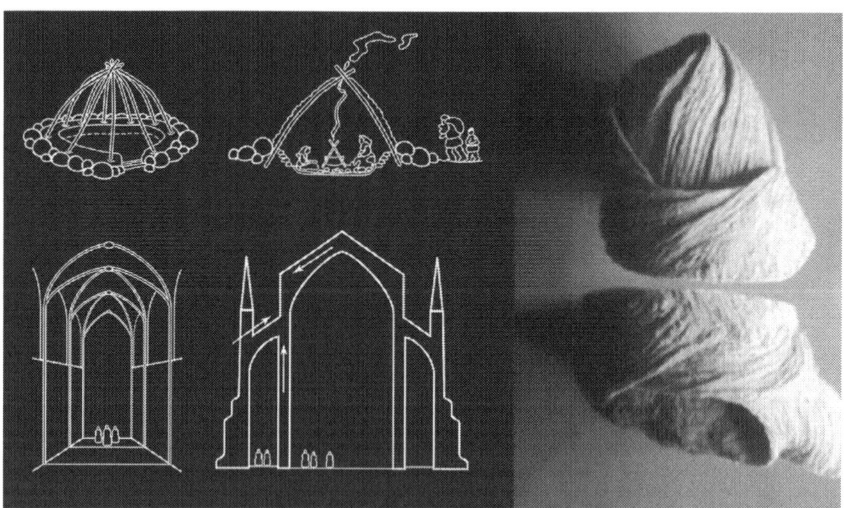

Figure 9a: Top is architecture of hut, with a conical dome and a wrap like a buttress, while bottom shows a cathedral with a dome and flying buttresses for external support.

Figure 9b: a heart with a similar conical component that is surrounded by a buttress.

Moreover, I found that creating larger tent-like structures to bring in even more people had required construction of an *external buttress*, which formed a brace. The Gothic arch then evolved. Its support simulates (**Figure 9a**) the heart's "wrap" in the form of external flying buttresses that support the classic Gothic domes of grand cathedrals. How astounding that this man-made construction of a place to worship *exactly parallels* the cardiac dome containing an apex, which is braced by its surrounding and supportive *basal wrap*. (**Figure 9b**)

This architectural similarity underscores my whimsical question, "Which was first — the church or the heart?" No answer is needed, since "truth" evolves from recognizing this *unified game plan* (incorporating nature, human, and the heart).

The Heart of Nature's Majestic Plan

By this point in the research, I was certain that the heart fit within nature's overall scheme. Yet this helical structure serves different functions in different natural realms. Yes, it gives the eland's reciprocal spiral horns incredible strength and durability. But particularly important to our attendees' understanding — was that this powerful helix structure is also responsible for the heart's narrowing, shortening, lengthening, widening, twisting, and uncoiling motions. I planned to show a video clip during my lecture to reveal the overall splendor of these clockwise and counterclockwise movements of the *working* heart — motions that Paco called the "cardiac dance."

As often the case, each piece of new information is accompanied by a new question. I began to wonder about the right and left spiral arm muscles interweaving in the helical heart — that create the beautiful twisting and uncoiling actions of Paco's "cardiac dance." Could they be in the same ratio as described for other spirals?

That thought spurred me down to the lab, where I eagerly unraveled Paco's rope-like model of the heart. Nobody had ever made these measurements.

I couldn't believe what I found.

The left and right-handed sides (or arms) of the helix were in that same ratio of 0.618. This was nothing less than staggering! It demonstrated the same Fibonacci proportional dimensions that correspond precisely to the ratio that Pythagoras described within the golden section (**Figure 10**) — and further certified the unity of man, the heart, and mathematics. *It is there if you look, and then you see.*

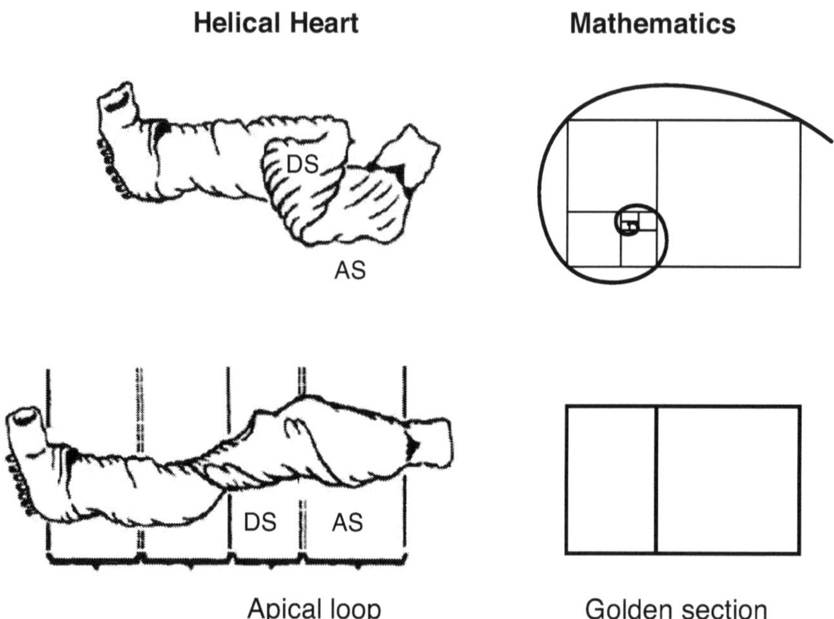

Figure 10: Relationship of helical heart to mathematics. Above, the helical heart whose spiral is partially unfolded, adjacent to the spiral of mathematics formed by golden proportion. Below, the helix is unwrapped, and the proportional size of the descending (DS) and ascending segments (AS) is in complete harmony with the golden section.

I could be only further awed at how the heart is part of this grand scheme. Cardiac muscle contains a hidden, yet remarkable harmony of spirals, beginning with the DNA double helix that provides the blueprint of life. Its reciprocal spiral configuration is similar to the heart's clockwise and counterclockwise muscle arrangement. These double spiral muscles are the same ones fully active in a beating ventricle of a normal person without heart disease... providing the natural *twisting and uncoiling movements* responsible for ejection and suction.

These natural motions are easily evident from the magnetic resonance and echocardiographic imaging scans that our patients may routinely undergo.

This principle — that motion will be produced by its underlying architectural structure — emphasizes the credo that *we must understand structure* to treat heart disease.

The Lecture

The day of the presentation arrived. Here was the test of whether the fascination that had captivated me during my preparations could be transmitted to the 4,000 curious cardiac surgeons that attended this Basic Science Lecture.

I asked them a fundamental question as I began: "Why would a heart surgeon get so involved in looking at spirals?"

I posed this query because its answer addresses the foundation to our specialty: structure is the absolute centerpiece of surgery. Our approaches differ from medical ones that use drugs or electrical stimulation (pacemakers) to address specific ailments. Instead, our job is to restore the heart's structure. We view disease as a distortion of normality, and our goal is to bring normality back. Our ability to succeed in this pursuit stems from how deeply we understand natural structure.

This was the first time I had ever publically discussed the helical heart and explained why the helix is critical. I described that its structure contained two arms composed of oblique (slanted) fibers that cross each other at 60° angles. This form allows the normal heart to pump out 60% of its volume (percentage of blood in the heart's ventricle that is ejected out into the body per beat — the ejection fraction).

Further, I explained that congestive heart failure develops because of a loss of the heart's natural spiral shape. This distortion by heart attack or disease will make the normally conical or elliptical helical shape (like a football) become dilated or stretched as its form becomes spherical (like a basketball). The disrupted architectural pattern makes the angles of muscle fibers change to closer to 30°, which impairs function — causing the ejection fraction to fall to 30% or less. Again, I made an analogy to the high school quarterback who can throw a perfect spiral pass 50 yards, while the premier basketball player is inaccurate from only 20 yards. Performance is independent of the player's underlying talent. Performance is related *to form*, and this is dramatically true for treating heart failure.

I knew that unraveling this relationship was central, since conventional treatment options *have never been aimed at fixing the distorted ventricular form.* Rather, their primary objectives (by means of bypassing obstructed coronary arteries, or repairing or replacing a defective valve) have *only* focused upon correcting the *reason* behind why the elliptical ventricle became a dilated spherical shape. Missing was the understanding of the need *to correct the dilated ventricle itself.* Instead, heart transplantation or mechanical assist devices were used to *replace the heart* if the dilation was extensive. The valid (and preferred) treatment option of using a surgical procedure that *returns the natural conical shape* to the dilated heart... was never considered.

Yet I pointed out that the spherical shape remains following conventional treatments of all ventricles stretched beyond 60 ml/m 2. This easily explains the often dire outcome of progressive heart failure — regardless of whether the cause was a heart attack, leaking heart valves, or disease in the heart muscle itself. I further noted that the alternate approach of heart replacement by transplantation was not common due to the limited donor pool, and that mechanical ventricular assist devices were problematic due to infection and abnormal blood clotting.

These well-known limitations led me to introduce the phrase "fix the ventricle" — a novel strategy I believed would be an essential part of all future treatments of congestive heart failure.

I saw a new world before us: we must return the spherical chamber to its natural elliptical form.

Restoration = Rebuilding

My Helix and Heart lecture was delivered before the STICH Trail began, and had a dual purpose. Our international RESTORE team (whose membership was described earlier) would present our findings on approximately 1,200

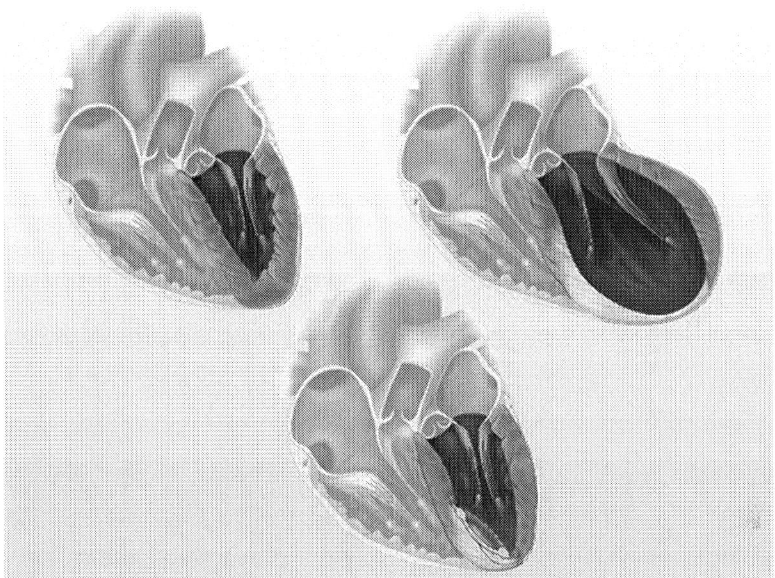

Figure 11: How ventricular restoration rebuilds normal shape. Upper left is normal conical or elliptical shape. Upper right is failing heart with spherical shape, caused by scar (in white). Below is restored heart configuration, with return to normality.

consecutive congestive heart failure (CHF) patients for the first time at this AATS meeting. Their surgical approach to rebuild the stretched ventricle was based on the breakthrough work of Dr. Vincent Dor of Monaco — who taught how to restore the natural elliptical form by excluding the heart attack scar that had created the dilated spherical heart. (**Figure 11**)

Connie Athanasuleas would report on our team effort, his presentation describing the astounding success achieved in congestive heart failure patients after their ventricular shape and volume was rebuilt into a normal configuration.

During my basic science lecture, I would additionally focus on my reasons for beginning the RESTORE team, a group that stemmed from my asking, "Who are we, as physicians, to invent the rules on how the heart should be treated? Instead, it seems most important to follow nature's design — and thus dedicate our efforts toward rebuilding the natural architecture."

Treasured Tradition: Learning from Others

My exploring the grandeur of this cardiac architecture — in particular, the heart's apex and surrounding wrap — led to intriguing analogies to other aspects of human existence. This proved to be especially moving for me due to a personal experience in 1982. I recalled a visit to Jerusalem, Israel where I purchased a prayer shawl, or "tallis," for my dad. Every Saturday, he would take it with him to worship. Returning home on one of those occasions, he told my mom, "While wearing this tallis in synagogue, it felt like Gerald's arms were around me." Tears still well up in my eyes each time I recount this. I picture my father surrounded by my gift... and me. Yet the broad parallels of the helix and wrap even mirrored this undeniable human quality. (**Figure 12**)

Helix and Wrap

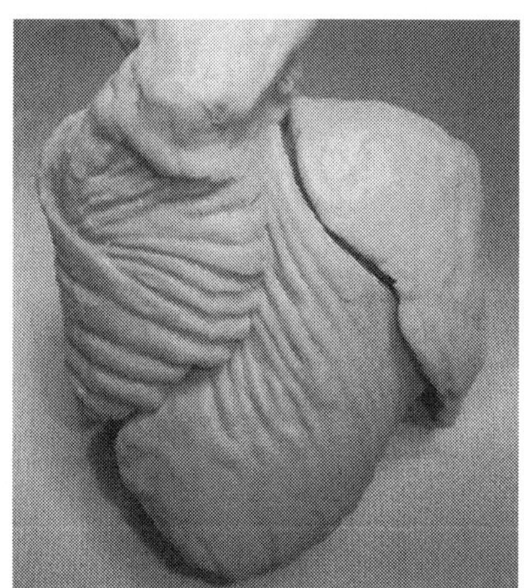

Heart

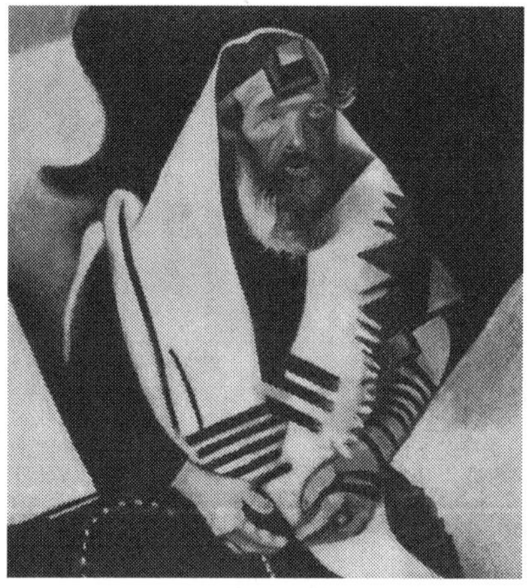

Human

Figure 12: The helix and wrap and the human.
On left is heart with a conical apex, surrounded by wrap.
On right, a painting from Chagall showing a rabbi, who forms the conical part as he is wrapped in a prayer shawl for heavenly support.

But there was even more to the connection.

When I visited my mom during her final illness, I learned you ultimately gain the traits of those you love and respect by recognizing their special qualities. When they depart, these characteristics become yours completely. While your arms and shoulders may have been what literally embraced them, it is your receiving their gift of guidance… that allows you to see further than you otherwise could.

For me, this was not only true of my father and mother, but also of the many mentors who have impacted my life. You love, admire, and ultimately learn from them. You take on their best qualities, and hopefully honor them by passing those along. As our teachers advise and serve as a source of wisdom, they become a focus — an apex — from which we, whose arms wrap around them, then emerge to teach others. A proper legacy is when your students will take what you offer, and then give it to their students.

This tradition of learning, teaching, and guiding is something I strive to continue.

"My Apex"

I hoped to pass along such wisdom during my basic science lecture at AATS.

As I've said, the origins of this presentation came from my transformative meeting with Paco Torrent-Guasp three years earlier. Paco had developed his ideas 40 years earlier as a medical student. But despite their truth, these ideas were discarded by "experts" in anatomy and cardiology. This age-old dilemma was discouraging to Paco, but my eyes opened anew as I suddenly saw how his wisdom might become a legendary contribution.

Fortunately, all his findings were recorded in a book in Spanish that he gave to me (copies were not available in the U.S.). It was captivating. One exciting and notable detail was that the description of the vortex formation at the apex of the heart also corresponds to the tip of a hurricane… where its

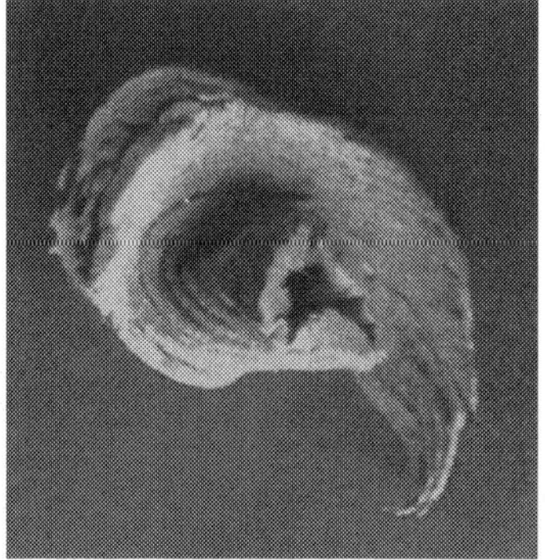

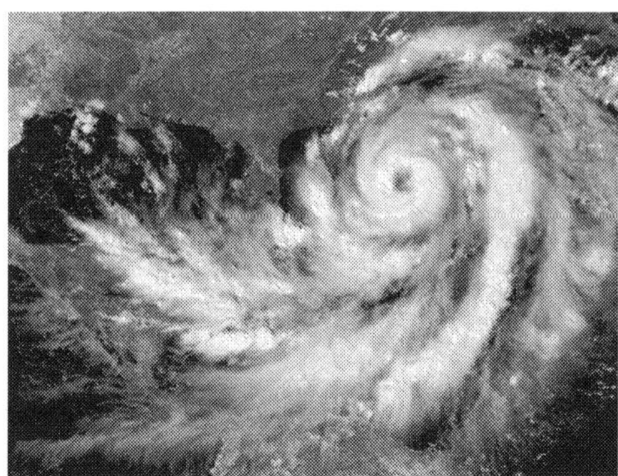

Figure 13: On left is view of heart that shows the whorl shape that starts at the spiral in its apex. On right are the whorls of a hurricane that have the same configuration as exists within the heart.

powerful spiral movements mirror the same rotations that exist in the heart as it produces efficient ventricular function. (**Figure 13**)

Recognizing the importance of similarities *and differences in related forms,* I had my lecture include the previously mentioned contrast to the hurricane (like the tornado) that does not contain a *circumferential buttress* or wrap to contain its energy. As a result, its top portions make larger and larger whorls, causing its trajectory to expand many miles wide. The wrap brace allows the heart to expend its energies into producing blood flow to the body, rather than allowing lateral explosion of its forces.

Conversely, I pointed out that the heart has the basal wrap around it, and this buttress maintains its physical integrity (otherwise, the heart would literally explode or implode when ejecting or sucking in blood). With this wrap harnessing its power, the heart pumps blood through *over 60,000 miles* of vessels, over 100,000 times a day, and 35 million beats a year throughout your life.

Yet there was something else even more profound that I needed to address.

I had found Paco's unraveling of the heart miraculous when he first unfolded it like a rope or worm for me, and I asked, "How did you come upon that idea?" Paco replied that he had studied the evolutionary development of humans. He described how we evolved from worms over one billion years ago, with a vascular tube (rather than conventional heart) that looks much like a rope. By 400 million years ago, a fish had evolved, with gills and a single pumping chamber (heart). Then by 200 million years ago, amphibians and reptiles developed, leaving the water to walk, having a two-chambered heart with just a single atrium and ventricle. Then by 100,000 years ago, the human emerged, with our recognizable four-chambered human heart. I was astounded by this knowledge, and certain my surgical colleagues would be equally delighted as I shared it. And I would find there was still more that was just as extraordinary.

Recognizing a certain familiarity to these different stages, I reviewed the development of the heart's anatomy during the brief gestation period of the human fetus — and found something quite stunning. At 20 days, the blood vessel system of the human embryo looks just like a worm. At 25 days, the first generation of a heart appears with a single pumping chamber, as occurs with a fish. At 35 days, the heart appears like that of the amphibian and reptile. Finally, at 50 days, the human heart is now formed. During this 50-day gestation period in all humans — we have each bridged one billion years of history.

The Essence of Learning

I gained important insights in preparing for this presentation, not only about how the heart functions and its deeper connection to nature's grander scheme, but also how the world responds to such new knowledge. Harvey's landmark writings from the 1600s taught us a wonderful lesson about our masters — they may be superb, but are not perfect. Yet the "experts of today" closely mirror those who wrongly believed Harvey — those who had cast away the valid concepts of Erasistratus and Galen about twisting and sucking. Sadly, critics continued to create barriers that curtailed others from properly recognizing Paco's legendary contributions to cardiovascular medicine.

History is the ultimate determiner of when truth will win. Yet along the way, new ideas, and most importantly, *the subsequent human reaction to them*, will create dynamic contrasts. It always has. A perfect example can be seen in the *responses* to theories about how the heart fills.

Opposition to both new — and old — medical concepts has pervaded history. We've already cited that Harvey *contradicted Galen* by saying the heart filled by pressure and was not a sucking cup. Galen had made his fundamental observation of the ventricles suctioning blood long before, in AD 180, when reporting the "violent sucking of blood" from the vena cava (two large veins) as he looked within the chest of a gladiator whose injury exposed the heart's biology.

Yet even though Erasistratus (the previously mentioned father of physiology) had also observed this same suction used by the heart to achieve venous return, *Galen was dismissive of him.* Galen freely notes that he did not like Erasistratus as he felt him dishonest in how he came to his theories. In fact, Galen disliked Lycus of Macedonia (an anatomist with additional theories) even more. He thought Lycus was pompous and not worthy to be considered alongside many other wonderful Greeks.

But Galen also made the most wonderful and insightful comment on the concept of learning. Despite all of this criticism, he said that Lycus "...is not to be disregarded; he may, perhaps, be stating some wonderful truth, unknown to any of his predecessors." Galen knew that no matter how much we personally like or dislike someone, or accept or reject their overall approach — we must continue to listen in order to learn.

This affected me profoundly, and led to my own observation: *Ignorance is being unknowledgeable, but able to learn... while arrogance is being knowledgeable, but unable to be taught.* It characterizes the pundits that believe in the yesterdays of tradition, but fail to look toward the future.

Symbol of Medicine... More than a Symbol

To advance medicine, we must retain our student-like ways. As we do, we enter what I call the "spiral pathway of learning."

This caduceus, (**Figure 14**) the symbol of the medical profession, is fittingly composed of two reciprocal spirals. These are interwoven, and from my perspective, this shape reflects a path to learning and then to wisdom. Near the top where a spiral is largest, we gather and enlarge our knowledge. As we

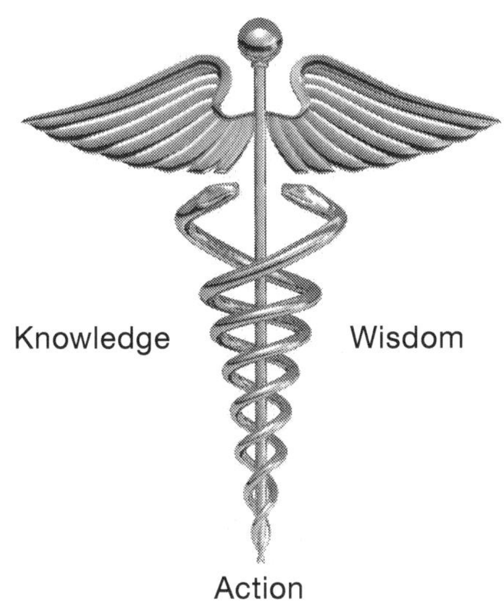

Figure 14: Caduceus, the signpost of medicine, displays the same reciprocal spirals as in the helix, but contains a staff between them, conveying the need for action.

move down one spiral loop, we interact with this information to analyze and differentiate it. Simultaneously, in the other spiral, we synthesize these facts and bring them together into a concept. We develop *wisdom.*

But that is not the end point. We must *do something* with this wisdom. A surgeon cannot be like a monk sitting on a hill. There must be movement of knowledge. A concept, an approach, or a technique must be created and then tested. As cardiac surgeons, we are particularly fortunate because we can learn, we can understand, and we can act on the behalf of our patients.

Recognizing this progression, and the absolute need for us to always remain willing to learn, led me to what became the final statement I would make in my presentation. It would be another quote from Albert Einstein, who said:

"There exists a passion for comprehension, just as there exists a passion for music. That passion is rather common in children, but gets lost in most people later on."

I would supplement my hero by saying: *"I hope not!"*

The Presentation at AATS

All of this thought went into the preparation for my basic science lecture at the AATS, which went extremely well. After I made my last remark and departed the stage, there was a ten-minute standing ovation from the audience of 4,000 surgeons... which I heard from my seat in the audience.

Francis Fontan, a dear friend and legend within our cardiac surgery profession, later asked me why did I had not remained at the lectern to receive the ovation. I simply told him I left because I was finished. Looking at me knowingly, Francis said, "You gave them your mind, and took your body away."

While I was elated to give the lecture, it wasn't about my receiving glory or applause. I was not looking to take credit for being a great lecturer. What was astounding was the information and correlations presented. Nature is the actual presenter and should get all the credit.

Francis and I both knew the true worth of science is only appreciated when the mind of the listener begins to accept new knowledge, after which they test this novel information to verify it, and a fresh view of reality then follows to create a new biological truth. That was my intention and hope behind delivering the talk.

Of course, people will respond however they respond. Andy Wechsler, who was the editor of the *Journal of Thoracic and Cardiovascular Surgery* for eight years, once described me as the "Intellectual Provocateur of Heart Surgery."

That portrayal may have been accurate, but I preferred the comment made by a physician from Russia who remarked, "You saw the invisible and taught it to us." It was the nicest thing anyone has ever said to me.

Yet I am not the first, nor will I be the last, to teach "the invisible." Our basic observations of cardiac suction began with the Greeks, were altered by Harvey, and are now changing back again to authentically reflect what occurs in nature. The reason for such progress — this "revolution" — is that the truth always wins. New knowledge changes the thinking of the listener, who in turn changes their actions.

Circling Around

While writing this book and reflecting on my experience of creating this lecture, I came to a fascinating recognition. Looking again at Monet's series of paintings cited earlier, I noted all his haystacks had a wide base and an apical tip like an inverted heart, while his cathedral possessed lateral support from flying buttresses. These are the two primary components of the heart — its base and helix.

Was this Monet's mindset, or did it reflect my imagination? What is certain was that Monet saw a new world every time he looked. It is just like the experience I shared with my daughters as we walked down the same street and saw new things. That is what Monet did. He played the game of discovery.

And so, the tradition of learning continues.

The Helix and Heart lecture can be viewed at:
www.youtube.com/watch?v=ArZ8GEFUQaw

Further, the talk was formally written up with greater detail in the *Journal of Thoracic and Cardiac Surgery,* which can be accessed at:
http://www.jtcvsonline.org/article/S0022-5223(02)00169-1/fulltext

CHAPTER 20

The Helix and Heart Failure: The Dilated Heart, Footballs, and Basketballs

Curious colleagues often ask me why this memoir is being written for the non-medical public, since until now, all of my publications have been directed exclusively at the medical community.

I recall a conversation I had with another colleague and friend, Connie Athanasuleas, who related a discussion he had with his mother. While sharing their time-honored traditional Greek salad, his mom, who had congestive heart failure, asked her heart surgeon son about a new procedure she saw on the television news (three years before our RESTORE team was formed). A surgeon from Brazil had removed a piece of heart muscle in a dilated heart in order to change its size and shape. Connie's mom, despite her lack of medical knowledge, thought this seemed like an interesting idea. Connie was unaware of the procedure, but immediately appreciated the approach, and agreed that it introduced an intriguing solution to an otherwise lethal problem.

The surgeon was Randas Batista, who I've mentioned before, and whose work will be described in this chapter. When confronted with new knowledge like this, a person can respond in one of two ways. Inquisitive physicians like Connie may not be aware of novel treatment breakthroughs that might solve conditions previously thought unsolvable, but they listen and are spurred to learn more. On the other hand, there are physicians, unlike Connie, who might know of some new procedure, but are hesitant to change. Their own traditional viewpoints are so limiting that they dismiss innovations that could have life-changing and life-saving importance.

My hope is that readers will mirror the curiosity of Connie's mother and welcome new discoveries such as those described in this and other chapters. Discoveries that might lead to compelling, persuasive conversations with their doctors to potentially open *their* eyes to new possibilities.

I believe patients must inform themselves. They should not just wait passively for someone to tell them what to do. Whether it is for their own life, the life of a loved one, or simply from intense curiosity, we all need to pay attention to forward-looking treatments. Groundbreaking advances are constantly being made in all areas of medicine, as pioneers search out new solutions to age-old problems. Fresh answers must be encouraged and outmoded mindsets changed. Sometimes it is the patient that instigates the reversal of medical inflexibility.

A New Angle on Dilated Hearts

After learning of Paco's discoveries, I grew even more fascinated with the heart. Paco presented glorious new information when he unveiled its true structure. This deeper understanding of how the heart becomes distorted would provide answers about how to treat the world's greatest health hazard: congestive heart failure.

We had already recognized the structural and functional differences that occur when heart failure causes the heart's size and shape to enlarge from the normal elliptical *football* shape to become spherical like a *basketball* (**Figure 1a and b**). We knew the changed heart shape was the source of the problems generated by heart failure. But the full understanding of *why* had eluded us... *until Paco's structural analysis furnished that answer.*

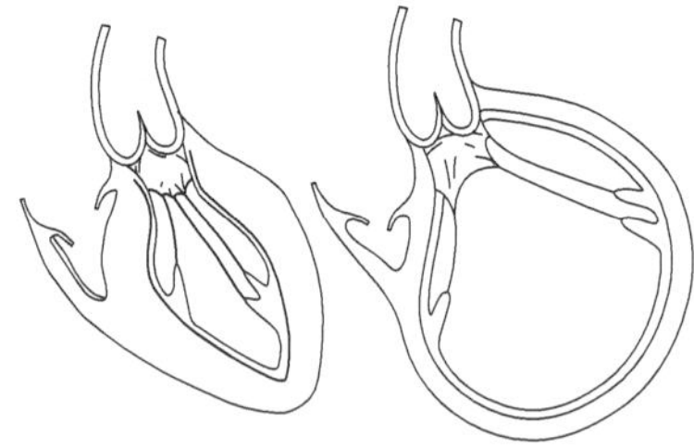

Figure 1a: Normal conical heart on left, compared to the dilated spherical heart in heart failure on right.

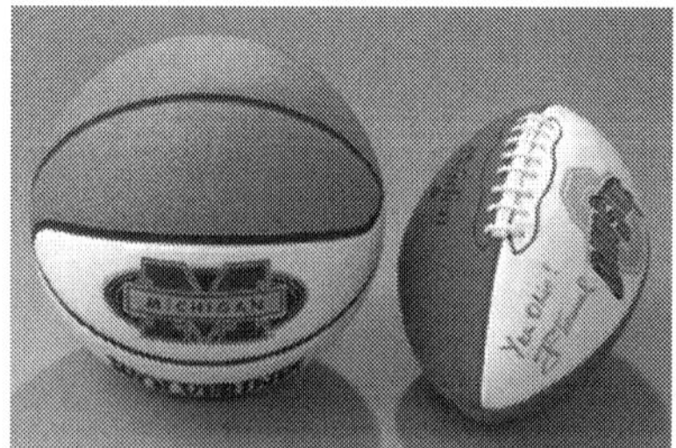

Figure 1b: Shows sports analogy, with spherical "heart" on left and conical heart on right.

Paco let us explore the *mechanical reasons* behind the problem of heart failure by revealing that heart musculature is formed by a helix and a basal wrap. (**Figure 2 upper**) We learned that the transverse (horizontal) muscle fibers of the wrap caused squeezing or compression (like a blood pressure cuff on your arm). Conversely, the diagonal fibers of the helix permitted the predominant function of *twisting* — as they crossed each other at 60° angles. The simplicity and elegance were astounding.

It suddenly was clear that as heart failure alters the cardiac structure to make the elliptical heart become spherical — this shape change makes its oblique (slanted at 60°) helix fibers *more horizontal* — to now resemble the wrap's flatter fiber angles. (**Figure 2 lower**)

But *why* does this geometric change create such a functional problem?

I discovered a breathtaking study by Edward Sallin that explained the relationship between the angle of muscle fibers and function. Sallin was a bio-mathematician, who in 1969, identified how the orientation of heart muscle fibers determined the heart movement. He showed that each individual

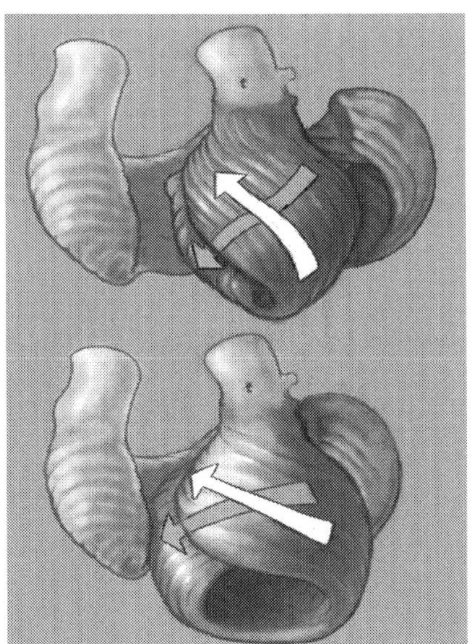

Figure 2: Upper drawing is normal architecture, with the helical arms reciprocally crossing each other at 60° angles. Lower drawing of dilated heart as fibers become more transverse (horizontal), at approximately 30° angles.

heart muscle fiber shortens by only 15% during compression at each heartbeat — yet in a heart with an *oblique (angled) fiber orientation* — the heart will eject 60% of its blood to circulate into the body (the normal response) during each heartbeat. Conversely, performance is impaired when these same fibers *have a horizontal orientation* — as *their contraction yields only a 30%* ejection fraction.[109]

Sallin's contribution was enormous because he had structurally solved the missing gap, as he used form to explain function!

I now fully understood *why* heart performance worsens when the cardiac form changes from the normal elliptical shape that contains obliquely angled fibers — into a dilated spherical shape where fibers are more horizontal. These observations validate the fundamental objective of rebuilding normality: we must return the fibers to their expected 60° angles in order to permit recovery of the heart's natural function. (**Figure 2**)

Different Heart Diseases — Same Focus

What a revelation! Yet while I now had the complete explanation behind the need to restore the heart's natural shape, I also knew that all conventional medical efforts were still totally aimed only at solving the illness that caused the heart to dilate (such as restoring adequate blood flow and preventing leaky valves) — rather than restoration of ventricular structure. Now more than ever, the spotlight needed to shine on correcting *the dilation itself.*

The medical community needed to realize that this missing knowledge leads to a critical error in judgment. The circular shape *is the consistent detrimental factor* in the three major causes of heart failure with dilated hearts:

- The heart attack — in which the ventricle has a scar the causes the remote muscle to stretch as it dilates
- A leaky valve — that makes the ventricle dilate
- The heart muscle itself — when infections or viruses cause dilation, despite the presence of normal blood vessels and valves

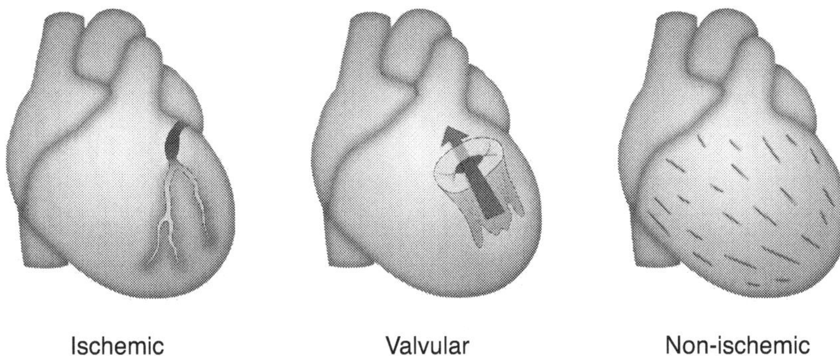

Figure 3: The three causes of a dilated heart include: on left, a heart attack due to a closed coronary artery; in center, a leaky aortic or mitral heart valve; and on right, direct damage of the heart muscle.

These three origins of heart failure are shown in **Figure 3**. They all share the same inescapable destructive spherical shape. *A circle is a circle is a circle*, regardless of the basic underlying disease causing this globular shape.

Heart failure cannot be cured until you convert the failing heart's spherical shape into its natural elliptical form. However, this is never the singular solution. Successful treatment *must also remedy* the disease that produced this shape distortion (such as coronary disease or leaky heart valves). Embracing these dual goals can have an immense impact — because dilated hearts exist in half of the 15 million patients with heart failure.

Heart Attacks — New Ideas, Old Resistance

Heart attacks are the primary cause of heart dilation in the United States. Before exploring the focus of this chapter, let me review how such dilation is now typically treated — and how the development of rebuilding natural ventricular shape has restored the heart's function.

The first prior approach was angioplasty by cardiologists, since this treatment restores blood flow and corrects the surface bulge (aneurysm). But it leaves a non-contracting, thickened muscle in its place. Cardiac surgeons sometimes participated in the initial treatment response by performing a bypass graft to renew flow in obstructed arteries, and also correct leaky mitral valves. Despite satisfactory early survival of patients, the long-term outcomes are problematic when the heart becomes dilated.[86] Patients with such stretched spherical hearts have a worsened quality of life due to heart failure or may develop lethal arrhythmias. Yet this fundamental cause of heart failure remains untreated.

Dor's concepts got me thinking about the geometric reasons for heart failure. The target area of our thinking was his focus upon the scar. While this is what causes the heart to stretch, conventional medicine ignores it. The role of the heart is to contract and support the circulation, and while the scarred region stops working immediately, the patient is kept alive by the still-functioning remote muscle that compensates for the dead scar. But we must now focus upon how to improve its function, because heart failure will develop progressively, despite such compensation. The reason for such impairment is linked to understanding the heart's anatomy, because cardiac performance is determined by how the heart's muscle fibers are oriented within its structural form. Healthy function occurs when they are slanted (as in a normal heart shaped elliptically like a football), but performance is dramatically diminished when the fibers become horizontal (as when the heart is stretched like a basketball).

These lessons were not only illuminated by Dor, Paco, and Sallin. Richard Gorlin stated in 1967 that the *prelude to heart failure* was having a scar that occupied more than 20% of the ventricular muscle.[77] He also observed that this structural change stretched the functioning remote muscle, which then compensated by contracting more forcibly. Returning a more normal shape was the objective of the surgical breakthroughs in 1983 by Dor[79] and Jatene.[83] Each observed that their patients fared much better, characterized by vastly improved cardiac function — when their ventricular approach excluded the scar by restoring the natural elliptical shape — to a previously failing spherical heart.

The Dor and Jatene surgical solutions departed from tradition... and a revolution was in the making. Validation of their approaches was powerfully shown in the superb clinical successes reported by our RESTORE Group, and in the 5,000 other patients described in the congestive heart failure chapter.[94]

But still, no one listened.

Not the Whole Answer

I was undaunted that traditionalists blindly held onto conventional treatment. Rather, I was exhilarated that our international confirmation of the Dor procedure in dilated hearts might help set a new standard for treating heart failure.

However, my enthusiasm was incomplete. Another dilemma confronted us.

As good as our outcomes had been, they were not always perfect. Only limited recovery occurred after rebuilding *very dilated ventricles.* I pondered the reason for this failure. Was the operation incorrect? Or was this technique simply less effective in very stretched hearts?

This much was very clear to me: *these pivotal questions needed answering!*

The Batista Solution

We started by making a "logical" guess that we had waited too long before intervening and the muscle had stretched too much. We assumed that a rebuilding procedure could not improve such an expanded muscle.

Yet that conclusion came from a deduction. It was not an answer.

That's when I remembered something. My visit to Randas Batista in Brazil blazed into my thoughts, as I recalled how I had been riveted while watching him geometrically return a very large dilated heart back into its natural shape. Until then, our focus was on the heart that became spherical after developing a scar after a heart attack, but Batista addressed the same circular shape that was due instead to a disease in the heart muscle, or secondary stretch from leaky heart valves. The credo of "a circle is a circle is a circle" rang true. Batista simply approached a different disease that also produced the same amount of spherical heart dilation.

As I thought back to what led up to my visit, I recalled that a cardiac surgical colleague, Tomas Salerno, who was Brazilian, had phoned me from his office at the University of Miami to tell me that a surgeon named Randas Batista had achieved phenomenal results after treating heart failure *by removing a part of the heart* in patients who hadn't had a heart attack.

Needless to say, I was eager to go to Brazil to meet Batista and learn about what he was doing. Coincidentally, Batista turned out to be the same Brazilian surgeon that Connie's mother had seen on a TV news program, as mentioned at the beginning of this chapter.

My quest began as I flew to Curitiba in southern Brazil, where Batista worked in a private hospital near the jungle. He described to me how he returned the natural elliptical shape to a dilated ventricle. The method involved removing a wedge of ventricular muscle from its side wall to allow him to reshape the heart as he closed the ventricle. Most operations were done in patients suffering from a chronic heart muscle infection, called Chagas Disease.

This educational experience was uniquely inspiring. I initially watched Batista perform this procedure, then assisted him, and finally did two of the operations with his help. I recognized that this novel procedure that *reshaped the heart back to its natural elliptical form* was absolutely unheard-of!

And it worked.

Opening the Door on the Dor Procedure

Batista's success had far reaching implications, since it took a circular heart that had no scar, and rebuilt the natural ventricular shape. This Brazil visit opened a huge door in my thinking, as I now understood why Dor's method was less effective in very large and dilated ventricles. Instead of only zeroing in on the rebuilding goal of excluding the scar... Batista introduced the *core concept of changing the ventricular form back to its natural form.* This groundbreaking development refocused me into establishing a new primary objective: to restore an elliptical shape in a dilated heart... independent of what caused its stretching.

This appreciation stimulated my revisiting the ground rules for doing the Dor procedure. That reevaluation was certainly needed, as many other surgeons from around the world had encountered less favorable results after rebuilding very large ventricular chambers. Exclusion of the scar was properly performed, yet the stretched remote muscle *stayed stretched.* The ventricular chamber was made a bit smaller *but remained spherical.* The gap in our thinking became apparent, as we had only looked at the scar *but failed to see the persistent and detrimental circular shape.* (The Batista visit had preceded the RESTORE group formation by several years.)

This newly found vision made me refocus upon the role of simple geometry. For a new breakthrough to emerge, form needed to take center stage. This did not contradict the critical importance of excluding the scar. Instead, it made us begin to understand that in *very enlarged ventricles,* the scar occupies a relatively small portion of the cardiac wall. Consequently, scar exclusion alone does not substantially change the spherical chamber's shape.[110] Thus, our failure to sufficiently restore the remote muscle's oblique (slanted) 60° fiber angles — resulted in the limited improvement that consistently followed our performing SVR in very dilated hearts.

The new focus needed to be reshaping the ventricular form — not just addressing the disease (scar) that caused the ventricular stretch. (**Figure 4**)

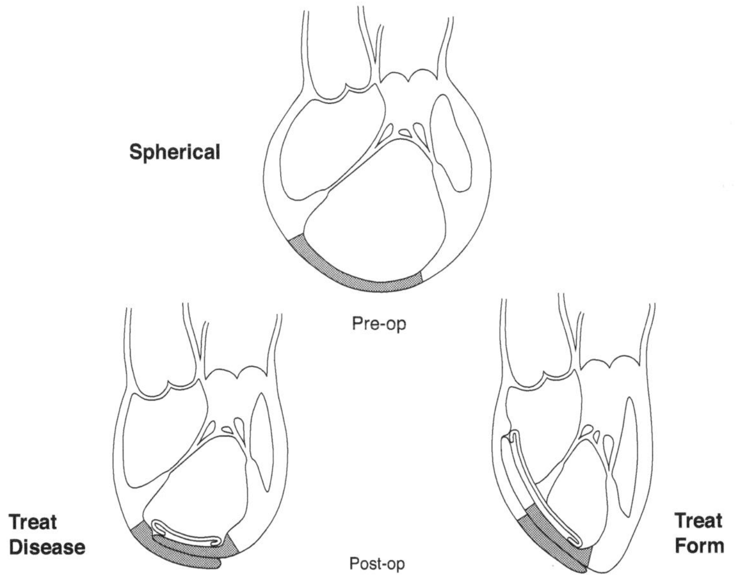

Figure 4: Surgical restoration for a failing spherical heart (upper image) after a heart attack. Lower left is treating the scar (disease). Lower right is treating form to rebuild natural ellipse.

This expanded range of thinking made me wonder if we had now fully replicated nature. I looked forward to testing whether bringing the very enlarged ventricular shape back into a normal configuration could deliver widespread positive results. Such a prize would yield the ultimate reward for patients and affirm the benefits of my traveling along the discovery pathway.

The Batista Solution Was Not Consistent

The basic tenet of science is that while ideas stimulate action, their validity only comes from proving they are correct. Reports of Batista's approach had begun to appear in various medical journals, describing the same excellent outcomes that I had witnessed during my brief visit to Curitiba, in which the seemingly incurable patient became dramatically healthy by reshaping the ventricle.

There was great excitement about this breakthrough among the medical community. Some cardiac surgeons realized they could finally approach the failing dilated heart (where the spherical shape was due to disease in their cardiac muscle rather than from a scar after a heart attack), and began to apply Batista's technique to very sick heart failure patients.

But results varied greatly, as 50% of patients either did not initially survive or died within the first two years. A powerful adverse response followed. Batista was called "A surgeon from the jungle who did a useless procedure." No one believed his sensational results, and he was uniformly repudiated.

It got worse when statistical reports tabulated results from many international centers and "certified" the high death rate from the Batista procedure. This account followed traditional medical guidelines in which a statistician provides conclusions after using the algorithms that everyone believes to be essential for determining the meaning of the data. Yet something very powerful is missing: the understanding that "statisticians deal with numbers, but have no knowledge of where these numbers come from." For example, did they arise from suitably selected patients? Or are they certain the operations were done properly?

Nor did the statisticians comprehend the full medical meaning of their numerical observations. In this case, the dramatic *reversal of a terminal disease* in 50% of patients would confirm a vital and profound finding. Such a dynamic outcome simply cannot happen "by itself" or by "accident." Yet the statistician's never-ending response is, "Show me more patients to see if I can come up with better numbers to sanction this procedure."

It is this disparity that provides the seeds for my imagined scenario below, in which I respond to this single-minded view of the statistician by saying, "I'd like you to meet my talking bear."

"A talking what?" this statistical analyst would skeptically reply.

I would take this person to the zoo, and upon arrival, we go to the bear's cage. The statistician looks through the bars, and so does the bear from his side.

The bear says, "Welcome, Mr. Statistician, I really appreciate your visit."

Shocked, the statistician exclaims, "Astounding — that is a talking bear!"

"That's right," I answer. *"How many do you need to see before you believe it?"*

This allegory rings true for the terminal heart failure patient, where the Batista procedure allows 50% to recover and live a normal life. Their survival tells an overpowering tale.

Glass Half Full

Looking at those 50% death rate results leads one to ask if a physician is a pessimist or an optimist.

All of the patients operated on were very sick, in NYHA Class IV heart failure — with an expected mortality of nearly 100% within two years. And yes, while 50% of the patients who received Batista's procedure died relatively quickly...

...50% did not. They returned to normal.

The medical community's response — to abandon all consideration of this procedure — could be described as having viewed those results like the half empty glass, pessimistically renouncing his work as having no value. Conversely, appreciating that 50% of these otherwise terminal patients *were normal* at two years, introduces a potent positivity. It mirrors seeing the very same glass as half full.

That latter brand of optimism is my approach. Yet that doesn't mean I was completely satisfied. Instead, these results ignited my burning question: "What caused the other *50%* of patients to succumb?"

"Was there an inherent problem with the concept behind the operation?" I wondered. "Or with how the operation was performed?"

I then remembered something Batista had said when I visited him. He acknowledged that he was not always successful in these dilated ventricles, and he was not sure why. On the other hand, he noted excellent success occurred in patients with enlarged dilated hearts *from valve disease.*

Was that the clue?

As I thought about this further, I recognized that conventional thinking (including Batista's) — was that enlarged ventricles that expanded from a chronic heart muscle infection, occur as that disease is evenly distributed throughout the entire ventricle wall. *But what if it were not*? What if *only part* of the ventricle wall was unhealthy? What if sometimes the surgeon — Batista or others — removed a wedge of muscle that *was not* diseased?

If true, this means that the concept of the operation was correct... but that it was performed on the wrong part of the heart.

This theory made sense to me, since Batista had superb results in valve patients — where no infection was present within the heart's muscle mass. Because of this, any part of the ventricular wall can be removed as an elliptical form is rebuilt.

I suspected this reasoning could explain why some patients had a better outcome.

Wheels of Progress

But this conclusion was only a deduction. The prevailing question became: could this lead us to develop a better way to treat patients with large ventricles?

Discussion, questioning, brainstorming — are standard activities for everyone from writers and musicians to educators and politicians. Why not for surgeons?

The crucial components include open communication while making sufficient time available to see if such conversation can be productive. This happened in southeastern Italy in 2000. I had attended a heart failure meeting and was returning to Rome by bus with Hisa Suma, a renowned Japanese surgeon who was part of our RESTORE Team. We both lamented that the Dor operation did not always work in very large hearts.

"I have an idea you might find interesting," I offered.

We were the only passengers on our small bus and for the next two-and-a-half hours, we paid little attention to the exquisite Italian countryside sweeping by our windows, as we discussed possible solutions to these previously unsuccessful treatments.

I brought up what I had learned while visiting Paco, about the helix and the wrap, and that the ventricle must be a V shape in order to function well (which helped explain our overall successes with the Dor procedure). I noted that Paco did not focus on what disease may have caused a distortion — his only concern was the structure that makes the ventricle and heart function properly.

Intrigued, Hisa concurred that, "With the Dor procedure, we concentrate on excluding the scar, to reduce remote muscle stretch and try to return the heart to a normal elliptical shape."

"That's right," I continued, "But what if we do that with very large ventricles?"

Hisa nodded, now understanding my curiosity. "It is less effective because the spherical shape remains, but just a bit smaller."

I then questioned, "So should we focus less on treating the disease [scar], and more on treating the form itself — by whatever method works best?"

Hisa was intrigued. I offered my solution to how to make this happen in the operating room.

"Instead of attaching one end of the patch at the heart's apex [the tip at its bottom] and the other up at the top of the scar like we do with the Dor procedure... what if we attach one end of the patch at the apex and the other to a site near the top of the heart? Such a baseline change in strategy..."

"...will not only exclude the scar, but will also *reshape even very large ventricles back into a V configuration,*" Hisa said, finishing my thought. We looked at one another and realized *a new solution was now before us.*

We were entering uncharted waters yet again, for nobody had ever done this. Here we were, two cardiac surgeons, from the East and West, seeking novel horizons while our bus wove through picturesque scenery. Yet our excitement magnified as we envisioned a promising new way to improve outcomes in the very dilated hearts of patients who'd had a heart attack.

Bringing Up Batista

Delighted as we were, we both knew our conversation was not over.

We realized this dilemma of impaired heart performance also affects patients whose enlarged ventricles — have no scar. The disease was in their muscle, as they did not suffer a heart attack.

So I cited, "Batista has his unique approach that might work."

Hisa was familiar with the Batista procedure, and agreed it was an extraordinary operation. Then he noted, "But Gerry, I'm sure you know it only works in about half the cases."

It was time to reveal my new theory.

"Yes, and we know that Batista and others remove one area of the ventricle to reshape it, believing the underlying disease is evenly distributed [homogenous] throughout the ventricle. *But what if it's not?"*

Hisa's eyes lit up. "That... is fascinating." I saw his mind working, sorting together pieces of the puzzle as he continued, "If it is only in certain portions — that could explain why procedures are only sometimes successful! If the surgeon elects to remove tissue that happens to be where the disease is — the operation is effective and the patient improves. But if the surgeon removes a healthy portion that has no disease..."

"...then the patient dies," I said, now finishing his sentence.

Hisa was as captivated by this possibility as I. He contended, "Gerry, we need to discover if such disease is throughout the walls of the entire ventricle, or only in one portion. Most importantly, if only a portion is diseased — we must find a way to locate it — so we only remove the diseased region."

The two of us were in agreement. We knew we had the right questions. Now we needed to find the right answers.

Guys Talk. But Men Act.

One of my favorite books, by the architect Gyorgy Doczi, is called *The Power of Limits*.[110] It deals with harmony in nature, art, and architecture. Doczi describes "knowledge" as analysis and differentiation — to take apart. He defines "wisdom" to mean integration and synthesis — to put together. Finally, "wholeness" reflects *the action taken* that will unite knowledge and wisdom.

This exactly describes surgery. Surgeons have to act. They can't ponder all day long, "What would happen if I did this or did not." The surgical credo involves taking such action, and this principle stands behind my describing this section as essentially, "talking by boys and actions by men." Often, you must go out and do something that nobody else has done before.

During our bus journey, Hisa asked further how I learned about the helix and the idea to reshape the ventricle. I told Hisa more about Paco Torrent-Guasp and his being a stupendous resource for revolutionizing our concepts of ventricular form and function. Hisa listened — and subsequently acted — by taking his own trip to Spain to visit Paco. He reported afterward, "You're right. This is unbelievable!" Hisa came back as impressed as I had been. He and I are dear friends, as we share a world of curiosity — the bridge to translating our ideas into new actions.

Hisa's concern about the oddly high death rate that others had witnessed while doing the Batista procedure, led to his next step. Taking a page from Leonardo da Vinci, who inspired us by stating, "First I shall do some experiments before I proceed farther," Hisa designed a beautiful clinical study to find the answer. (da Vinci's advice to first conduct experiments had not been followed by those surgeons who tried doing the original Batista procedure). Hisa's inquisitive nature led him to find out *why something happened.*

Hisa took small pieces (biopsies) of a diseased ventricle's lateral wall and septum. What he found was remarkable.

He discovered that the total amount of diseased tissue was about 19%, but that the *concentration* of this diseased tissue varied in different areas from 4 to 60%! For example, in one-third of cases, it was most pronounced in the lateral wall... yet in another third, it was greatest in the septum.[111]

The disease was not uniform throughout!

These findings showed that the conventional belief of even distribution of the disease over the entire ventricle was completely wrong.

The ramifications of this knowledge were gigantic because Hisa solved a worldwide question that had confronted many surgeons. It now became clear that the patient might die — if the surgeon unknowingly removed the healthier portion (that maybe had only 5% diseased tissue). Mistakenly "taking the good while leaving the bad" was the unequivocal answer that explained the inconsistent results after the Batista procedure.

The incorrect assumption was that all parts of the ventricle suffered a uniform disease. They did not! The Batista procedure was not faulty. The problem was that it was done on the wrong part of the left ventricle.

This was incredible information. But how to use it?

That led to a critical question that still had to be answered: was there a way to determine (without a biopsy) *which area is heavily diseased* and needs to be excluded?

Action is the driving force of the surgeon, and Hisa Suma dove in to search for a way to define the answer. His creativity bloomed as he developed an ingenious method to sort out which ventricular area should be excluded.

In the operating room, Hisa started the heart-lung machine to decompress (vent) the stretched and poorly contracting dilated heart to bring it to normal size and shape. He then used an echocardiogram to watch the heart contract — and found that after the stretch was temporarily taken away by decompression — the area that contained healthy muscle would immediately regain strong contraction! Conversely, the decompressed *diseased* muscle remained non-functional.[112]

Hisa used this unique observation to introduce a new technique called the "site selection process." This echo analysis provided a perfect functional equivalent to using the biopsy method. By revealing this uneven disease distribution, the surgeon could now safely choose to exclude only the unhealthy and non-working region.

The New Patch Approach

Ideas are great starting points. But truth comes from testing.

Our central mission was to change the ventricular form, and Hisa applied his new approach in two patients with large, dilated, non-ischemic hearts (that did not have heart attacks). The normal elliptical shape was rebuilt — using the patch approach we had discussed during our bus ride to Rome. The outcomes were superb! This procedure was either called The *Pacopexy* (the term I coined to honor Paco), or the *Septal Anterior Ventricular Exclusion* or *SAVE* procedure (Hisa's name).[108, 112]

Hisa called me to report on his successes with both the patch procedure, as well as using site selection to determine what portion to exclude. Our joint exhilaration was palpable as we shared this thrill, undaunted by the 6,000 miles of ocean between Japan and UCLA.

Sharing with the World

While two surgeons brainstorming ideas during a ride through pastoral Italy proved fruitful, the real value is when discoveries are shared and adopted by the larger medical community.

I introduced this new step in thinking, along with my discussing the helical heart, when I delivered the Basic Science Lecture at the American Association of Thoracic Surgery in 2001 as described in the last chapter.[108] The audience of approximately 4,000 cardiac surgeons listened intently as I explained how form was the centerpiece of correcting the spherical world of dilated heart failure — whether caused by scar from a heart attack, valve disease, or diseases in ventricle muscle. The cornerstone of "treat the form, not the disease" was new and seemed well-received by those in attendance.

At this same meeting, Hisa described our new procedure for treating patients with an enlarged ventricle due to cardiac muscle disease, which returns these failing dilated spherical chambers to their natural smaller elliptical form. He reported that heart failure symptoms were dramatically relieved and mortality was diminished — a landmark finding as many of these patients would have otherwise succumbed within the first year from only traditional treatments.[108] Hisa further presented his triumphant initial clinical experiences in 36 consecutive patients using site selection with the Pacopexy / SAVE procedure.

There was substantial interest in Hisa's outcomes... yet his manuscript was *rejected* by the reviewers of the *Journal of Thoracic and Cardiovascular Surgery*. This was an astonishing reaction since no data like this had ever been presented in the world medical literature. Hisa had introduced a revolutionary method to identify the site of disease in the heart, and described a breakthrough operation that rebuilt normal ventricular shape. I read the responses of the reviewers. Their rebuffs made no sense. I suspect the reviewers disregarded how he had avoided the problems of the Batista procedure (by site selection), and failed to appreciate his ingenuity in designing a whole new operative procedure with stunning outcomes.

The open mind met rigidity, and as so often occurs, tradition trounced innovation.

Undaunted by the journal's spurning of his paper, Hisa's continued work has shown a 69% five-year survival rate for patients who previously would have had a 50% two-year death rate. *Truth wins, not editors.*

Such new ideas are fuel for the future.

And Hisa took them even a step further.

Using the Patch Procedure with Heart Attacks

The concept of "treat the form, not the disease" was reinforced again, as Hisa now also applied this approach to *treating heart attack patients* with large ventricles — in those patients he knew would not respond well with the normal Dor procedure. Together with his colleague, Tadashi Isomura, Hisa utilized the Pacopexy / SAVE procedure in end stage heart failure patients with enormously dilated hearts. The data tells the story, as the seven-year survival rate was 72% — versus 61% if the ventricular size was surgically reduced, but its shape was not made elliptical.[113] Additionally, eight-year survival rose to 84% when the reduction in ventricular volume was more substantial. A wonderful contribution and highly significant improvement for those with very sick, very dilated hearts.

Restoring Geometric Structure Works!

Overall, the results following restoration of the ventricle's normal form for *both* heart attack and direct muscular disease were vastly superior to those from traditional medical treatment, as the numbers make very clear.

Following conventional medical treatment, 50 to 70% of patients in NYHA Class III and IV categories will succumb during the first two years, and their quality of life is awful, as it was in my father's case. In contrast, when patients in these same categories undergo ventricular restoration, their condition improves to a Class I and II score. This spectacular and unheard-of change translates to a *70% survival*, when measured at five years (further follow-up is needed to observe survival rates for even longer intervals).

On top of this, ventricular restoration adds another significant benefit to this functional improvement — by counteracting sudden death — which otherwise is a fatal event in 50% of all congestive heart failure patients. The stretched ventricle is the primary cause of this lethal arrhythmia, and this terminal event is nearly entirely avoided by reshaping this expanded ventricle. This approach also surpasses conventional methods of implanting a defibrillator to circumvent sudden death, as these patients will still die of congestive heart failure. So returning ventricular shape toward normal by ventricular restoration offsets both sudden death and heart failure.

Valve Disease Results… Not Yet In

The final breakthrough involves the third major cause of producing severely dilated hearts: the leaking heart valve.

How this dilation (expansion) happens is straightforward, as a leak in the *aortic valve* (between the left ventricle and aorta) or *mitral valve* (between left ventricle and left atrium) will make the heart work harder. For example, a heart might normally pump out 100 cc of blood, but the leaky valve may allow 100 cc to flow backward into the ventricle each time. So now, the heart *must pump 200 cc* during every heartbeat to effectively eject out 100 cc. That causes the ventricle to enlarge. In doing so it must stretch in order to squeeze harder to compensate, but this dilation can make it wear out, resulting in heart failure.

Though the leaky valve heart becomes spherical, this change is different from our earlier situations. There is no scar or infectious tissue in ventricular walls — so that excluding *any portion* of the ventricle will safely rebuild the heart's normal elliptical shape and offset heart failure.

Unfortunately, awareness of this approach has still not impacted current thinking for treating patients with valve disease who have dilated hearts. This absence of interest continues, despite clear evidence that valve replacement alone, fails to improve long-term survival in patients with large ventricles (when ventricular volumes are greater than 55–60 ml/m2).[114, 115] They succumb from the same heart failure and sudden death complications as patients whose heart dilation is caused by a scar or from heart muscle infection.

So data is not yet available on the effectiveness of rebuilding a normal elliptical shape in patients with leaky valves, as this treatment has not yet been recognized, embraced, or even studied. The nature of this opposition is twofold: a lack of acceptance (due to the faulty STICH trial results) *that changing the ventricular shape* can dramatically improve function after a scar forms from a heart attack... and doubts regarding the Batista Procedure (as it was considered dangerous). These false conclusions caused the medical community to reject out of hand that ventricular restoration of a normal but stretched muscle — can be life-saving in patients with valve disease.

Yet these barriers are not unassailable. Someone saw this truth, evidenced by Batista's excellent success operating on the enlarged dilated hearts of patients with valve disease. My term for this concept is a "valve ventricular approach," which I believe should be further explored. His findings may yet establish a new method for treating dilated hearts in patients with valve disease.

However, interest in such an approach is particularly slow in the United States. Ventricular stretching from leaky valves is progressive (meaning it continues to worsen as time goes on), and valve repair or replacement is usually performed on patients here before such extensive stretching has time to occur. So the need for ventricular restoration is less common.

But many patients in Asia, Africa, and the Middle East die because of large dilated ventricles from rheumatic fever (which produces valve damage). They don't have our timely medical follow-up examinations to check how the ventricle is responding. By the time of their first examination, there is sometimes a severely dilated ventricle from a leaky valve. So they may be more likely to benefit if their ventricles were restored to an elliptical shape, at the same time as their valves are treated.

Wake-Up Call: Restoring Hearts, Restoring Lives

It is now clear that returning the heart's normal elliptical shape and dimensions will improve symptoms and survival in heart failure patients far beyond the expected outcomes when correction of the spherical heart is not performed.

But these approaches have still to be accepted. Resistance to them is due in part to residual effects from the flawed STICH trial. These misguided outcomes resulted in keeping the cardiologists and surgeons from even considering an approach to heart failure that rebuilds the ventricle. This is frustrating because we have the answer, while no one is willing to consider the question.

Wake-up calls are needed to counter the medical community's inability to successfully treat such terminal heart diseases. Yet the driving force for this change may come from the greater awareness of suffering patients — who rather than passively rely upon "confident experts" that continue using unsuccessful traditional treatments — *may instead strongly encourage their physicians to look beyond* what they already believe and practice.

Too often, our medical leaders have blinders on. They are unwilling to admit that knowledge can come from unexpected places: from a cardiologist in Spain who uncovers the authentic architecture of the heart, or from a surgeon in Brazil or Japan that does innovative operations. One needs an open-minded approach that pursues the truth. This can bring healing to hearts... and significantly better quality and longer lives to our patients.

New knowledge and effective treatments exist now! The prevailing short-sightedness must be tossed aside and replaced by the passion to learn about and then use these innovative ways to overcome the devastating effects of heart failure.

This sea change may indeed start with the reader.

Yes, with you.

CHAPTER 21

Art and Science:
The Helix and Heart Video

The positive and enthusiastic responses to the Helix and Heart lecture at the American Association of Thoracic Surgery Association conference made it clear that I needed to bring my marvelous voyage with Paco Torrent-Guasp to a wider audience. I knew others would also be captivated by the unraveling of the heart to show its structure. My goal was to encourage greater awareness and acceptance of his findings, which would lead to unprecedented improvements in cardiac care.

This quest to both learn and teach flourished after my initial return from Spain, and is delightfully illustrated by how I further explored Paco's discovery. I played a video of Paco unfolding the heart to a UCLA colleague, Carmine Clemente, who is a renowned anatomist and author of an anatomy textbook used by over 1,500,000 students worldwide. Carmine was so impressed by this first exposure, that he invited me to the anatomy lab to see if we could unwrap a heart.

We set out to duplicate what Paco had done. The scene was remarkable in another way. The world's most famous anatomist and an internationally recognized heart surgeon, began to work in the same place that the freshman medical students start their professional journeys. We were alone at the exact tables where the first anatomy courses start — the perfect location for two curious professors to pursue their constant search for new knowledge. Our passion to understand was just as exuberant as that of someone new to the field.

Unfortunately, we failed in our task, as we did not possess Paco's technical facility at dissection techniques. Yet neither of us was dissuaded. Pausing a moment to appreciate our quest, I simply asked Carmine, "Why don't all of the university faculty act just like us, pursuing our endless journey into learning?"

Six months later, Paco came to Los Angeles and we used my laboratory for him to demonstrate his heart dissection. He taught us his method and we were both intrigued and astounded by its simplicity. The depth of Carmine's interest became evident when he requested drawings of Paco's dissection for use in his anatomy text. His excitement became transmitted to other anatomists, as the Moore and Dalley text, another major anatomy volume, delayed its publication until images of Paco's dissection could be added. Carmine also asked me to give a one-hour lecture at the upcoming meeting of the American Association of Clinical Anatomists, which I gratefully accepted.

I was pleased that we'd seen some acceptance of Paco's findings, as now two major anatomy texts — one written by Clemente and the other by Moore and Dalley — included images of his unfolding the heart. Yet the importance of these findings was even more powerfully imprinted upon me when I heard Dalley's comment after he first watched the helical heart dissection.

He stated, "New findings change many things, but not anatomy; today Torrent-Guasp has changed anatomy."

Unfortunately, newer anatomy textbooks are hardly ever read by those that provide continuing education courses to physicians after they leave medical school. These teachers include pathologists, cardiologists, and specialists in echocardiography. Yet they rarely re-examine the basic anatomy that forms the source of what they're teaching. The older anatomy books do not contain Paco's breakthrough findings — and as a result, very few in clinical medicine know about it. This discrepancy exists because our teachers and mentors often believe they already know what they need to know. My recommendation is that they should always remain students.

Yet among those who did know of Paco's work, vehement opposition to the utter simplicity of his discovery arose from some leaders in the pathology and echocardiogram imaging communities. Efforts to discredit his theories included claims that Paco had used incorrect tissue planes during his efforts to separate the heart muscles. His critics could not envision how he found the connective muscle sheath surfaces that allowed him to prove his concept. Additionally, leaders in echocardiography refused to accept there was a circumferential wrap around the helix.

But proof must come from action, not words. The only important test is whether the finding can successfully explain the relationship between form and performance. Coming up with possible conceptual arguments against a new point of view is not helpful. There is one simple yardstick: watch the heart function and then describe mechanically why it happens. This task is made easier by using new imaging tools like advanced echocardiography and magnetic resonance imaging that provide a 3-dimensional dynamic view. If your concept explains everything we see the heart is doing, *you have an answer that merits serious consideration*.

Unfortunately, this theme of resistance to changing traditional thinking is ongoing. That obstruction is particularly true in this case because of certain inbuilt limitations — since *pathologists* observe structure in the dead heart during autopsy and then *deduce* function in the living one — while *imaging personnel* observe function in the living heart and then *deduce* its structure. But reality demands that you must *understand* structure, so you can use the correct form to *explain* function.

For reasons that are not evident, some medical authorities believe that something exists scientifically — simply because it's what they said. Their word becomes the law, rather than their having proved it. This approach is indelibly imprinted within the many major journal publications that presumably define "state of the art" information.[116, 117] Yet astonishingly, they exclude mentioning the wrap around the basal loop, a circumferential muscle that has been a centerpiece of every anatomic description dating back 400 years![118]

Spreading the Word

The truth is that many people knew about the helix, just as many were aware of the basal loop. But nobody understood how they functioned together. What Paco did was unfold the entire structure in a way that could now identify how the heart's structure explained all of its major functions.[104–106]

My goal now was to spread this understanding to others so it would become a game-changer in the medical world's view of cardiac care. I realized that this was not unlike the transformation attempted by French impressionists in the art world, nearly 150 years ago. They faced harsh opposition from the traditional art community, for until then, art reflected a realistic representation of what you were seeing. Impressionists changed that by rendering and dramatizing the *feeling* of what you're looking at. They portrayed the brilliance of its brightness, the elegance of its beauty, and the passion of its exultation. The grandeur of its artistic meaning exploded from the canvas, differing from what others had seen before. The heart now parallels this, as its power erupts from our having learned the grand design of the cardiac motor.

The wonderful reception of my Basic Science Lecture at AATS became my springboard for now introducing this information to cardiologists, to those working in the other medical fields, as well as to others who wanted to understand the heart. A starting point had been established, as we had shown the impact of this knowledge in dealing successfully with congestive heart failure. The potential for sweeping applicability now became possible.

But how to do that?

My curiosity toward developing inventive ways (ones I never used) to educate others, led me to consider making a *video presentation*. Its artistic medium, coupled with animation, seemed ideal to allow us to communicate these groundbreaking scientific discoveries. (**There will be a link to view this Helix and Heart video at the end of this chapter.**)

New Territory

The creative voyage of Paco Torrent-Guasp would be the focal point of this video production, as his unmasking of the previously hidden cardiac structure provided solid evidence of my belief that "elegance is simplicity" — instead of the "confusion is complexity" concept that had previously prevailed regarding the heart.

While being involved in such a production was a new experience to me, I had the good fortune to connect with a team called the Vesalius Group.

They created medical videos and took their name from the Flemish anatomist considered to be "the father of anatomy." How perfect. Their team included a director, medical artist, video specialist, narrator, and a producer who together could dramatize the story of Paco's scientific milestone, while integrating current technologies like magnetic resonance imaging and radionuclide studies to furnish visual proof of his concepts.

Paco welcomed the prospect, as he could now provide commentary, along with observations from myself and other physicians, that would explain the new truths brought to light by his breakthrough.

Production Commences

We met in Jim Cox's office at Georgetown University in Washington, DC to make the video.

A brilliant cardiologist named Cecil Coghlan introduced the video, by first confirming the phenomenal contributions of William Harvey's theories about the circulatory system. Cecil then stated that Harvey's understanding of anatomy was incomplete. He had incorrectly deduced that the heart constricted and dilated to circulate blood, a concept that prevails in medicine to this day. In this way, Cecil introduced Paco into the video, noting that 400 years after Harvey, Paco's discovery of the architecture behind cardiac shape had initiated the revolutionary understanding of how cardiac structure can now explain all of the heart's motions.

Paco Presents: Seeing is Believing

Early in the video, Paco traced his excitement back to when he was a medical student in Salamanca, Spain. His passion flowed from his words as he described the extraordinary simplicity of cardiac construction — one that resembles a helically-coiled rope. The concept of universality of form became evident as he disclosed this helical design was common to the hearts of many different species of animals that he studied in postmortem examinations.

Paco then visually demonstrated his concept as he used only his hands to dissect the heart (no instruments) and expose its rope-like configuration. The drama and grace of this presentation remains eternally etched in my mind. Yet this totally innovative look at the heart's architectural configuration was accomplished during only three minutes of dissection.

He then crowned the demonstration by refolding it to rebuild the intact heart. We watched him unveil the utter simplicity and beauty of its mystery... an astonishing experience.

Making the Invisible Visible

Even before production began, I knew that we needed to bring the "dead model" to life, so we could dynamically display the helical heart's sequential movements to all viewers. Toward that end, I was privileged that Lowell Offer, a dear friend and my swimming partner, who had just retired from Disney Studios, invited me to seek their counsel. We visited the Walt Disney Studios, and Paco (who was in town), Lowell, and I met with Andy Henry, who headed the audiovisual department. Andy joined us in being spellbound by the possibilities of Paco's discovery, and found us an animator who could use Paco's model as the guide to dramatically reconstruct the heart's actions. The excitement of finding our next step seemed contagious, and I was thrilled with Andy's team joining the project.

Paco's concept showing cardiac motion would be demonstrated by photographing three-dimensional moving images of the heart from different perspectives: top, bottom, and side. A visually engaging animation would then be created to portray its rhythmic patterns of twisting and uncoiling — the drama of true cardiac motion.

First Contact with Paco

I was the next physician to appear on screen. Of course, I had to describe my colorful first meeting with Paco. After all, I was the professor, and he was someone few people took seriously. Yet after my explaining to him some thoughts about structure, his response made quite an impression. He boldly asserted that I had no understanding of cardiac anatomy, despite my 30 years as a heart surgeon! But *I listened and learned*, rather than being offended.

I was definitely curious about Paco's novel information, particularly because I already knew the heart's natural shape was conical, and also that when the helix's normally slanted muscle fiber angles change to a more horizontal configuration... heart failure will follow.

So Paco's perspective intrigued me as it suddenly made clear that these natural fiber angles became horizontal as the heart stretches to become spherical. This helped me understand how our rebuilding a normal shape would counter heart failure (as performed by our RESTORE team).

Stated simply, you cannot fix what is wrong until you know what is right, and Paco's work provided that knowledge.

I additionally cited in the video that my search to learn about the heart revealed how its structure falls into the grand design of the helical spiral that exists throughout nature. As I had related in my AATS presentation, this is apparent in a series of natural spiral examples ranging from the tiny helical images of our microscopic DNA to a macroscopic spiral galaxy — riveting into place the breadth of commonality in nature's universe.

"Evolving" Process

The video also illustrated how Paco's striving to better comprehend how the heart developed compelled him to explore the human phylogenetic code (which describes the evolutionary development of a species).

He theorized that our evolution began as a worm one billion years ago, with a vascular tube (rather than a conventional heart) that looked much like a rope. The video used animation to illustrate that 400 million years ago, this evolved into a fish with gills — and a heart structure containing a helix and a single pumping chamber. This helical configuration continued when the amphibian / reptile developed 200,000 years ago with a heart where the two atriums and the ventricular septum each had a hole in their walls. But these internal cardiac holes closed as the ape/ human developed about 100,000 years ago — giving us the two separate atriums and two separate ventricles that form our four-chambered heart.

The video then highlighted the startling discovery I made while preparing my AATS lecture. This transition from worm to fish to amphibian / reptile to man took over a billion years. Yet a *most remarkable similarity takes place* when one looks at how the human develops during the first month and a half of embryonic gestation. The heart of the human fetus undergoes this same billion-year transition from worm-like heart, to fish-like heart, to amphibian / reptile-like heart... to finally the human heart. All within 50 days. Astounding!

Pictures Worth a Thousand Words

When Paco initially uncovered the anatomy of the heart, he had yet to determine how it functioned. One day he saw an MRI sequence that captured the dynamic motions of the functioning heart and it all came together for him. Our video replicated this stunning clarity of the heart's sequential movements by including a multi-gated acquisition (*MUGA*) *scan, which* showed how components of the helical heart caused sequential cardiac motions —*just as Paco had theorized.*

This superb connection between structure and function was further dramatized in a video segment of a beating human heart during a surgical procedure... that demonstrated the harmonic rhythms that Paco fondly called the "cardiac dance."

Stimulating the Helical Heart

The other physician to appear in our video was Jim Cox, the distinguished cardiac surgeon and electrophysiologist (a field that focuses on the heart's electrical system). Jim was fascinated by the straightforward solution to cardiac anatomy that became apparent as Paco literally uncoiled the Gordian knot of heart structure. Jim always believed there had to be a simple architectural answer (unlike many mystified others who concluded that heart design could never be fully understood). Jim delighted in learning that Paco Torrent-Guasp had untangled this "complex" mystery.

The validity of the helical heart was further reinforced when Jim described how the electrical, physiological, and functional data that he collected over many years — *supported* how impulses would be delivered throughout a ventricular band — the central component of Paco's helical heart concept!

In fact, the video reported that credibility of this helical design continues to grow stronger, despite physicians having long been taught that the heart constricts and dilates (squeezing like a fist to eject blood and opening to fill). Instead, the spiral formation of the heart actually makes it twist and uncoil to eject and fill with blood — with these motions clearly confirmed by MRI studies demonstrating this movement during each heartbeat — caused by the heart's helix and wrap configuration.

Importantly, this new knowledge of normality further sets the stage for understanding why deviation from the heart's natural elliptical form into a spherical shape leads to the problem of congestive heart failure.

Heart Reflected in Architecture

This concept of healthy (and sick) hearts relating to structure — was expanded upon when Cecil Coghlan then related them to examples found in architecture, much like I had during my AATS lecture.

He highlighted that we can certainly marvel at Romanesque design, where circular structures offset stresses by using a centerpiece (or keystone) placed at a central focal point on the top of the arch. Forces that could cause disruption will be directed upward toward this centerpiece. Yet serious limitations exist in these Romanesque structures, whose circular form correlates with the spherical heart of congestive heart failure. They become unstable if their constructed arch is too high or wide, so that their strength is augmented by stacking individual arches in layers to gain the necessary height. This is evident when looking at Roman aqueducts in Segovia, Spain... or the Roman Coliseum (**Figure 1**).

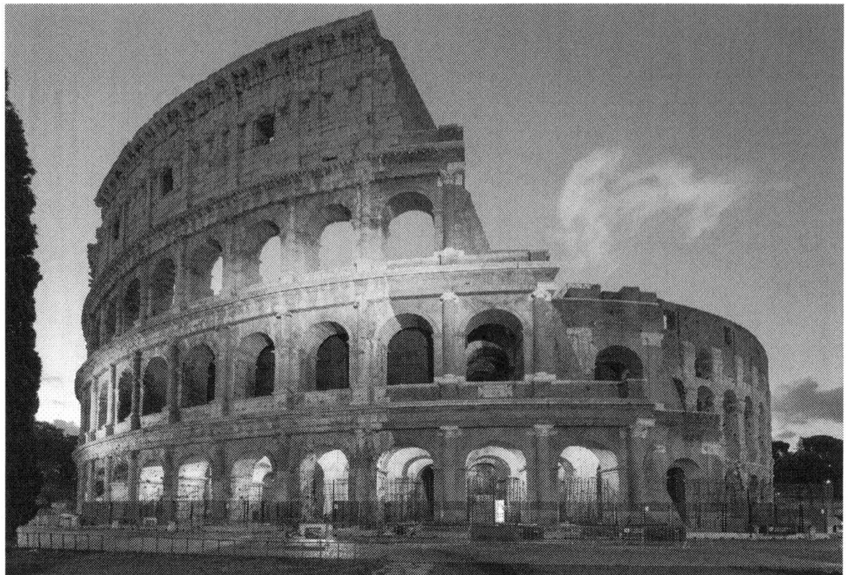

Figure 1: Romanesque design contains many circular arches, with forces directed to the central point on top of each arch, called a keystone. This limitation means that many layers are needed to increase height.

Cecil elaborated that to achieve a greater height and width, architects subsequently used the gothic design, as exists in Notre Dame Cathedral (built in 1345) and others, whose external buttresses brace the arches whose structural forces would otherwise move downward. (**Figure 2**)

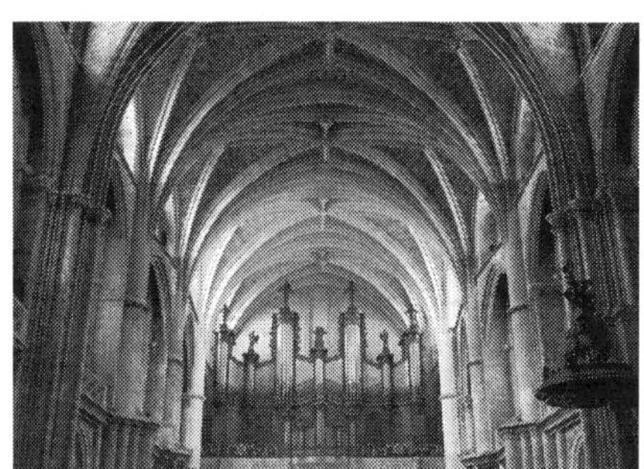

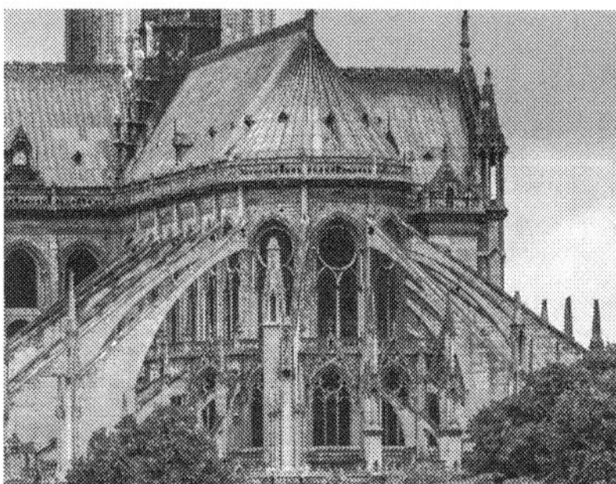

Figure 2: Gothic dome on left, whose great height is maintained by support from external (flying) buttresses on right.

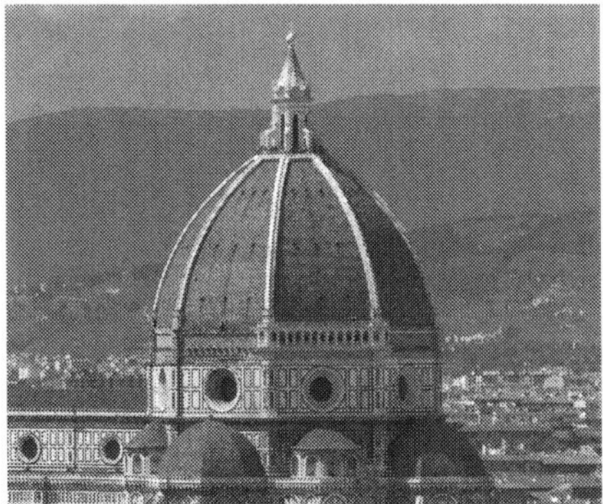
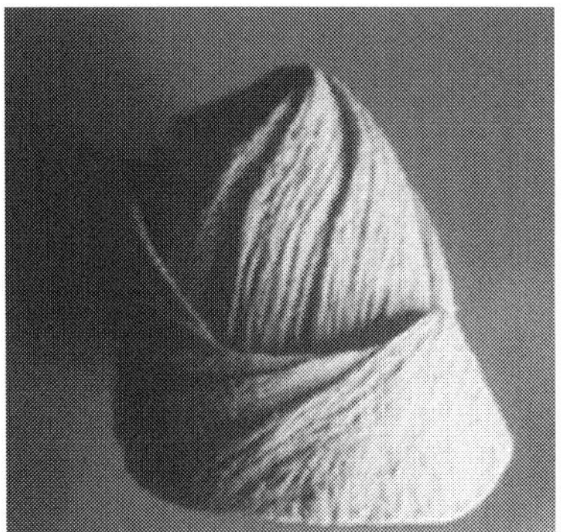

Figure 3: The similarity of the cathedral on left, and the heart on right where the basal wrap is the buttress.

Cecil then presented an amazing juxtaposition, whereby he showed the parallels between gothic architecture and the healthy elliptical heart as he held Paco's model upside down — its apex on top (like the gothic dome) and circumferential wrap (the *heart's buttress*) below — precisely forming the cathedral design that we know so well. (**Figure 3**) They became one as both shared a powerful and stable form.

Ironically, gothic architects had copied the heart's design many centuries ago, yet the heart's own geometry was only "just discovered."

Such types of comparisons help us to better understand the heart, including grasping the reasons for problems that develop during congestive heart failure. The sporting metaphor mentioned before was used again in the video to create a clear visual example, as we contrast the football (for normality) against the basketball (for heart failure). From Paco's discovery, we now understood how ventricular stretching within this poorly functioning spherical form will distort the fiber structure within the helix. The resulting architectural change in these dilated hearts becomes the geometric cause of heart failure.

The video includes an operation done by the RESTORE team that shows them reconstructing a normal ventricular shape in a patient with heart failure — improving heart performance as this changes the basketball shape back into a football form.

Acknowledgment of a Major Contribution

Paco's revelations of heart structure are so far reaching, that Cecil Coghlan compared their impact to William Harvey's groundbreaking discovery of the body's circulatory system in 1628. Cecil felt (and Jim Cox and I concurred) that Paco's novel understanding of cardiac structure may exceed the contributions of William Harvey.

Appropriately, the video's final scene involved only Paco, who reappeared with the helically looped rope to emphasize the straightforwardness of his spectacular findings. He concluded by declaring his contribution was "simple, not complicated."

Of course, that is its beauty and power. *Paco's discovery reaffirms the elegance of nature.*

The Freddie Award

Copies of the video were sent to anatomists worldwide and to directors of every cardiac surgery residency program.

I was subsequently invited to visit Lake Louise in Canada to present this video at their Canadian cardiology meeting. A highly enthusiastic response followed the video presentation, and one of the staff came up to ask if I was interested in submitting the work for the "Freddie Awards." Apparently, this was the competition of the International Health and Medical Media Awards for health and medical videos. The biomedical equivalent to the Oscars and the Emmys, it was to be held in New York City as a black-tie event.

We submitted our video and won the Clinical Science Award. I could not attend the prize ceremony in New York because I was in Argentina. Richard Craig, the writer and producer from Vesalius, attended in my place. In addition to the awards for individual categories, a final Surgeons General Award was to be given to the best submission within the entire competition.

Soon after the conference, Richard phoned me. "Gerry, are you sitting down? You're not going to believe this. We not only got the Clinical Science

Award... but our Helix and Heart video received the Surgeons General Award as well!"

I was deeply gratified by this, not because we had "won," but because to me it meant that the video *had meaning.*

The Legacy

How our video, and the information it presents, impacts the medical field in a profound and lasting way is still to be seen.

I am reminded of a commonality between Harvey and Paco, both legendary masters of the cardiovascular system. Harvey had brilliantly described the systemic circulatory system, overturning 1,800 years of how medicine looked at the heart / body connection. Interestingly, Harvey could only postulate the existence and role of the body's capillary network, due to scarcity of measuring instruments. It wasn't until three years after Harvey's death that Italian anatomist Marcello Malpighi actually detected capillaries using a microscope.

In a similar way, Paco's *helical ventricular myocardial band* has provided the mechanical functional basis to accurately explain cardiac actions, resolving 400 years of limitations due to anatomic misconceptions. Yet the importance of his discovery only started to become clear eight years following his death (2005), after others were able to fully correlate his architectural discoveries with the movements that exist in the functioning heart. I wrote papers and delivered lectures on it while new imaging tools (including advanced velocity vector imaging, MRIs, and 3D echocardiograms) unequivocally confirmed how heart motion precisely matches what Paco proposed.

I had a remarkable experience in Birmingham, Alabama, where I traveled to meet with Navin Nanda, the editor of the *Journal of the American Society of Echocardiography.* When I told him what Paco had uncovered, Navin said, "Gerry, with velocity vector imaging, we should be able to see what you just described." This was my first exposure to VVI, which takes rapid pictures of the heart lasting just microseconds, and each image details every directional movement. Navin could break down one heartbeat into perhaps 150 photographs or "slices." I was amazed. Why? It was not because the technology was impressive (it was). But rather, because I was able to look at those slices — and tell Navin exactly what was causing every single muscle movement at every moment.

Navin was astonished, and frankly, so was I! With Paco's work, I had finally found the "secret formula," and suddenly could explain everything occurring during each heartbeat!

Changes Ahead

Indeed, the enormous contributions of William Harvey and Paco Torrent-Guasp do parallel each other, as Harvey discovered the circulation... while Paco illuminated the functional heart anatomy that occurs during both health and disease.

People are finally getting interested in learning about Paco's findings. Yet there can be great distance between what *is known* and what *is accepted.* New ideas make you think differently, and as has been the case in the world of art, there will almost always be initial opposition. These hurdles cause scientific acceptance to be a far-off goal. Yet the truth will win.

The world resisted the early French impressionists, but now long after they have passed on, the world looks at art in a different and grander way because of their efforts. So it will be for Paco and the grand contributions he made to understanding our hearts. He allowed the medical field to look at the heart differently, and use this knowledge to uncover new solutions to illnesses.

Svetlana Alexievich, winner of the 2015 Nobel Prize in Literature, captures this potential. She writes, "History records the lives of ideas. People don't write it, time does."

An exciting future lies ahead.

Link to Helix and Heart video: www.youtube.com/watch?v=R-aPVWOmBjg

CHAPTER 22

Diastolic Dysfunction: Contracting Longer but Not Better

Fifteen million patients in the U.S. and Europe suffer from heart failure. Our RESTORE team addressed this problem in the 50% of patients where the cause was a dilated and stretched ventricular muscle that could not contract properly and ejected poorly — a condition called *systolic dysfunction*. We showed that a surgical solution to this dilemma was possible for these 7.5 million patients.[94] We were frustrated that ventricular restoration was not embraced by the medical community, which failed to accept that it could be used to reverse heart failure in patients with a dilated heart.

At the same time, we were also aware that the other half (7.5 million patients) who develop heart failure — do so despite having a normal ejection fraction. Their hearts *have normal size and shape, but cannot fill properly* when the ventricle relaxes (diastole) — a condition called *diastolic dysfunction*. But no one knew why this happened, which meant the key to developing a proper treatment was missing.

Yet I knew that the helix is the centerpiece of the heart, as its two arms determine efficient ventricular ejection and filling. When compromised, it can likewise become inefficient. I believed my new understanding of the helical ventricular band design could serve as the springboard toward discovering fresh insights to counter *diastolic dysfunction*, which shortens the life of the other half of high-risk heart failure patients.

The "Other 50%"

I began looking for clues.

Patients with diastolic dysfunction develop clinical problems when their lungs become congested. But their complaints of, "I'm having trouble breathing... It's interfering with my walking... I can't sleep at night," similarly occur in patients with failing *dilated (stretched)* hearts. But diastolic dysfunction patients are different because they have a *normal heart size and shape,* together with *normal ejection fraction* (percentage of blood the ventricle pumps into the body). For this reason, the disease is called "Heart Failure with Normal Ejection Fraction" (HFNEF).

While they describe *what happens*, I knew these words failed to hint at the *mechanical cause* behind it. Perplexed cardiologists and surgeons echo each other's lament by asking, "Why can't they breathe if their heart size, shape, and ejection fraction are normal?"

Without that answer, conventional treatment can only relieve the symptoms of heart failure. Generic medications are given to slow heart rate, relax blood vessels, and decrease heart wall stiffness, while diuretics drain the fluid congesting lungs. Yet the lives of the 7.5 million patients continue to be impacted by this devastating form of heart failure.

As said before, the frequency of congestive heart failure caused by dilated hearts — or from *diastolic dysfunction* in normal hearts — is comparable (50% in each category). I knew of other similarities, after reviewing data from both forms of heart failure in an outpatient study of 556 patients[119] — as each caused the same 16% mortality within six months of treatment, and identically lowered the quality-of-life in survivors.

Yet to my surprise, *both* types of heart failure are also managed by the *same generic treatment* (drugs) — even though their failure developed from completely different mechanical causes.

Along with so many other physicians, I too was at a loss for the reasons behind diastolic dysfunction. Yet my motto "disease is a disruption of normality and its treatment must return normality" would continue to guide my efforts to understand diastolic dysfunction — an explanation that had eluded everyone.

Until now.

The Start of a New Search

Colleagues, especially cardiologists, often ask me, "Why does a surgeon study what is essentially a medical issue [that does not strictly aim at solving a surgical dilemma]?"

I am reminded of comments from Dr. Comroe during my training at CVRI (Cardiovascular Research Institute). He would say some outcomes from surgical procedures may generate unique problems — that will stimulate the need to perform new studies to search for their solution. Indeed, my attention became riveted to this issue as I recognized that *surgical patients* sometimes developed diastolic heart failure after a successful heart operation. I followed my mentor's suggestion to find out why.

But more than a need to know was compelling me to understand the reasons that heart failure developed in a normal sized and shaped heart. *I believed I possessed the tools needed to search out the answer.* I could apply my newly acquired knowledge of the helical heart structure and function — to develop novel investigative methods that may finally let us understand this mysterious condition.

A Door Finally Opens

Fortunately, new imaging tools had already opened the way to discovering why hearts with diastolic dysfunction failed. With the development of the echocardiogram, cardiologists by the late 1980s could watch the rate and flow of blood into the heart during its natural sequence of *early rapid filling* of the ventricle (the interval before it is expelled into the body) — and found that about 70% of the filling occurs during the first third of the diastole (relaxation-filling) phase.[120]

Those studies were central to exploring the reasons for diastolic dysfunction. They confirmed there was normal ejection during "systole" (when the left ventricle contracts to eject its blood out to the body)... yet identified that the ventricles *could not fill properly* during their "relaxation" in "diastole" (when the left ventricle fills). Hence the name *diastolic dysfunction* was coined, and we had our first clue as to *what* was happening. But still no one knew *why*.

Or how to counter it.

False Beliefs

The key to developing a proper treatment would grow out of recognizing how this diastolic disease process departs from normal function — since rebuilding normality is the only proper remedy. The starting place must be to understand what determines normal ventricular filling — since ventricular filling was the problem.

It had long been thought the reason that the ventricle fills with blood from the atrium is because of a pressure difference that exists between them. Atrial pressure (pressure in the atrium) is greater than ventricular pressure (pressure in the ventricle). But this explanation seemed unlikely to me, because the pressure difference between the 7 mm Hg atrial pressure and 5 mm Hg ventricular pressure was very slight. It just seemed impossible that this tiny pressure difference would cause the ventricle to receive 70% of its blood during the rapid filling phase that occurs within the first third of diastole.

I believed that *suction* seemed the most likely cause of filling. After all, the ventricle *twists* to eject blood during ejection... and then *uncoils* to suction (or aspirate) blood from the atrium for rapid filling. The dynamics of this suction motion are beautifully evident on magnetic resonance recordings (MRIs). Exploring this movement became the foundation of our new studies to understand why suction occurs — *and then to use this knowledge to reverse diastolic dysfunction*.

Unrecognized Reality

As I looked deeper into this... the truth began to reveal itself. I reviewed a spectrum of different studies on diastolic dysfunction that had tried to pull together isolated pieces of the puzzle. They showed that the heart size is normal, *but for some reason*, the heart wall stiffens (could this imply that excess calcium may exist in the ventricle's wall?).

Most importantly, these studies consistently demonstrated that ventricular suction is impaired.

When faced with such adverse events, our body compensates to keep us alive. Studies showed that when suction is absent, a *higher* pressure difference *is needed* to drive blood from the atrium into the ventricle. Atrium pressure rises to 15 to 20 mm Hg or more to stretch this now stiffer ventricular wall (rather than the normal 7 mm Hg atrium vs. 5 mm Hg ventricle difference).

Unfortunately, this is not "a free ride"... because this higher atrium pressure *is also transmitted backward into the lungs*. This produces their congestion by making fluid fill the air spaces, which causes the patient to experience shortness of breath. Conventional treatment addresses this symptom of breathlessness, but fails to address why it occurs. ...And so it continues.

This failure is due in part to the ongoing belief that the normal heart compresses to eject, but is then followed by passive filling due to a pressure difference between the atrium and the ventricle.

By this point, I was convinced that suction was the key element behind solving this riddle.

New Exploration

My search toward uncovering the answers to this puzzle seemed straightforward, since cardiac performance involves the interaction of only three muscles: the surrounding wrap, and each arm of the helix. Each muscle starts and stops at different times — and the "dominant" one at any given moment determines the heart's movement[104] — since that muscle is contracting most powerfully. It's like when you move your arm. The biceps and triceps are both contracting, but the arm's direction is governed by which muscle is strongest during its contraction.

Similar interactions between the helix and wrap occur during each cardiac motion. Therefore, every heart movement we observe can become explained by understanding which muscle is dominant at that given moment.

Heart's Four-Phase Cycle

There are four phases of motion that occur during every heartbeat. They are:

- prepare for ejection
- ejection
- prepare for suction
- suction

Phases one and three have more classical medical names (isovolumic contraction and isovolumic relaxation), but using the phrase *"prepare for"* may aid your understanding of their roles.

My knowledge of the helical band now allowed me to understand the reasons for each of their movements.

The first phase, "prepare for ejection," involves contraction of the wrap and the inner arm of the helix to *build pressure* in the left ventricle (before it ejects blood into the circulatory system). This narrows the ventricle *and* rotates it counterclockwise. This immediate rise in ventricular pressure also shuts the valves in the atrium so blood does not move backward during ejection. The first part of the classic heart sound of "lub-dub" that everyone knows — the "lub" — is generated during this "prepare for ejection" phase.

The second phase is "ejection." It happens just 60 ms (milliseconds) later, and begins when the outer helical arm starts to contract. This creates twisting — as the apex (cardiac tip at bottom of heart) *rotates counterclockwise* while the base (top of the heart) *turns clockwise*. This movement causes blood to be "wrung" (ejected) from the ventricle, much like wringing a towel expels water.

The third phase is "prepare for suction" — and is what we will chiefly focus upon in this chapter.

This "prepare for suction" phase begins immediately after the ejection stops. It happens as the "dub" (of the "lub-dub") sound occurs that reflects the closure of heart valves in the aorta (main artery that sends blood into the body) and pulmonary artery (that sends blood to the lungs). During this third phase, the wrap and inner helical arm *both stop contracting,* but the outer helical arm movement *continues.* The circumferential wrap unwinds, which triggers a dramatic shift in the heart's motion: its twisting is abruptly replaced by rapid *uncoiling* of the whole ventricle (producing a clockwise motion).

A whorl is generated. This whorl creates a centrifugal force that produces a vacuum effect, which occurs as the fourth phase starts and permits suction to begin (as the rapid clockwise motion continues).

Finding the Key

My knowledge of the helical heart allowed me to dive deeper into uncovering the crucial element of why diastolic dysfunction mystery happens: *it appeared to be the uncoiling motion, a movement that starts during the "prepare for suction" phase.*

This uncoiling happens during the gap of time between the end of contraction by the inner helical arm — and the end of contraction of the outer helical arm. (**Figure 1**) This interval (that includes the subsequent suction) lasts about 120 ms.

I then realized the key: successful uncoiling will be *compromised by any reduction of this time period.*

We needed to find out why this would occur.

Which brings us to the fourth phase, "suction," which rapidly fills the ventricle — and is heavily dependent upon this prior "prepare to suction" interval. Suction only starts when the outer helical arm *uncoils* — an action that can only begin when it stops contracting.

I finally had my clue.

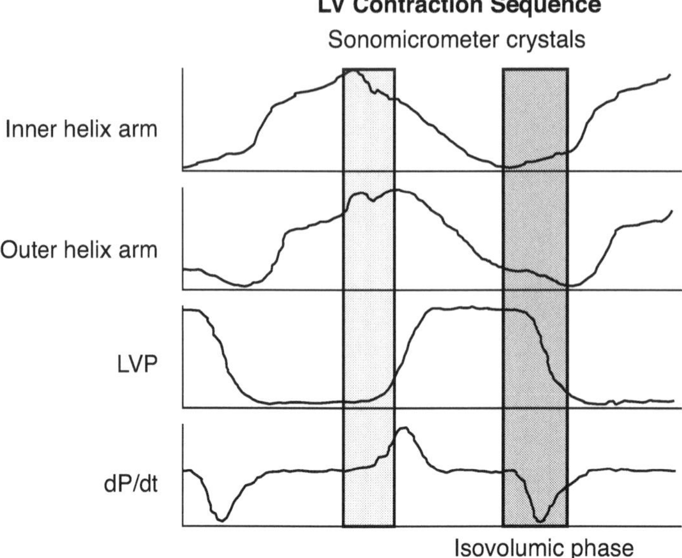

Figure 1: Experimental evidence of timing sequence of inner and outer helical arm contracting and relaxing, as revealed by sonomicrometer crystals. Outer arm starts after inner arm (shown in left column), and contracts for 90–120 ms more after inner arm stops (shown in right column). LVP = left ventricular pressure, and dP/dT means change in pressure divided by change in time.

The Saga of the Siphon

As I reflected on what I had just discovered… I realized that while diastolic dysfunction describes the ventricle's inability to properly fill, there has been a glaring failure to recognize that *its basic cause* is the inability *to develop suction*. This chasm is in no small part due to the ongoing resistance to recognize that the normal heart must develop *suction* to fill itself with blood.

Yet such reluctance is surprising because suction is not a new finding.

In AD 180, Galen observed that "the overlying heart, at each diastole, robs the vena cava *by violence* of considerable quantity of blood." This action was dynamically apparent as he looked into the chest of a wounded gladiator, to observe the atrium suddenly deflate just after ejection ended — as its blood becomes sucked away to rapidly fill the ventricle. Galen's introduction of this "ebb and flow" action (that reflected the ventricle sucking in and subsequent ejecting of blood) mirrors the relationship between ocean waves and their undertow.

Galen's concept remained a common belief for 1,400 years, until Harvey described his theories of circulation in the 1600s. Harvey believed the left ventricle filled due to gravity (the passive process I described where blood transfers due to high atrium pressure and low ventricle pressure). This explanation unfortunately replaced Galen's concept, and created a misbelief that has persisted for 400 years... *until now.*

Yet even before now, Harvey's speculation was not universally accepted, as Gerhard Brecher, a renowned German physiologist, challenged this pressure-related concept in 1956. He declared that the passive ventricular filling explanation was incorrect.[121] His experimental studies dramatically documented that the ventricles *sucked in fluid themselves.* He proved this by connecting a tube from a beating heart to a reservoir placed below the heart, and recording that blood flowed *upward* into the more highly positioned heart during every beat. The reservoir was below the heart so that pressure could not account for this; suction was the only explanation for rapid filling!

Brecher demonstrated these findings by removing a still-beating heart from a frog and observed it "hop" across a tabletop as it contracted to "eject," and then "relaxed" to develop suction between beats.

Despite all this, Brecher's science was not accepted. Physiologists criticized him as they repeated the same condemnations that the "learned critics" had hurled at Galen in the 1600s, when Harvey discovered circulation.

Yet progress inevitably takes place. Some 40 years after Brecher's denunciation, acknowledgment of suction began to re-emerge as the reason that blood moved rapidly from the atrium into the left ventricle. This was due to the 1996 introduction of three-dimensional MRIs, which affirmed that during its rapid filling phase, the ventricle exerted a vacuum-type effect on blood coming into it from the atrium.

Nature did not change between 1956 (Brecher) and 1996 (MRIs) or between Galen's AD 180 observation and today. It was our failure to recognize the limitations of our prior investigative imaging tools (2D echo and ventriculograms) that allowed the truth of heart suction to remain camouflaged. Still, most in the medical field continue to pantomime the opening and closing of the fist to represent "ejection and suction." Yet I know that progress is only possible when we can accept the shortcomings of previous beliefs.

Fortunately, the helical ventricular myocardial band provides us with the gift of understanding because it unmasks the reasons for normality, provides new insights into suction's mechanisms — and possibly reveals ways to combat the ravages of diastolic dysfunction.

Correct Words → Correct Understandings

There is another factor that leads to confusion about heart function.

Proper words to describe the heart's individual motions are guideposts toward understanding the reasons for diastolic dysfunction. But confusion springs out of the inaccurate vocabulary that exists for describing diastolic dysfunction.

A prime example is the frequently used medical phrase, "isovolumic relaxation interval" (IVR), which describes the 90 ms interval that includes the "prepare for suction" phase between the end of ejection and the start of filling. But "IVR" is not correct, because ultrasonic crystal recordings (the same ones that confirmed the validity of Paco's model) — demonstrate that the outer arm of the helix does not "relax" during this interval. Instead, it continues to *contract.*

I realized that the key to comprehending diastolic dysfunction *rests on truly understanding what occurs in this vital* "prepare for suction" period. Calling this phase "relaxation" is misleading since some of the heart is still contracting. Appreciating this distinction is critical — since the treatment of what goes wrong during this interval is essential to overturning a disease that affects 7.5 million people.

Another deceptive word that hampers this quest is the universally used "untwisting." The normal heart muscle does not untwist (a movement where the apex would rotate clockwise and the base would rotate counterclockwise). Instead, the *whole chamber* (apex and base) rotates clockwise during this "prepare for suction" period.

It seems especially strange that "untwisting" continues to be used, since the MRI, our gold standard of imaging, reveals a *whole heart clockwise motion*. So "untwisting" should really be replaced by "uncoiling," "recoiling," or "unwinding." These correct cardiac movements must be named and recognized — since understanding the mechanics behind them is fundamental to solving why diastolic dysfunction occurs.

With the right words comes the right understanding, along with the passageway toward our long-sought answers.

The Secret of Suction

My pursuit of solutions to diastolic dysfunction is steered by my belief that nature provides us with the clues to resolve medical conditions.

We can begin by looking to the natural harmony of waves in the sea created by the balance of their "ebb and flow." Imagine standing on a beach, watching the normality of a wave's crescendo followed by its rapid withdrawal. Then envision a disruption of this natural balance. Interrupt *either* one of these functions, and their *interdependence* will cause the other to be dramatically altered. As said before, this ebb and flow analogy to the body's circulation came from Galen, who described it in AD 180. Could this return of its relevance now help us uncover the cause and treatment of diastolic dysfunction?

Focusing only upon the diastolic phase (when suction occurs) has been the traditional approach to determine what goes wrong during diastolic dysfunction. But no solutions could be found from that. This is what set me wondering: could it be shortsighted *to only* study diastole? Could *interdependence* between the systolic (ejection) and diastolic (suction) phases define the root of the problem?

After all, the heart cannot prepare to fill... until it completes its twisting.

Here is what I realized: the action of the ventricle uncoiling — a motion that is essential to the suction for filling — *is made up of two steps.* First, there is what I have called "prepare for suction," during which 50 to 60%[122] of uncoiling occurs to make the ventricle ready for suction. Second, the remainder of uncoiling (the other 40 to 50%) then provides the suction needed for rapid filling of the ventricle.

Both of these two phases of uncoiling are needed for optimal suction... yet the *cause* of diastolic dysfunction *really* takes place during the *"prepare for suction" phase.*

This interval occurs between the end of contraction and extends to the beginning of suction. I could now easily see a dilemma arising if the ejection twisting period (contraction) became prolonged beyond normal. Why? Because that would then delay the start of this *"prepare for suction" phase,* and shorten this vital period for uncoiling. *There would not be sufficient time to develop the centrifugal force needed for suction.* Instead, ventricular filling would suddenly depend only upon pressure differences between atrium and ventricle.

These observations felt like clues, and this "prepare for suction" phase took top billing for my attention!

The Answer: Delay = Diastolic Dysfunction

It had become clear to me that the *uncoiling* during this "prepare for suction" phase, a motion that prepares the heart for suction, becomes pivotal for its success — and thus is the key element to solving diastolic dysfunction.

Fortunately, I had the tools needed to explore this new realization.

We could readily calculate the duration of the "prepare for suction" phase — by measuring the interval between when the *inner helical arm* contraction ends (when ejection stops) — and when *outer helical arm* contraction ends (suction starts)![104] I further realized this "preparation for action" phase has artistic and sports analogies. For example, rehearsals always precede a show, and warm-up before a sporting event is essential. Performing well in acting, dancing, and sports is not possible without such a preparation. Yet no one had appreciated that compromise of this "prepare for suction" phase set the stage for development of diastolic dysfunction.

This would now become our research focus.

Manuel Castella (the Spanish research fellow who helped test Paco's model) collaborated on this study. We needed first to cause diastolic dysfunction in a test animal. This could be readily done by temporarily limiting blood flow to the heart by closing a nourishing artery for 15 minutes. Diastolic dysfunction predictably followed, providing us a perfect chance to evaluate the "prepare for suction" phase.

What we found was very specific — *and very revealing.*

When diastolic dysfunction developed, *the contraction of the inner helix arm (twisting for ejection) lasted longer than normal.* This delayed the start of uncoiling — and *significantly shortened* the interval between ejection and suction. It compromised the crucial "prepare the heart for suction" period needed to prepare for developing suction. This *awful persistence* (of the prolonged twisting phase) became the central dilemma in the process! Quite simply, *the heart cannot get ready to fill — if it is still twisting* (contracting).

This observation contradicted the conventional belief that "all is well, since there is a normal ejection fraction," a concept that is simply incorrect. Instead, this longer time of twisting (or torsion) curtails the "prepare for suction period." The warm-up period is compromised. In fact, evidence of this is apparent in patients with impaired suction, as their hearts consistently have prolonged systolic torsion (taking longer for ejection).[123] This unmistakable connection has escaped detection by most of those that treat diastolic dysfunction. Consequently, contracting longer does not yield a better outcome. Said differently, torsion is important, but its prolongation promotes diastolic dysfunction.

Getting Closer

Recognizing that the systolic issue (prolonged contraction during ejection) is responsible for diastolic dysfunction, led to my asking two fundamental questions: Why does prolonged ejection happen? and How can we fix it?

I realized we could not develop a treatment until these questions were answered. This is particularly true since patients with a variety of different diseases can develop diastolic dysfunction — *but each of them shares the same underlying problem of a prolonged ejection interval.* These diseases include restricted coronary blood flow (just as we simulated in our experimental study), high blood pressure (hypertension), aortic stenosis (narrowing of the opening of the aortic valve), the aging or elderly population, and finally those with a stretched and failing dilated heart.

Despite this commonality, the impact of prolonged contraction (ejection) has not been addressed, except in patients with high blood pressure or in those who had aortic valve narrowing.[124–126] We know that diastolic function improves after either lowering blood pressure in patients with hypertension or after correcting a narrowed aortic valve.[123] Yet it wasn't known *why* these treatments worked, largely due to an absence in understanding of the mechanism causing diastolic dysfunction (they happened to offset prolonged contraction, and restore normal twisting and uncoiling).[123] The lack of effective treatments for diastolic dysfunction in aging patients, or in younger patients without high blood pressure — is due to this same void in understanding of *why* it happens.

This was the challenge facing me.

Luckily, I had knowledge of the helical heart — a starting point to search for the answer.

Calcium, the Diastolic Warlord

When I recognized that a prolonged contraction (ejection) would compromise this "prepare for suction" interval and lead to diastolic dysfunction — I recalled my own experiences with patients who'd had post-operative muscle damage after cardiac surgery, in which the heart took a longer time to eject. This brought me back to the experience at the beginning of my career, when John Kirklin told me the heart muscle became stiff when its blood supply was returned after being absent (ischemia). I suggested it might be like a charley horse, which led me to reduce calcium as I tried to prevent reperfusion injury in surgical patients.

It now dawned on me that diastolic dysfunction stemmed from this same problem: prolonged contraction of the inner helix arm was the culprit. Normally, contraction happens with high cell calcium — and relaxation happens when calcium is pumped out. But if excess calcium remains — the contraction persists. This scenario would match well with possible causes for diastolic dysfunction in the older population, as their ability to pump calcium out of cells is less efficient.

Because of this, I wondered if excess calcium could be the indisputable warlord of diastolic dysfunction, causing the "awful persistence" that allows prolongation of systolic contraction (ejection) — and prevents the ventricles from filling properly. Moreover, I knew that calcium retention also stiffens the heart, which further inhibits its ability to suction.

While this theory was based upon our past experiences and made sense, testing was needed to confirm it. Once proven, our subsequent goal would be to answer these two questions: *why* does excess calcium occur in the cells, *and how* can this problem be remedied?

Fortunately, fresh and unexpected answers came to light as I followed my motto: "traveling to teach allows me to learn."

Pharmacologist Unlocks the Mystery

I had a fascinating experience during an international conference at the University of Western Ontario in Canada, where I'd gone to give a talk. There I was taught about a chemical reaction I had never heard of. It describes a natural sequence that allows the body to avoid accumulation of acid that damages its tissues. Morris Karmazyn, a luminous physiologist and pharmacologist, educated us by explaining the *sodium-hydrogen exchange mechanism.*

This is a normal process that occurs in the tissues of all within the animal kingdom. A cell becomes acidotic (excess acid) if too many hydrogen ions accumulate within it. The cell tries to get rid of the acid by pumping it out, using this sodium-hydrogen exchange mechanism in which it actively exchanges hydrogen for sodium. Then, because a sick cell cannot develop the energy to get rid of the sodium in the normal way, the cell — *exchanges sodium for calcium.*

The problem is, if too much sodium amasses in the cell — this cell then *becomes overloaded by the calcium that enters to replace the sodium* — and the high intracellular calcium drama begins.

I sat there listening... absorbing. The sequence he described made sense. I now understood why people accumulate excess calcium in the cell.

What got me even more excited was that Morris reported a pharmaceutical company had worked with him to develop a unique way *to inhibit this sodium-hydrogen exchange mechanism.* I realized if their new drug prevented this devastating sequence, it would counteract the awful calcium persistence that may produce prolonged ejection — and may solve the basic mechanism behind diastolic dysfunction!

Could this be the answer I was searching for?

The findings Morris presented had an extraordinary impact upon me. I learned that Cariporide (Morris' drug) successfully reversed calcium-related damage in the eye, brain, lung, gastrointestinal system, thyroid, prostate... and heart. It was remarkable, and astoundingly, a discovery few had heard of. Not cardiologists. Not surgeons. Yet here was this incredible drug that changed all these different diseases in all these varied areas. The importance of this was overwhelming, since the role of this exchange mechanism was universal and existed in all tissues. Yet this concept is not taught in medical school and its remedy is never used in patients.

I took a walk with Morris after his presentation.

"What you're doing is unbelievable!" I told him. "I consider this to be a landmark finding, one that rivals the discovery of nitric oxide — that won the Nobel Prize for Lou Ignarro, my colleague at UCLA."

A twinkle flashed in Morris' eyes as he quietly admitted, "I think the benefits will exceed those of nitric oxide."

I knew he was correct, but this reality could only be possible if someone listened, tested it, and started the ball rolling.

Getting Involved

My discussion with Morris would turn out to have a unique outcome. I soon received an invitation to participate in the drug studies for Cariporide. I had previously demonstrated that reducing calcium would limit reperfusion damage, so the drug company asked me to now evaluate if this new pharmaceutical agent would limit calcium buildup after coronary artery bypass surgery.

I also saw this as an opportunity to explore whether this drug could combat the probable excess calcium component of diastolic dysfunction.

Fortunately, an established framework to test a solution to diastolic dysfunction was already soundly in place. Our prior experience using ultrasonic crystal probes could now allow us to detect the timing of the end of the inner and outer helical arm contractions, and determine if this drug could counter any prolongation of the ejection phase (the action that shortens the preparation for suction phase and causes diastolic dysfunction).

I was eager to start.

Experiment Begins

In the first portion of our testing, the blood supply to a region of the heart was closed for 15 minutes (duplicating the condition that exists in coronary artery bypass surgery). As expected, this lengthened the period of ejection, as the inner helix muscle contraction was prolonged due to the awful calcium persistence.

Cariporide was studied during part two. It was administered just before closing off the blood supply for 15 minutes. Diastolic dysfunction again occurred immediately after new blood supply was restored — *but by the end of one hour, all measurements had returned to normal.* Diastolic dysfunction completely disappeared, natural twisting recovered, and uncoiling returned to normal![126] These observed findings were consistently repeated.

It was absolutely marvelous. We now not only understood the muscular reasons for diastolic dysfunction. We also had successfully tested a remarkable new drug to reverse it!

The Next Step

How exciting that a medical remedy to this dilemma now existed. This drug reflected the potential for a monumental breakthrough. Next, we'd need to confirm these expectations in a clinical trial with patients.

My involvement in the study continued as I served on the Medical Steering Committee that established the parameters for a clinical trial, which would study whether heart damage after coronary artery bypass operations is reduced by this drug. I was optimistic, though wary, since the validity of such studies depends upon the credibility of the investigation. I was still deeply troubled by the highly flawed STICH trial that tested ventricular restoration as a counter to heart failure,[94, 99] and terribly saddened that their tragic failure to maintain credibility had produced results that adversely affected the lives of countless sick patients.

Recognizing this drug's potential as a game-changer, the pharmaceutical company (instead of the NIH, in this case) sponsored a very large, very expensive, prospective randomized trial for Cariporide. The steering committee defined the dose and duration strategies for use of the drug, emphasizing that it should be used only during the period of reperfusion in the operating room, and perhaps during the immediate stay in the intensive care unit.

Each steering committee member was thrilled about the significance of potential positive trial outcomes.

However, a problem developed.

I suspect the drug company's desire to sell great quantities of their product may have been what caused them to alter the steering committee's recommendations. They changed our guidelines to extend drug delivery *to 48 hours and added a high dose delivery* — instead of using a lower drug concentration during a much shorter post-reperfusion period. They did this despite our emphasizing that these patients did not need elevated doses.

Trial findings showed clear cardiac improvement, but slightly increased neurological damage was evident as well. This adverse outcome resulted in the non-marketing and abandonment of this drug.

These mishaps caused their own major tragedy, as the potential expansion of these findings might have allowed many diastolic dysfunction patients to receive a potentially life-saving treatment. Plus, Cariporide could offer massive benefits that go beyond those with heart failure, as I previously cited its role in reversing related calcium damage in the eye, brain, lung, gastrointestinal system, thyroid, prostate, and other organs.

So Cariporide is not available. But this does not preclude others from viewing the collected data. This information may help future pharmaceutical research solve diastolic dysfunction by modifying how calcium is exchanged... rather than only employing approaches that aim at its symptoms.

The Future

Diastolic dysfunction is still not viewed as a muscular disease, and this glaring error underlies the gaping inadequacies of current treatments. From what we found, successful managing of this disease requires understanding the form / function relationship behind it. The mechanism relates to the prolonged inner helix contraction during ejection, which in turn shortens the "prepare for suction" phase. This basic knowledge is essential as drugs may be developed to rectify this process (we used a sodium-hydrogen exchange blocker, but other calcium mobility agents may also accomplish this goal).

Unfortunately, neither fundamental concept (the helical ventricular myocardial band or the sodium-hydrogen exchange mechanism) is taught in medical schools. This vital information remains unknown within the fields of cardiology and cardiac surgery. A lamentable problem, as we may have the means to solve diastolic dysfunction, but nobody is looking at the two basic issues that might explain and reverse it.

Fortunately, science is not like politics. The truth wins, not popularity. Understanding these essential building blocks will eventually prevail and may generate a groundswell of exploration. Hopefully sooner rather than later, since the high mortality from diastolic dysfunction has remained constant for over three decades.[127] It is certainly time for a change.

The triumph of truth is the cornerstone of history.

CHAPTER 23

Art and Science: The Cardiac Dance; Spirals of Life

I received many invitations to speak after showing the Helix and Heart video. Organizations were intrigued by this new perception of the heart, which sprung from observing the simplicity of design after the heart was unwrapped. I believed this new knowledge might usher in a fresh understanding of heart structure, one that could — and should — lead to a revolution of how we treat the heart.

My educational goal widened, and I began to wonder if there was another means to reach an even broader audience.

I have always been captivated by the rhythmical movements of the normal helical heart, motions that Paco called the "cardiac dance." I reasoned, if it looks like a dance, why not create a ballet? Something that could enhance the understanding of the beauty of the normal healthy heart, demonstrate what happens when something goes wrong, and finally, reveal how restoring natural structure will return its natural harmony.

I again entered uncharted territory, but now in art rather than scientific endeavors. I'd only seen ballets performed on TV, except for one performance in Paris while attending a conference, which happened to be Baryshnikov's first public performance after he left Russia.

But I knew that ballets always told a story, and there was no more wondrous tale of movement than the one told by the beating heart. Good fortune for this pursuit prevailed, as I had maintained a close relationship with my alma mater, the University of Cincinnati, which had an outstanding College-Conservatory of Music. Their dean was Doug Lowry, whose vision of leadership was dynamic, inspired, and eager to explore new avenues of expression. I visited Doug there, and he was enchanted by the elegant simplicity of this helical heart discovery. He arranged a meeting with several of their teaching staff.

Their professor of dance was Shellie Cash, a graceful, creative, and committed person. My excitement and joy about the possibilities of looking at the heart through dance was infectious, as it ignited her flame by describing how the heart lives within nature's world of spirals. Shellie was thrilled, as spirals connected to nearly all that she does within the choreography of dance. The freedom of imagination flourished during our brainstorming on how to use movement to express this new heart concept. How exhilarating to join these intensely inventive people to develop a variety of ideas as I entered another new world (of dance). I loved it.

We set the ground rules of our collaboration, as Shellie and her staff would be in charge of generating the performance, and I was their consultant. My job was to ensure the dance truly embodied how the helical heart functioned.

A New World for *Everyone*

As it would turn out, this became a production unlike any they had ever done. Prior performances had nearly always been of classic ballets, relatively straightforward with the lighting and staging that would naturally be used to highlight the show. When you perform *The Nutcracker*, for instance, you essentially use the same music, sets, and dance moves to tell the same tale that has always been told. The similarity of a current performance to one given 25 years ago is predictable.

But our production had to be totally innovative. We would start from scratch. We needed to demonstrate the normality of the helical heart, show its failure after becoming spherical following a heart attack, and celebrate its rejuvenation upon restoring normal heart shape. Our team incorporated different departments at the College-Conservatory of Music: set design, multimedia, lighting, sound, music. All brought their best talents, and Shellie's skill as a leader allowed her to blend the gifts of these individuals from various disciplines into one integrated production. The College-Conservatory of Music had never put on such a multi-dimensional performance, in particular one that inextricably linked art and science.

I learned again that *interdependence* created an environment in which we could thrive. Independent efforts could not have achieved our collective goal. In truth, working with others has defined my entire career. Interdependency is crucial when a trained surgical team performs an operation, or when my research fellows take the lead in conducting our studies. The power of working collaboratively brings about something much grander than is possible by pursuing individual accolades. The reward is exponential, not additive.

Working in Tandem

Shellie was the producer. She coordinated all the different pieces of the whole, thereby placing an even greater demand upon her beyond the simultaneous chore of choreographing an original ballet. She boldly took on the job.

Her teamwork with grad student composer, Jenny Merkowitz, was spectacular. Jenny was equally fascinated by the project, and was also a dedicated student of the concept of golden proportion, which is so integral to the heart as well as to nature. The design department constructed a 20-foot model of the helical heart by placing fabric over an architectural framework that followed the simple design of Paco's rope-like model. This gargantuan replica became the distinctive backdrop that would stay in place during the first, second, and final acts of the ballet. Its simplicity and intrinsic elegance were awesome.

The same exceptional commitments to revel in the splendor of the helical heart existed in teams responsible for sound and lighting design, those creating multimedia projections of spirals on the stage floor and backdrops, as well as costume creation, and of course, within the talented student dancers Shellie's casting had selected. The power of her leadership was palpable during rehearsals, as was her unwavering dedication.

As my availability to travel back east to the College-Conservatory of Music was limited, Shellie would record videos of rehearsals and send those to me for review. In turn, I would respond when I saw things that might be incorrect, such as how to portray the bulging of the ventricle that develops from the non-contracting region after it is damaged by a heart attack. My personal experience with patients led me to sometimes make additional recommendations, such as having the two featured dancers wear grim expressions and slump their shoulders to exhibit the human experience that follows the development of heart failure after a heart attack. Likewise, when the heart returns to normal, they show the exhilarated smiles that express their newfound grace. So my "science focus" fused with the artistically presented human response that characterizes the tumultuous world of congestive heart failure. Such personal drama is portrayed throughout *The Cardiac Dance; Spirals of Life.*

I attended the final rehearsals for the show. Sitting alone in the empty wings of the theater, I marveled at the interweaving of each of the departments of dance, music, lighting, multimedia, etc. The devotion and caring that each had brought to the production was brilliantly apparent.

My global view of the heart, and of the production, allowed me to introduce further suggestions as the ballet was taking final form. I helped define how the dancers' motions represented actions of the normal heart, and especially after they are strikingly distorted by a disrupted heart form. But I also found myself posing ideas of a more aesthetic nature to enhance the message. For example, I worked with the multimedia person to ensure that background imaging was not emphasized in a manner that drew attention away from the dancers.

Along the way, I learned the scope of effort needed to put on such an ambitious production. I began to appreciate the pivotal roles played by those individuals we never see (much like those participating in a cardiac operation). I became aware of how much planning it took to change scenes with the large helical heart fabrication, as it needed to appear, collapse, and then later fully reappear as it became re-erected and regained its vibrancy. I could otherwise never have appreciated the smooth coordination required of a stage crew to silently raise it back up with pulleys — all managed covertly while the dancers carried on.

The cardiac surgical team of my world had now become the ballet production team, as this novel treat became a scintillating experience.

Showtime!

The day of the opening performance finally arrived: May 25, 2007. I was there with my wife, Ingeborg, along with a packed house from all over the Cincinnati area. There would be three public performances (all to capacity crowds). A professional videotaped version of the production would also subsequently be made (**and can be viewed via a link at the end of this chapter**).

Before the live performance, a brochure was distributed that not only described the show's background and cast, but also provided audience members an introduction to the helical heart concept. It revealed that even 400 years ago, there were scientists who believed the heart had a helical structure with a surrounding horizontal wrap. However, unwinding the structure to define this configuration had not been possible until Dr. Francisco (Paco) Torrent-Guasp used dissection to successfully unfold this "Gordian Knot" of anatomic architecture — and amazingly demonstrate that the heart unfurled like a rope.

I quoted Paco's memorable remark that "Nature is simple, but scientists are complicated." The brochure contained a drawing that showed how to recreate the heart's helical configuration from a piece of paper in less than ten seconds. (**Figure 1**)

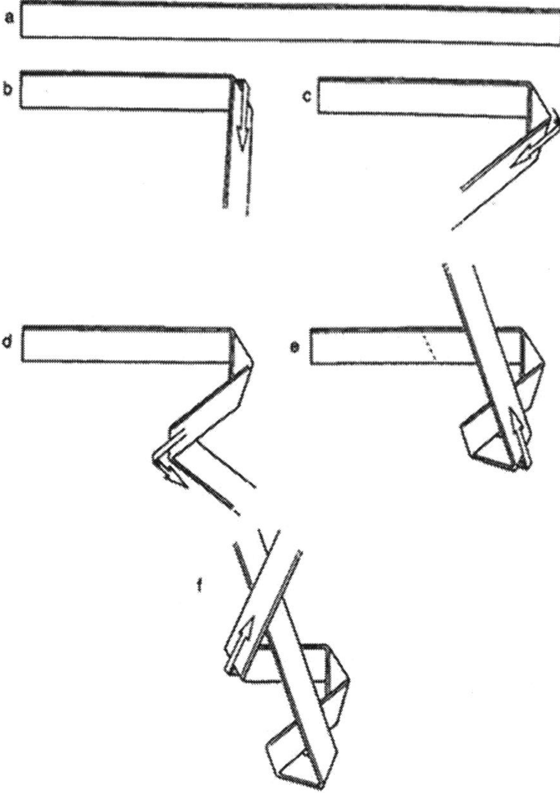

Figure 1: Helical heart design made from strip of paper.
Its beauty is its simplicity.

Pre-Show Video

Education was the goal of this *The Cardiac Dance; Spirals of Life* presentation, so we preceded the ballet with a nine-minute video, in which I cited the long-believed misconception that the heart basically constricted and dilated to function, instead of its proper twisting and uncoiling movements.

Paco Torrent-Guasp was introduced, together with his simple design of a helix and a wrap. The astonishing unraveling of the heart was shown both through animation, and with a video recording of Paco unfolding the rope-like heart by performing a dissection using only his hands. This pre-show video also included animation from the Helix and Heart video that demonstrated the heart's twisting and untwisting motions, along with its narrowing, shortening, lengthening, and widening movements.

We then described the disease of heart failure, which is poorly understood by the general public despite its affecting 5 million patients just in the U.S. alone. Actual footage of beating hearts showed the contrasts between the normal elliptical form, and the spherical shape that occurs when there is heart failure. We amplified this by contrasting the "healthy shape" of the University of Cincinnati football, to the "unhealthy form" of the Xavier University (the cross-town rival) basketball.

Following this, a clinical demonstration showed how heart failure changes *both form and function*, by first showing an MRI of a normal heart exhibiting its natural rhythmic action, and then contrasting it against the poor contractions of a dilated heart in congestive heart failure. The path of a heart's journey from normal, then its disruption, and finally returned back to normal — was illustrated by an animation of the surgical technique of opening the *now spherical* ventricle, and rebuilding it to restore the normal and healthy *elliptical form*.

Finally, the audience learned this was not some conceptual approach, as the video unveiled the results on heart performance following a cardiac operation that accomplished what the animation had portrayed. This was dynamically shown by using paired MRI images, which contrasted the dilated failing heart on one side of a split-screen... against the other side's image of a patient's *reconstructed ventricle* that had undergone this Surgical Ventricular Restoration procedure.

This pre-show video provided the audience with a background that would enhance their understanding and appreciation of *The Cardiac Dance; Spirals of Life* performance that was just about to start.

The Lights Dim....

As Act I began, the corps of dancers interwove, linking together as each held onto an 18-inch wide meshwork cloth that started as a straight line. They proceeded to move into a spiral configuration. The narrator's voice-over described the wide spectrum of spirals occurring in nature, ranging from the microscopic DNA to the macroscopic galaxy. The meshwork's spiral configuration then blossomed into a helical heart configuration, as the dancers interwove this lengthwise "rope" in a manner that mimicked the helical design that Paco had demonstrated with his heart dissection.

The concept of form affecting function was demonstrated in energetic fashion in Act II, as the dancers mirrored the heart's joyous rhythmical twisting and uncoiling motions. These movements were later elegantly featured in the video made of this ballet production by using an overhead camera, a creative move reminiscent of Hollywood director Busby Berkeley's elaborate musical productions in the 1930s. The elation, fluidity, and power of normality within the moving heart were thrillingly evident.

This happiness was then highlighted by a pas de deux of jubilant movement by the two principal dancers, who are portrayed as lovers. The vigor and merriment of being enraptured by healthy normality, exhibited by their shining faces and upright shoulders... would then collapse as a heart attack disrupted cardiac form and function. The magnitude of this dysfunction was dramatized by a startling collapse of the background's gigantic natural helical heart structure that was constructed by our design team. A brilliant conception by our creative group that had breathtaking impact. Simultaneously, the spirals of the multimedia presentations on stage became circles and the devastation of dysfunctional movement in the dancers took hold.

Dis-Harmony Heartache

In Act III, the dancers portrayed the consequences of this dysfunction. The heart attack and ensuing heart failure erased the ecstasy of the healthy heart's normal rhythmic function. It sapped away their merry smiles and replaced them with dismal expressions. These glum faces were married to slumped shoulders and irregular body motions as the heart's spiral helical shape was replaced by a circular form. The dancers showed that as a result of the heart attack, part of the heart contained dead muscle that no longer could squeeze, and now bulged as the heart contracted. At the same time, they displayed the limited function of the remaining living muscle that was undamaged by the heart attack.

The group movements representing this affliction provided a prelude to the second pas de deux performed by the two lead dancers, who portrayed the sadness stemming from the burden of a troubled heart. The duet ends with the dancers wrapped in each other's arms, a sorrow within them, within the music, and shared by the audience.

Then, slowly... a bright light shines upon them. The beam signifies their entering the anesthesia area, just before the female dancer is lofted and then carried into the operating room to undergo the left ventricular restoration procedure.

(Astonishingly, Jenny Merkowitz, our composer, was later analyzing the musical timing track of the play, and found that this bright light had occurred exactly at a point that was 0.618 of the play's total length. She could not believe it! Somehow, this numerical golden proportion ratio had made its way into the play... in the same way that it became evident when I unwound the heart to discover this identical proportion between the lengths of the two spiral muscles creating the helix).

Restoration Rejoicing

A reappearance of the meshwork material linking all the dancers opened the fourth act. The dysfunctional heart shape was represented by this circular cloth wall, which showed an irregularly contracting muscle with a circular form containing a bulge where the heart attack had happened.

But then our dancers simulated cardiac surgery, and this poorly functioning circular segment was opened at the heart attack's scarred region. Individual dancers entered the chamber, carrying a patch-like structure to demonstrate how surgeons rebuild cardiac shape. The irregular heart motions that had been coupled with the sad-faced corps de ballet (the "chorus" of non-soloist dancers) were now repaired. The dancers' gleeful demeanor resurfaced as the heart's harmonic rhythmic twisting motion returned. *The heart and the human became one.*

Revitalization

The last act captured the rejuvenation both within the heart and within the person. The spherical heart with irregular action returned to the elliptical configuration that brings normality. This marvelous wonder that flows from coordinated and cohesive heart motion was embodied by the dancers, whose movements seemed to explode from their happiness as they reveled in their newly found energy and joie de vivre. Their smiles, proud stance, and rhythmical motions became a source of dignity within themselves as their blissful rendering of completeness captured the audience, who joined them in the thrill of normality restored.

This resurrection was accompanied by restoration of the immense helical heart backdrop behind the dancers, whose structure reflected the exquisite symphony of normalcy. Moreover, the cardiac reciprocal spiral shape, initially performed by the dancers when they first formed a natural helix, returned as well. Their encore of healthy motions portrayed the marvels of the hearts' natural narrowing, shortening, widening, lengthening, and twisting movements.

The performance was met with resounding applause. The dancers' faces gleamed as they took their bows. It was clear that Shellie and the rest of her team were equally gratified.

Personally Fulfilling

The creation of *The Cardiac Dance; Spirals of Life* was profound for me. Not only did I witness Paco's concept of the heart transform into a beautiful work of art, I was also required to play a totally different role than I had as a cardiac surgeon and researcher. I became part of a new world of inventive individuals, each blending their unique ideas with others to generate something visibly pleasing. It was exhilarating.

Shellie said it was the best, most creative thing she had ever done. Additionally, the background set manager told me how thrilled he was to have participated in the College-Conservatory of Music's most collaborative production, as artists from so many disciplines merged toward a singular lofty goal.

I was equally grateful to have been a part of it, and extremely appreciative that everyone put forth their best efforts to realize this vision of telling the heart's story through dance.

"Touring" the Show

The primary thrust of this ballet was to create a teaching project — a means to enlighten others about the helical heart. So we restaged the ballet and recorded it. The video turned out beautifully, and copies were sent to all divisions of cardiac surgery throughout the United States and Canada.

Response was positive, and I was invited to present the video at the American Association of Medical Colleges meeting in Boston. The educators raised thoughtful questions after the presentation. They recognized that a powerful part of this educational format was to capture the imagination of the students, many of whom are not yet burdened with the information of yesterday, and whose thoughts will create a fresh tomorrow. My goal was successful in using art to stimulate a new awareness and understanding of the human heart. The "student's mind" of everyone who viewed the ballet became stirred, regardless of age or professional status.

Validation of this helical heart concept — and of the other advances presented in this book — has already been demonstrated. Yet the step of further scientific confirmation remains. This must be done by open-minded members of the medical community. We need them to endorse additional study and testing. This will lead to greater medical refinements of these approaches, and greater acceptance in the community.

The staging for this promising future has already taken place. The only question now is, when will the curtain go up?

Link to video of The Cardiac Dance; Spirals of Life:
www.youtube.com/watch?v=8ksNlYfgeRw

CHAPTER 24

Case of the Missing Link: The Septum

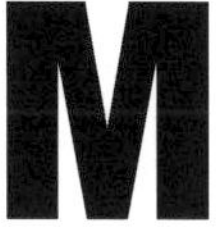ysteries abound in medicine. Many persist for centuries, until new discoveries and understandings can reveal the truth.

There is no portion of the heart more enigmatic than the septum.

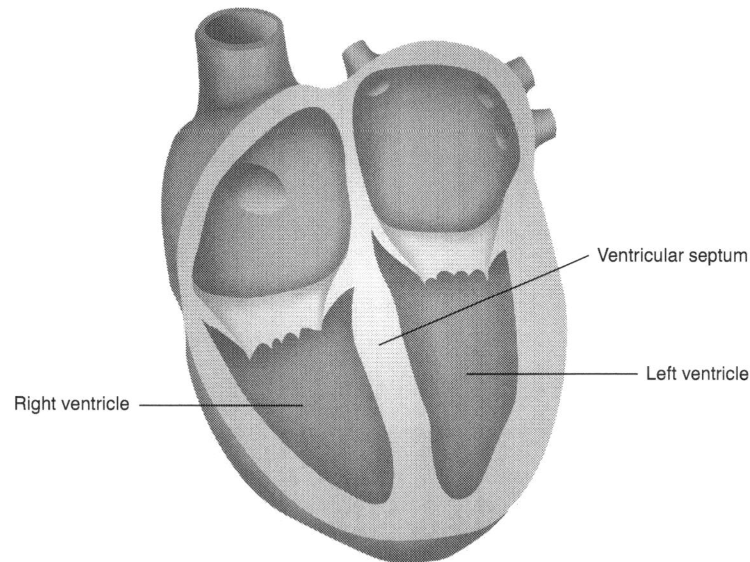

Figure 1: Typical image of heart, showing the right and left ventricles and septum separating them.

This thick curtain of muscle separates the left and right ventricles. (**Figure 1**) Yet understanding its function has long remained a puzzle. This is not simply an academic concern. It has real-world consequences for vast numbers of patients. For example, a common occurrence after open-heart surgery is that the septum does not work properly — while the ventricles seem to function just fine. The effects that this abnormality has on the heart are often underestimated. Its occurrence may be life-changing.

We know that disease develops when normal structure is distorted, and that the only valid treatment is to restore normality. Yet a dilemma exists when you don't understand what is normal. How can effective treatment be provided without this knowledge? This lack in understanding explains why so many treatments are ineffective.

Exploring the riddle of the septum takes us into a shadowy world of unanswered questions.

Clues from the Past

The medical profession has long attempted to understand what the septum does, since this knowledge could improve our ability to care for the heart. The origins of this quest stem back to when Hegar, a renowned anatomist and physician, asserted in 1865 that "Cardiac anatomy and function will be uncertain until the structure and function of the crossed angles of fibers in the septum are defined." Hegar's object of wonderment remained a mystery until Paco Torrent-Guasp taught us that *these are the oblique (angled) fibers of the helix,* and they make up the septum.

Despite this development, the age-old pursuit to understand the septum continues to be impeded by how those in medicine perceive the heart today. They persist in viewing it like a topographical map with three landmarks: the left and right ventricles, and a muscular septum between them. Hegar's warning was right. We cannot see truth if we're only fixating on what is easily observable.

But an alternative exists, one that lets us think of structure in a manner that can explain a wide variety of ailments. Our vision expands once we think of the heart's structure as the helix — as hinted at by Hager one-and-a-half centuries ago. This pathway suddenly carries us to dramatic new discoveries — ones that I will describe for you in this chapter.

As you will read, seemingly diverse issues (including right heart failure, infant cardiac procedures, ventricle assist devices, pacemakers, faulty valves, low blood pressure, and diastolic dysfunction) will encounter new breakthroughs all linked to a novel and comprehensive appreciation of the heart's structure. This involves developing an even deeper perception of how the helical ventricular myocardial band (comprised of an inner helix containing two arms and an outer surrounding wrap) will determine heart function. (**Figure 2**)

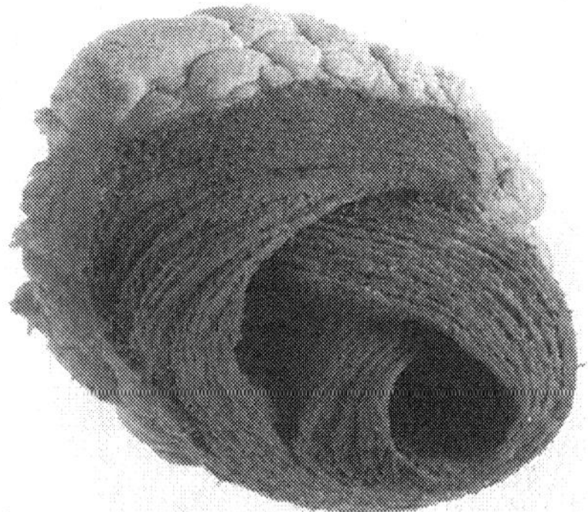

Figure 2: Displays how a heart's muscle fibers are oriented.
(The top light-colored area is fatty tissue on the heart's surface that is removed below.) The upper portion shows the surrounding wrap of circumferential muscle (called the basal loop). The septum is formed by the helical fibers displayed in the lower part of the heart's conical shape, which is made of a helix that has 2 arms of muscle fibers that cross each other at 60° angles (they form the apical loop, with a vortex at its tip or apex).

This is the beauty of Paco's contribution. His unfolding of the heart to reveal its structure changes everything we think about how *form impacts performance*. The cardiac world becomes simpler and clearer. Comprehending this normality would permit me to begin untangling the many mysteries brought to light within this chapter.

The Chase Begins

Exploring the secrets of the septum made me feel like I was in a detective story as I tracked down the "bread crumbs" laid out before us.

These clues begin with the heartbeat. Two of the biggest hints are the narrowing and shortening motions of the heart during contraction of the right ventricle. These two movements occur during each of the three billion heartbeats within our lifetime. Yet, the mechanism by which shortening is achieved has largely remained unknown until now.

So far in this book, we have only addressed heart failure in the left ventricle (that fills and then ejects blood to circulate through the body). But failure of the right ventricle (that pumps oxygen-depleted blood to the lungs to be re-oxygenated) has always been a perplexing predicament — especially because of our limited understanding of the mechanical forces that determine the right ventricle's performance.

The conventional view of right ventricular function insists that the surrounding thin right ventricle (RV) "free wall" (a surrounding wrap that encircles the outer wall of the RV, but not the septum) — compresses the blood in the right ventricular cavity against the thickened flat septum — to cause its ejection into the lungs. The action is similar to how a bellows might be used in a fireplace to compress air forward to feed the flames. This concept is unchanged from William Harvey's theories in the 1600s.

Further support for the bellows concept of the ventricles came from the more modern use of two-dimensional imaging tools (ventriculogram and echocardiogram) that show this narrowing action. Yet in addition to this compression... these tools also saw a *shortening movement* of the RV (right ventricle).

But they could not clarify *why* it shortened, or explain the importance of its shortening.

As we will soon find, the mechanism of shortening relates to the septum. This knowledge will shed light *on the true nature* of the right ventricle's function.

Deepening the Pursuit

My thesis, which you've heard a million times by now, is that heart anatomy determines its performance. This led to my need to understand structural form, so that the mechanical reasons for the heart's movements could be established.

This investigation made me feel a little like Sherlock Holmes. I recalled how Holmes would frequently ask Dr. Watson, "How often have I said to you that when you have eliminated the impossible, whatever remains, *however improbable*, must be the truth?"[128]

Popular medical belief said that right ventricle failure could be explained by the bellows concept. But I knew this theory was not true. Sherlock's *reductio ad absurdum* aphorism then leads us to look at *the septum* as the likely prime suspect in defining right ventricular performance.

"The Game is Afoot"

My quest to verify the role of the septum was successful. New deductions emerged after I used my knowledge of the helical ventricular myocardial band to put missing pieces together. Moreover, reports made by others were used to further build a solid case for understanding the function of the right ventricle.

I embraced the classic detective credo: "The simplest answer is often the correct one." The helical ventricular myocardial band concept identified that only two component parts make up the right ventricle's architecture. First, there was the surrounding wrap of the RV free wall, the one upon which nearly everyone had exclusively focused. The second was *the helix of the septum*. I reasoned that *it* may provide the simplest explanation for long-sought answers — because, quite simply, it was the only part left.

I believed that deductions could be made about the importance of each of these two parts (the circumferential wrap and helical septum) — by measuring how the right ventricle's function was affected — after each of them was injured.

The wrap was the easiest starting place because it is on the heart's surface. Prior researchers described extremely inventive ways to cause wrap damage: burning it by electrocautery, cutting the wrap completely out and replacing it with a patch that could not contract, or surgically removing it and then sewing it back (it subsequently would be made functionless by inducing electrical fibrillation).[129–131] Despite these devastating interventions, the right ventricle *always functioned properly*! This led to a stunning conclusion: the free wall *did not play* a significant role in right ventricular performance. No effect followed removal of its bellows action.

The power of the septum had finally captured the spotlight.

Step two was now needed. The septum must be made nonfunctional, while leaving a healthy wrap. The septum was damaged by impairing its nourishment (by closing the right coronary artery) and then either using electrocautery to burn its external surface... or by interrupting its electrical impulses... or by raising resistance in the lung blood vessels (by restricting the outflow of blood from the right ventricle). Each intervention made the right ventricular shape circular, which caused the septum to bulge toward the left ventricle cavity. In every instance, *distorting septum architecture caused right heart failure.*[132]

It became clear: the septum was responsible for most right ventricle performance. My realization that damage to the septum causes right ventricular failure led me to appreciate that "*the septum is the lion of the right ventricle.*"

The Secret of Shortening

The second riddle that needed to be solved was why the right ventricle shortened. There was no medical understanding for why this happened. Yet they did not know what I knew: Paco's helical heart model shows that contraction of the septum's helical muscle causes shortening. A valuable clue toward helping us understand the septum's performance.

This knowledge had not been recognized. Many believed the right ventricle shortens due to contraction of longitudinal (up and down) right ventricle muscles. While it seems natural to think that a longitudinal muscle pulls the base toward the apex (conical tip of the heart) as the heart shortens by 30% — *no longitudinal muscle fibers exist* in the septum! (The only exception is the thin papillary muscle that holds attachments for the heart valve).

Pursuing the cause behind this mystery motion exposed the weakness of the conventional two-dimensional imaging tools that had been relied upon for so many years. They record motion, but do not explain why it happens. Up-to-date three-dimensional tools reveal it's the heart's *twisting movement* that explains shortening. A coiling motion is generated by reciprocal contraction (rotating in opposite directions) of the helix's spiral muscles... with the direction of movement guided by that moment's dominant spiral arm.

Uncovering this connection allowed us to explain how the helical ventricular myocardial band determines right ventricle function. First, the RV *outer free* wall's bellows function is less efficient, as its transverse (horizontal) fibers only cause compression — accounting for just 20% of performance. Second, *the helical septum* produces twisting that generates the powerful RV ejection of blood into the lung. Its oblique (angled) fibers create twisting — a muscular action responsible for 80% of right heart efficiency.[133]

Key to Overcoming Counterforces

The importance of the septum's function becomes even clearer as we explore how its vigorous contraction gives the right ventricle its ability to push blood out of the ventricle *and past its opposition* — the natural "counterforce" of the blood vessels feeding the lungs.

What is this "counterforce?" During normal ejection, the vessels or arteries feeding the lung and the body will offer opposition to the blood flow directed at them from the heart — due to their progressively narrowing diameters. This is called "vessel resistance." It was known that the amount of such opposition by the vessels to the lungs is lower than that from those going to the rest of the body. In fact, lung vessel resistance is only one-sixth of the whole body vessel resistance — so the heart's work during right ventricular ejection (when it empties blood into the lungs) is substantially less than that for the left ventricle (which empties into the body).

This low lung vessel resistance means the less-effective wrap, which only causes compression (bellows), can by itself provide adequate RV emptying into the lungs. Septum twisting is not needed *under normal conditions.* However — *disease may increase* lung vessel resistance. When that occurs — right ventricular failure (as described later in this chapter) will develop if the septum is unable to twist and provide the added required force.

It's a straightforward concept that, once understood, brings unprecedented insight for a surprisingly accurate bedside diagnosis... far better than possible by use of the current sophisticated diagnostic equipment. The truth emerges because of a deep understanding of why things happen.

As an example, Saleh Saleh, a colleague of mine, was making clinical rounds with medical students, interns, and residents, when they encountered a patient with extensive coronary artery disease. The patient's major left and right coronary vessels were completely obstructed. Yet there were no signs of right heart failure — even though lung vascular resistance was high. Saleh told this cadre of students, "At least we know the coronary artery responsible for supplying blood to the septum was normal and without obstruction, since the right heart was functioning well" (given that right heart performance depends on the septum, he realized *the septum* must be receiving sufficient nourishment to function properly). His astonished listeners were leery that such a conclusion could be made without laboratory testing. But Saleh was confident.

So after rounds, these young doctors hurried to review the patient's coronary angiogram (pictures of blood flow through the coronary arteries)... and were flabbergasted to confirm the accuracy of Saleh's bedside assessment. But his decision was not capricious, as he was armed with the most powerful knowledge — an understanding of the helical ventricular myocardial band. He simply knew what to look for, rather than relying only on a test to give the answer.

Saleh is among the few to adopt the helical ventricular myocardial band explanation of heart function. While clues to identifying the septum's helical configuration *exist* — the concept is still not widely accepted, and the guidance it can provide toward better treatment is rarely used.

Peril of the Septum: Turning a Football into a Basketball

As I've said before, disease reflects a departure from normality, and its successful treatment rebuilds normality. It follows that negative outcomes with patients may be due to the lack of awareness of the heart's true structure.

Right ventricular failure is a perfect example, since it is difficult to manage, and medical teams consistently try to enhance the RV "bellows effect" to overcome it. They do this by delivering excess fluid into the right ventricle in order to stretch its free wall in an effort to expand the wrap. Yet improvement is either limited, or heart failure worsens.

The problem is the ongoing lapse in recognizing that this RV free wall contraction accounts for only a small percentage (20%) of its function. In reality, the septum is responsible for the majority (80%) of right ventricular function[133] — so it must always be the chief suspect behind causing (and then resolving) right ventricular failure.

This brought up a new query, one that had not been tested: Would the septum's vital role in right ventricular function be hampered if its helix shape was disrupted?

Clues were out there. We knew that *left* ventricular function crumbles if its elliptical helix shape (football) changes into a basketball-like form. Not surprisingly, my sleuthing revealed that the right ventricle suffers the same fate — including when excess fluids are given to "stretch" the bellows in an attempt to improve right heart failure. The right ventricle's portion of the septum also becomes stretched and its shape distorted into a more spherical form — its helical muscle fibers becoming more horizontal because of this expansion.

Knowing that the elliptical football is better than the spherical basketball shape for the heart, it became apparent to me that the direction of septum stretch did not matter. A circle is a circle. Similar dysfunction occurs when the septum bulges toward either the left or right ventricular chambers (since the septum's *now horizontal* helix fiber angles will impair its performance).

This discovery may be initially looked upon as bad news — but there is good news as well, since recognizing these mechanics is the stepping stone to a fresh approach. They tell us that *restoring normal septum architecture* could be a successful treatment for many different conditions.

Transforming Knowledge of Form and Function into Better Patient Care

Just as the classic detective gathers all of the suspects and clues together to reveal what he has deduced about the case, I will now present a series of real world examples that show how correctly understanding structure reveals remedies that will benefit patients who have right ventricle failure *from a variety of different causes.* The *septum* is the one consistent factor in each "mini-story."

Astounding Dilemma During Open-Heart Surgery: "Sweeping It Under the Rug"

Let me start by saying the mystery surrounding the septum has resulted in a "sweep it under the rug" approach to this injury when it malfunctions.

Echocardiograms, routinely used during open-heart surgery, sometimes reveal images of a dramatic change in normal septum performance — even though the heart seems to contract adequately after an operation. Yet a huge disparity exists if the septum is injured, as it does not contract, so that this midline muscle (between the ventricles) stretches to billow into the right ventricle. It now appears like an aneurysm inside of the heart. These adverse actions consistently take place after the septum is damaged (which is also called "septum stunning"), even though patients sustaining such dysfunction are consistently thought to be doing well.

Lesser damage will make the septum squeeze poorly or only a little — but a bulge is the worst injury of all. Surprisingly, this clear functional impairment caused by septum dysfunction, has continued to be considered *an acceptable complication of cardiac surgery.* This indifference to its presence may arise because the patient is discharged four to five days later, an end point that creates a sense of self-satisfaction for the surgical team about the operation's success.

But this is not true.

Hidden in the background lurks an injured septum. Consequently, serious potential problems can arise — including right or left heart failure, or diastolic dysfunction — because this part of the heart is not working properly.

So how frequently does this septum injury occur?

Disturbingly often. A recent survey of 3,292 patients showed approximately *40%* had bulging or "paradoxical motion" (the septum moving away from the left ventricle free wall during ejection, rather than its normal movement toward it). These incidences are even higher (about 60%) after valve surgery.[134]

Sometimes the septum never gets better. But even when it does, it can still be a significant burden to the patient. I have a friend that regularly swims with me, who had mitral valve repair and went home after five days. But then he could not swim for six months due to shortness of breath. He recovered, but unfortunately had to endure a preventable ordeal.

As we will discover, an ill-functioning septum has many ramifications. The ongoing failure to fully understand this septum problem has led to a unique fallback position for surgeons and their cardiology colleagues: it is disregarded and is conventionally judged as an acceptable post-operative complication.

Weighing the Reasons for Failure

My commitment to solve these "*whodunit*" mysteries of septum dysfunction grew after I asked a colleague, a legend of cardiac structure, about the size of the septum. I knew the answer when I posed the question, but wanted to find out what this leader thought. Carmine Clemente is a brilliant, world-renowned anatomist, whose textbook is used by over 1.5 million students worldwide. He guessed the septum occupied 10% of the total weight of the ventricles.

I had already weighed the septum after completing some experiments, and compared it to the weight of the free walls of the right and left ventricles. His guess was wrong, as the septum weighed *almost 40%* of whole heart ventricular weight (while it accounts for *about 50%* of just the left ventricular weight). (**Figure 3**)[135, 136]

This realization prompted me to accelerate my investigations, especially since the septum was often damaged during cardiac procedures, and this injury was simply accepted as a natural complication of heart surgery. It was astounding that incapacitating something that occupies *nearly 40%* of the whole heart's ventricular weight was not thought to be important.

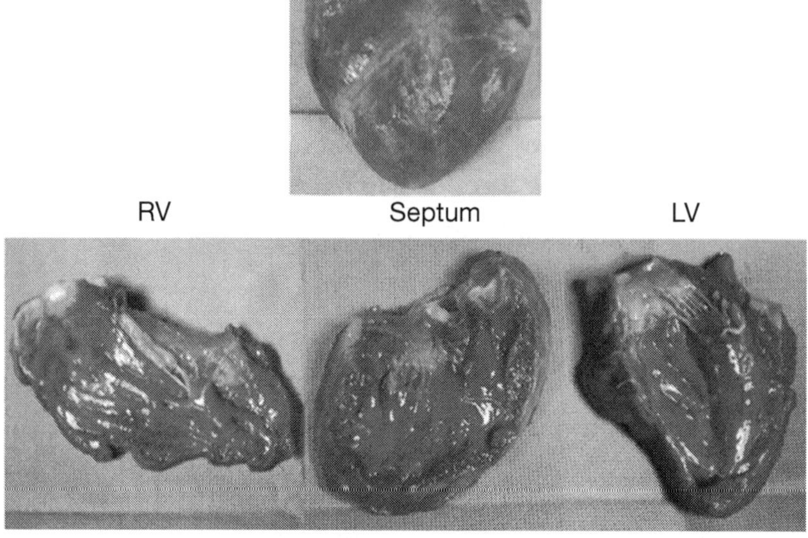

Figure 3: Upper image shows intact heart. Lower 3 images show separation of heart muscle into right ventricle (RV), septum, and left ventricle (LV). Note size of septum.

A trail of clues began to appear. I started by looking deeper into the previously described study of 3,292 patients. There was a tip-off right in front of me: the report indicated that septum bulging was *most common when aortic clamping was prolonged* while the heart was being repaired.

To me, that sounded exactly like a reperfusion injury.

My prior work showed our method of myocardial protection *avoids* reperfusion damage. I speculated that a surgical procedure shouldn't cause damage to the septum — if our methods to protect against reperfusion injury were done correctly.

But this theory needed testing. So we studied 119 consecutive patients to see if this was true. The result: *No septum damage* developed *in any* of our patients, despite aortic clamping times that extended up to 155 minutes.[136]

We next gained an even more powerful clarification.

We compared results following operative procedures that employed our full approach — to those performed by others who had used the same cardioplegic solutions — but *did not* follow our delivery methods. The result: *septum damage occurred if our delivery strategy was not followed, but was absent when it was.*[137]

The conclusion: success involves two components — the cardioplegic solution *and* adopting a proper delivery strategy. Avoiding septum damage does not result from addressing just one part of an answer (like only selecting a single instrument of the orchestra), but rather by using an integrated approach that enhances its effectiveness (the whole orchestra).

I believed the surgical community needed to know and utilize this information. So I submitted a report, "Cardioplegia: Solutions or Strategies?" to the two major American cardiac surgery journals. It was rejected by both. Yet incredibly, not one of these seven reviewers stated that their methods of myocardial protection avoided septum injury.

The sweep-it-under-the-rug attitude persisted, unaffected by truth.

At issue was not a suggestion that they only follow our protection methods. Instead, I recommended that they must always examine whether the septum's function was compromised. I advised that if there was *no injury*, then they should continue their current protection methods. However, *if there was injury*, their protection methods should change. The end goal is to avoid septum damage. The selection of what process to accomplish this is up to the surgeon. It seemed unconscionable to subject the septum, which comprises 40% of its ventricular muscle weight, to a preventable form of heart damage.

As important as it was to solve this avoidable septum issue in cardiac surgery, I realized this surgical problem is only one example of many issues that can arise from a damaged septum. It was this appreciation that made me recognize that avoiding septum injury may "crack the case" — and resolve *numerous* causes of right heart failure.

Baby Heart Surgery… The Hidden Septum Role

My search to better understand issues with the septum intensified when I came across a revealing and unsettling problem.

As said, the inherent interplay between the septum — and right ventricle function — is linked to high resistance within the lung vessels against the blood flow that comes from the heart. This situation is dramatized by the tragic development of sudden right ventricular failure, which can develop unexpectedly… shortly after doing a successful heart operation in infants.

Before the baby's operation, the beauty of the body's ability to adapt to obstacles is clear — since right ventricle performance is normal — despite many of these infants having a high resistance to the flow of blood into their lungs. In other words, the *uninjured* septum had adjusted its function to fully compensate for this high lung blood flow resistance — enabling the right ventricle to readily eject blood into the lungs.

But that "adjustment" ceases as soon as the septum is acutely injured due to ineffective myocardial protection during a heart operation in infants. A new drama unfolds, as the infant may now experience the same septum problems that had confronted the adult. But the existence of this problem *is initially hidden,* since the infant's right heart performance immediately after the operation may appear normal and satisfactory. Why? Because the surgical procedure had lowered the high resistance in those vessels going to the lungs by an operation that closed a congenital heart defect (a hole)… or one that opened a narrowed pulmonary valve to improve lung blood flow.

The infant looks fine at first, yet some babies, after they are in the intensive care unit, will quickly develop a problem called *vasospasm,* a sudden narrowing of their small lung arteries. The right ventricle will fail, as this unexpected obstruction of its outflow of blood (to the lungs) cannot be overcome by the heart, when the septum is damaged. A dilemma evolves that can turn into a life-and-death crisis.

The bewildered surgeon asks, "What happened? I repaired everything that was wrong. The infant was fine yesterday!"

The culprit is the septum.

What happened is the heart is again confronted with high pulmonary resistance from this sudden narrowing of the small lung arteries (vasospasm). Septum twisting is needed to powerfully push the blood past this higher resistance, but it cannot do so because of its injury during the operation.

A false conclusion had buoyed the physician's confidence on the first day — arising from the misguided thinking that the bellows action of the contracting wrap was all that was needed. While this is true with *low* lung vascular resistance — everything changes now if the cardiac twisting becomes compromised, as the septum can no longer be relied upon to combat the newly developed vasospasm.

Hopefully, understanding why this swift and sometimes life-threatening development of right heart failure evolves — may motivate selecting improved methods of protection that can avoid the aftermath of this awful complication.

Left Ventricle Assist Device *Impairs Right Ventricle...* But Why?

Spectacular advances have been made to support a failing *left* heart. *Ventricular assist devices* are put in left ventricles that are not ejecting blood well, their role being to suction blood from the heart and then pump it back into the arteries of the body. Impressive improvement frequently follows... but a major complication can also occur.

While the left heart performs better, the right heart now sometimes fails.

How can this be?

The problem is not with the device, but rather with the misunderstanding of how structure determines right ventricular (RV) function. The dilemma develops when the device may super-efficiently eject nearly all of the left ventricular blood — so that the left ventricle (LV) cavity shrivels to practically collapse. The septum (the muscular "wall" between the two ventricles) then bulges into the left ventricle to fill this now-empty space created inside it. The right ventricular cavity becomes more spherical as it stretches.

That expansion causes the septum's oblique (angled) 60° fibers to become more transverse (horizontal) — a geometric change that makes RV function worsen.

The telltale clue to again deducing the septum as a culprit arose from my realizing that most of the critically-ill patients suffering this setback — had very high pulmonary resistance (from narrowed blood vessels to the lungs). The counterforce to this condition is a "fully functioning (twisting) septum" that will ensure an efficient and robust right ventricular performance. But this cannot happen until the septum fibers return to their natural oblique orientation.

Understanding this sequence leads to a straightforward action to counter this problem: all you need to do is *decrease the suction* on the left ventricle assist device, as this returns a normal LV chamber size and shape. The septum promptly returns to a midline position and right ventricle performance improves.[138]

Unfortunately, the septum's role in this clear-cut solution has not yet been recognized, which needs to happen before better protocols for left ventricular assist devices can be developed to offset this problem. Yet anyone who has come to understand how the structure of the heart governs its function — including you, the reader — can easily grasp this need.

Electrical Ignition and Muscle Firing... Do We Have a "Concert?"

As you just read (and as I've often cited elsewhere as well), effective treatments are based upon comprehending normality, appreciating how disease distorts this, and finally using this knowledge to restore normality. For example, the septum that bulges is a serious dilemma, one that is solved by returning it to its natural midline position.

Yet the reason for abnormal septum bulging may be completely different from having a left ventricular assist device set too high. For example, problems due to uncoordinated *electrical stimulation* of the septum may cause it to billow. This happens when the septum's electrical stimulus is delayed and the left side of the heart contracts before the septum. As a result, the non-contracting septum bulges into the right ventricle.

Enter the world of *electrophysiology* medicine and its use of a device called a *pacemaker* to provide programmed stimulation. This method is used in the over 5 million pacemakers implanted in patients in the United States alone. This is a common way of "pacing" when normal impulses through the natural wiring system within the heart are slow.

Aside from its common basic function of raising a low heart rate, one that most people are familiar with, a pacemaker can also be utilized when uncoordinated electrical stimulation causes the septum to bulge into the right ventricle. This treatment is called cardiac resynchronization therapy (CRT). Electrical leads are placed in the atrium and into the left ventricle and septum. Its goal is to stimulate both ventricles together to synchronize their beats, so that the outer left ventricular wall contraction is simultaneous with that of the septum. The septum returns to the midline position when this is effective.

Yet while pacemakers successfully increase the heart rate and return the septum to its proper position, *the type* of muscular contraction they create must be considered. Direct septum stimulation does not make the left ventricle *twist*. Instead, the muscle touched directly by the pacemaker lead develops an irregular local contraction, rather than the sequential full heart contraction generated by the normal flow of impulses that arrive from its natural wiring system — the prerequisite for producing the heart's natural twisting action.

This difference motivated me to investigate how to use the *natural wiring system* to pace (electrically stimulate) the heart. I found this second approach had been established by other researchers, as pacemaker leads (wires) were instead placed into the area where the natural impulse starts — a site called the Bundle of His (pronounced "hiss"). The magnificence of nature reveals itself when this is done. These impulses travel *ten times faster* than those from direct muscle stimulation, and they produce twisting. The cardiac concert is restored by our pursuing normality instead of using the conventional pacemaker stimulation approach that cannot bring about the natural twisting beat.

While both types of pacing options are available, this second natural ignition pathway is rarely selected by physicians. It reflects a revolution in thinking, and very few cardiologists want to do it. Nor do the pacemaker manufacturers wish to redesign their currently widely used and profitable products.

Of the 5 million pacemakers implanted in the U.S.... the number of people who have been paced in this second manner is probably less than 1,000. (The possibilities of reproducing excellent normality with pacemakers will be further explored in Chapter 26).

Septum and Heart Valves... Leg Bone's Connected to the Knee Bone

The heart has two atriums (to receive blood) and two ventricles (to pump blood). Cardiac valves are located between each atrium and ventricle. They open to let blood into the ventricles from the atrium, and close when the heart begins to contract. Today, *the most common adult heart surgical procedure* is to fix or replace these valves after they malfunction.

But in some cases, disappointing outcomes follow successful operations.

This is because those procedures are directed *only* at the valve. Understanding why this is a dilemma requires an appreciation that a heart valve does not live in isolation. Yes, it is the "doorway" between atrium to ventricle, through which blood flows. *But the valve also has supporting structures* — such as the collagen tissue that are struts that hold the valve leaflets as they open and close, and the papillary muscles that connect the valve to the ventricle's muscular wall.

Leaky valves often happen because of issues with these supporting structures, and occur despite there being a normal valve configuration. So it isn't always a valve problem. This dilemma is common in patients with dilated hearts that are failing. Simply fixing or replacing the valve does not make the patient get better.[114, 115]

Why? Again, structure / function interaction becomes the crucial clue. The septum once more plays a pivotal role — since the valve's supporting apparatus is physically connected to it.

This dynamic relationship of *interdependence* stirs vivid memories of my time in medical school when I failed that first anatomy test. My study habits were fine. I had memorized every muscle, nerve, artery, and bone, but I had not considered the relationships among them. Reminiscing back even further, I recall a song we sang as children, "Dem Bones," the one that goes, "...the leg bone's connected to the knee bone... the knee bone's connected to the thigh bone...." It's a lesson that remains relevant today, as the septum is connected to these valve structure components.

Just as Sherlock Holmes would find clues that were hidden in plain sight, the secret here involves *seeing what you are looking at*. For example, the papillary muscle (attached to the valve) is connected to the septum in the right ventricle — *and it gets stretched* when the septum bulges into the left ventricle. Similarly, when the septum bulges into the right ventricle, the left-side papillary muscle (located adjacent to the septum) is pulled downward. This form of tugging has a fancy name (tethering), and produces the dangerous action of causing a leaky valve (called valve *insufficiency*) by preventing the valve leaflets from fitting together.

The solution? As Holmes might say, "The answer is elementary." Just take the stretching away — by bringing the septum back into normal position.

We followed this strategy in our studies to evaluate the interaction between the septum and the heart valves on the left and right sides of the heart. First, we made a test animal's septum billow into the right ventricle by delaying the electrical impulse delivered to the left side of the heart. As expected, there was leaking from the mitral valve. Equally anticipated, returning the septum to a midline position by cardiac resynchronization therapy (CRT) — decreased mitral valve leaking.

To test further, we next made the septum bulge into the left side — by inhibiting the ejection of blood from the right ventricle by narrowing its outflow artery to the lungs (pulmonary artery). The tricuspid valve began to leak. We then returned the septum to its natural midline position by using drugs or mechanical devices... and complete recovery of tricuspid valve function resulted![139]

In each instance, the leaky valve was caused by the supporting structures that were connected to the septum — not by a problem with the valve itself. Recognizing how the valves' architecture interfaces with the septum may generate new approaches for how leaky valves should be treated.

Treat the Low Blood Pressure... or Treat the Heart?

Nothing stimulates a prompt medical team response like a patient in an intensive care unit who suddenly develops low blood pressure. Fear of a heart attack or stroke rouses immediate action. A cascade of drugs like dopamine and epinephrine are commonly used to raise blood pressure and improve cardiac contraction. This includes instances when low blood pressure occurs in a patient with right heart failure.

As I considered everything I had learned, I questioned if this was the best approach. It made me ask a fundamental second question. What should be corrected first: the low blood pressure itself... or the heart that regulates it?

These inquiries surface because the drugs commonly used to raise blood pressure will *narrow* the body's blood vessels — *all* of the body's blood vessels. That means they *also constrict small lung artery blood vessels* — which raises lung vessel resistance — restricting the successful outflow of blood from the right ventricle into the lungs. So while raising the pressure is seen as a win, the heart may lose — since cardiac function worsens in the right heart failure patient when their lung vessel resistance is raised. Why? Because the right ventricle's efficiency (produced by the septum's ability to twist) is already impaired, and becomes further impeded if the septum's twisting capacity is strained even more. Our chance to treat and reverse this condition is worsened by escalation of this powerful downward cascade.

But a different approach can be taken to treat right heart failure and low blood pressure, taking advantage of a better understanding of the heart / function relationship. Simply stated — diminish this opposition to the right ventricle's pumping out blood to the lungs — to offset the septum's impaired ability to twist and challenge the increased lung vessel resistance.

Lung vessel resistance can be lowered — by drugs like amrinone and milrinone — allowing heart function to improve as the right ventricle can more easily eject blood. So now the ventricle shrinks and the septum returns to its normal position. Normal septum twisting and shortening recover, and the improved heart action makes it eject more blood, *producing increased blood pressure.* A vast improvement over the outcomes of using drugs that narrow all the body's blood vessels.

Better decision-making regarding patient treatment comes from the awareness that drugs that *dilate* (expand) lung arteries may be preferable to those that narrow them.

Unfortunately, persistent misunderstanding of anatomy and function relationships will allow flawed decisions to continue. *This must change.*

Septum and Diastolic Dysfunction

I then asked the most basic question I could ever ask: "Are we observing the heart properly?"

My new understanding that the heart is composed of only three parts — a circumferential wrap and inner helix (with two arms) — is a view that completely differs from the conventional "topographic" approach where the "classic concept of "left ventricle, right ventricle, and septum" commands our total attention. Yet it is our willingness to learn a fresh approach that can lead to developing new answers to old problems.

This concept becomes clear when an innovative look is taken toward addressing diastolic dysfunction (discussed two chapters previously) — that form of congestive heart failure experienced by 7.5 million patients just in the U.S. and Europe — caused by impaired suction for ventricular filling. This common disorder also perfectly reflects how the septum's geometry influences the function of both ventricles.

The important question of "what is the heart?" takes center stage. That's because the traditionalists' view of the three parts (left ventricle, septum, right ventricle)... considers the septum's function to be isolated from the others.

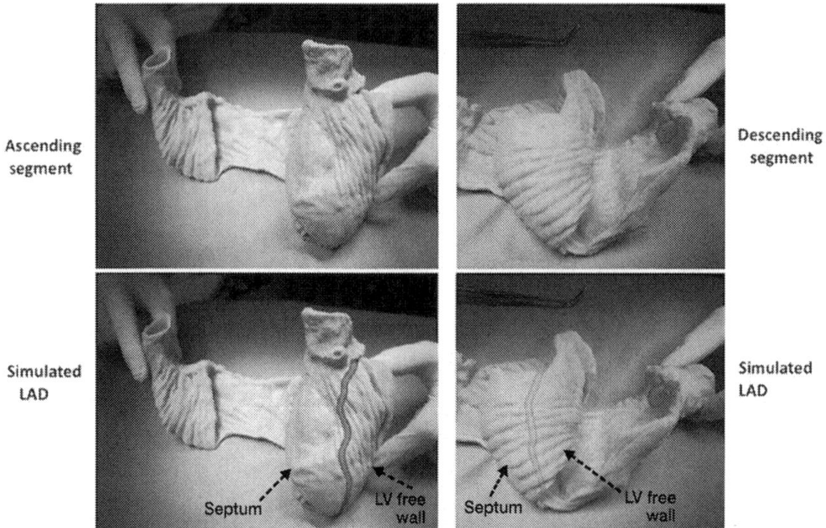

Figure 4: Upper two images show the anatomy of the helix containing the ascending (outer) and descending (inner) segments. The lower two images show a "simulated artery" that runs along (bisects) its outer and inner walls to demonstrate how the septum and the LV free wall are formed by the same outer and inner helix muscles.

Yet a more comprehensive view emerges when the helical ventricular myocardial band concept is applied — in which *the same inner and outer helix muscles* form the septum and left ventricle free wall (the "outer" wall of the ventricle opposite to that of the septum) as seen in **Figure 4.**

Suddenly an inescapable conclusion becomes apparent, as the septum is *no longer seen as an independent structure*: damage to one portion of the helix *must* affect all structures that are part of it. Consequently, an injury to the septum must also affect the left ventricular free wall. Said differently, diastolic dysfunction cannot be considered an isolated event that influences only one part of the heart.

A prime example is found in some heart surgery patients who return with mild left heart failure symptoms several weeks after being discharged from the hospital. Its cause has remained a mystery for many physicians. Yet I knew that *stunning of* the septum (reflecting its injury) is commonplace during cardiac operations (as described earlier in this chapter), and believed my understanding of helix structure might unravel its connection to these later problems. To my surprise, I found the frequency of diastolic dysfunction occurring after surgery ranges from 44 to 75% — which precisely matches how often a bulging septum motion is observed during such surgeries.[65] These dual observations of similar complications contrast sharply with the conventional conclusion that septum impairment is an acceptable outcome of surgery.

Because the helix involves the septum and left ventricle outer wall, when you impair one part, you will always impair the other. After all, it is all the same muscle. Thus, such a reperfusion injury (septum stunning) imparts the same damage to the left ventricle free wall — thereby impairing its ability to uncoil — which will reduce suction and cause symptoms of left heart failure.

This conclusion is easily missed if we only consider the conventional topographical view of three separate heart parts (left ventricle, the septum, right ventricle), whereby septum stunning and diastolic dysfunction (heart failure) are considered *independent* events. Such a lapse to appreciate the anatomy behind this devastating disease will hamper the evolution of new solutions.

Conversely, using the helical ventricular myocardial band to escape the confines of traditional thinking will give us a fresh way to look at the heart, granting us a portal toward discovery and new treatments.

Mysteries Solved

Our detective work solved the mystery surrounding the septum described by Hegar in the 1800s. There is now clarity for its major role in determining many cardiac treatments, including those for: right heart failure, open-heart surgery, infant heart surgery, left ventricle assist devices, cardiac electrical events, heart valve problems, low blood pressure drug selection, diastolic dysfunction... *and probably more to be uncovered.*

I am grateful to Paco Torrent-Guasp for unlocking this gateway to understanding the basic components of the wrap and helix that form the heart. The simplicity of this design represents a huge leap in knowledge, one that may allow us to successfully treat many different clinical issues that were previously and perplexingly insoluble.

Accordingly, I envision that wide recognition of "the motor of the septum" will provide new understanding and guidelines to enhance how we diagnose and improve treatment in areas that have until now baffled us.

CHAPTER 25

Arts and Science: Stonehenge and the Heart

To me, the most exciting part of the learning cycle is the way in which new knowledge launches the next educational exploration. This process occurred again when I created the Basic Science Lecture on the Helix and Heart. I was astonished by the unity of how the heart fit into a natural design of similar spiral patterns that stretched from DNA to the nebula of the cosmos.

Suddenly, the biologist mirrored the artist who observes an enriching blend of shapes and shadings in their surrounding world. *What changes is not so much where you look, but how you see.* My view now included the fluidity and efficiency of spirals as I watched them in the water swirling down a bathroom drain, the webs made by some species of spiders, and the gracefully carved scroll of a violin. And then, one day, I looked at a picture of Stonehenge — and saw something I never had before.

Stonehenge is the group of very large standing stones located on Salisbury Plain in southern England, presumed to date back as far as 3500 BC. (**Figure 1**) I visited it in 1990 with my wife while driving through England after attending a conference in Oxford. We knew that many theories had been offered as to why it was built, but none had been proven. Beyond that, I thought little about it, until I developed my Basic Science Lecture that taught me of a coherence among things... *if you look for it.*

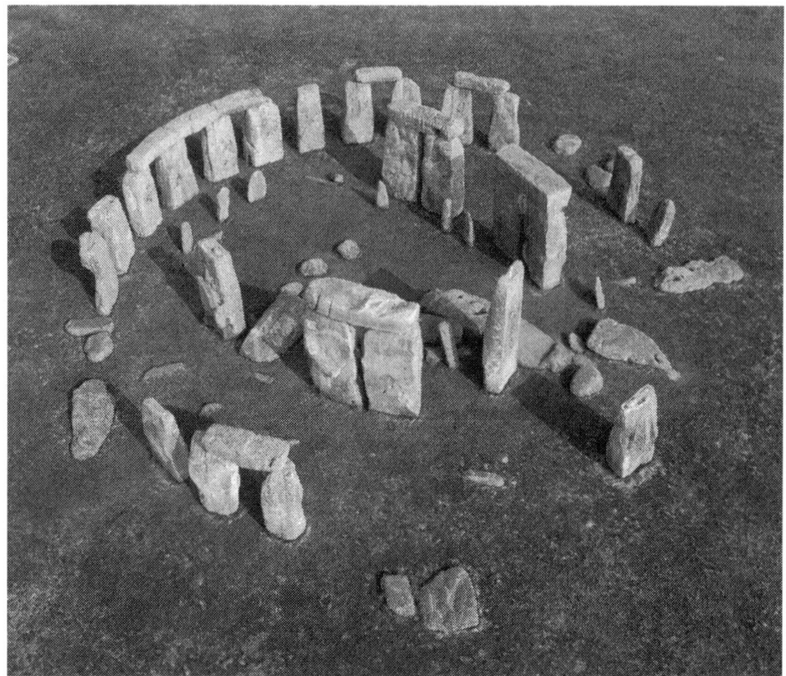

Figure 1: Stonehenge with Sarsen Circle and interior Bluestone Trilithon Horseshoe

Twenty-four years after my visit, I was mesmerized by an image showing Stonehenge's complete layout. I stared because I saw similarities to the heart.

This vision launched my new search to see if this correlation could be justified.

Exploring the Speculative World of Stonehenge

Construction of Stonehenge began approximately 5,500 years ago, and took *over 1,800 years* to complete. Its form continues to capture the interest and imagination. It is an ancient wonder of the world. Nearly everybody has heard of it, many have seen it, and some theories as to its origin and meaning exist. But no one understands it.

The harmony of its construction stretched over 50 generations of builders, suggesting that a powerful underlying architectural principle existed and had been passed down… yet nobody knows what that principle was. The tendency to offhandedly reject my suggesting a correlation between Stonehenge and so unlikely a candidate as the heart presents a typical response to any challenge of traditional thought — indeed paralleling what has occurred so often with results of my medical research. But evidence is the true determiner, not belief. So I began looking for data to test this comparison.

It wasn't long before I found it.

I became captivated by a book called *The Power of Limits: Proportional Harmonies in Nature, Art, and Architecture*, by Gyorgy Doczi, a Hungarian architect and scholar.[110] He explores some basic mathematical ratios that are common within natural structures — and within those that are human-made.

Doczi emphasizes that one pattern within this world of harmony stems from the golden section of Pythagoras. As described before, it defines proportionality, where the smaller portion relates to the larger portion in the same ratio as the larger portion relates to the whole (further detailed a bit later). This famously recognized "golden section" becomes the foundation of the Fibonacci ratio of 0.618… a proportion that also exists in all spiral structures.

The heart is neither described nor analyzed in his book, but the principles Doczi discusses are universal. For example, I previously found the proportions of the Fibonacci ratio in the lengths of the right- and left-handed sides (arms) that construct the helical heart segments. I was astounded to learn that Doczi found the same mathematical golden proportion relationship within Stonehenge's architecture. This intriguing observation further motivated my quest to find the structural commonality between the heart and this eternal megalithic structure.

Parts of the Whole

With help from Doczi's book, I began my investigation to better understand Stonehenge.

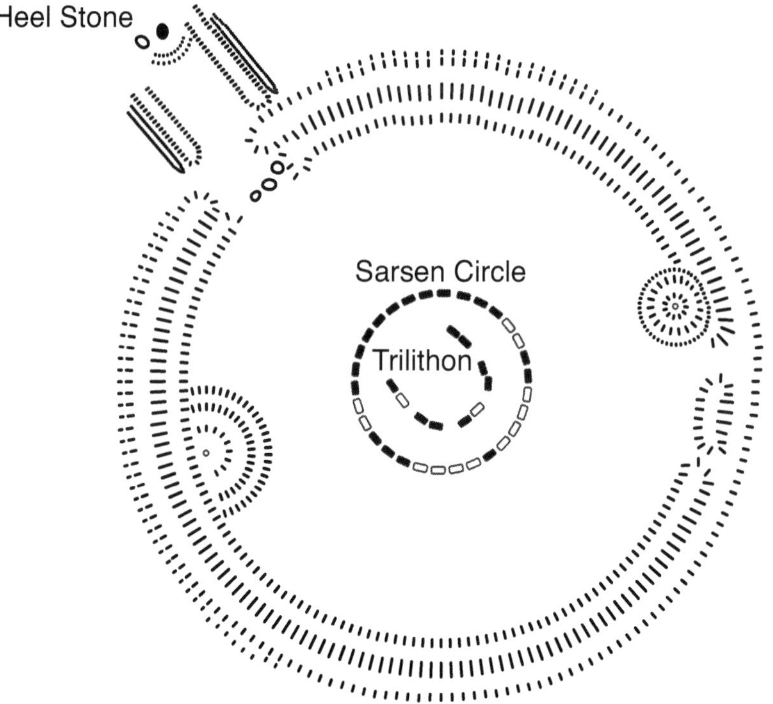

Figure 2: Overview of Stonehenge, within the outer circular rim.
The inner components include the Sarsen Circle and Trilithon Horseshoe.
The Heel Stone (small unshaded circular shape) is beyond the outer rim and the Summer Solstice is observed when viewed from these inner components.

Stonehenge's round outer wall of stones make up the Sarsen Circle. (**Figure 2**) Existing within this circumference is the Bluestone Trilithon Horseshoe with its U-shaped arms. Its open endpoints aim toward Stonehenge's four outer wall pillars that have three beams (or lintels) on top of them. These structures are associated with the two best-known "views" in Stonehenge. (**Figure 3**)

The first is the overall architecture containing its Sarsen circle, Trilithon horseshoe, and outer pillars. The second "view" reveals itself only once a year, at the summer solstice, when the sun's yellow disc rises between the pillars and beyond the Heel Stone. The observer witnesses this by sitting on a stone (called the "Altar Stone") in the center of the horseshoe. This perennial observation has intrigued scholars for centuries.

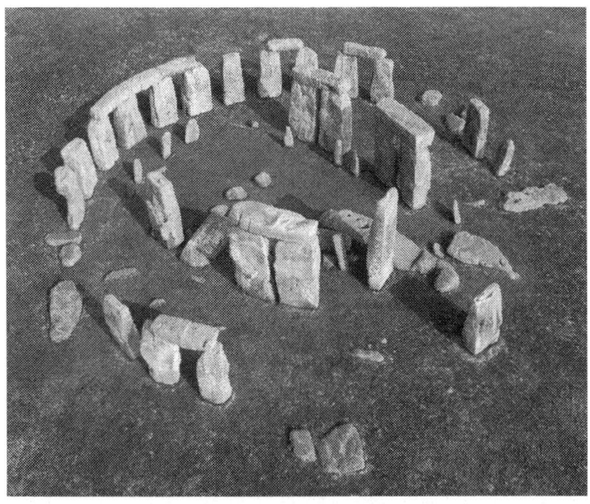

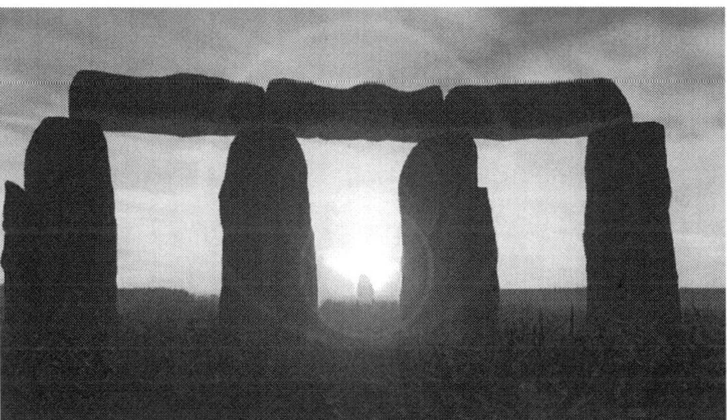

Figure 3: Classic views of Stonehenge. On top is Sarsen Circle and Trilithon Horseshoe. On bottom are the pillars and beams through which the summer solstice is seen behind the Heel Stone.

But my own fascination with Stonehenge stemmed from a different source — my knowledge of the design of the helical heart, whose structure contains a helix and surrounding wrap of muscle. (**Figure 4**) That awareness, along with my recent discovery of *The Power of Limits*, made me wonder about possible similarities between the heart and Stonehenge. I knew *parallels* existed, since the megalithic structure permits us to see the moving cosmos, outside us... while the helical cardiac structure is responsible for the moving blood, inside us.

But was there more?

The heart has a cone-shaped helical loop, with a vortex at its apical tip — and only functions efficiently if its conical shape is supported by a surrounding external buttress (the wrap).

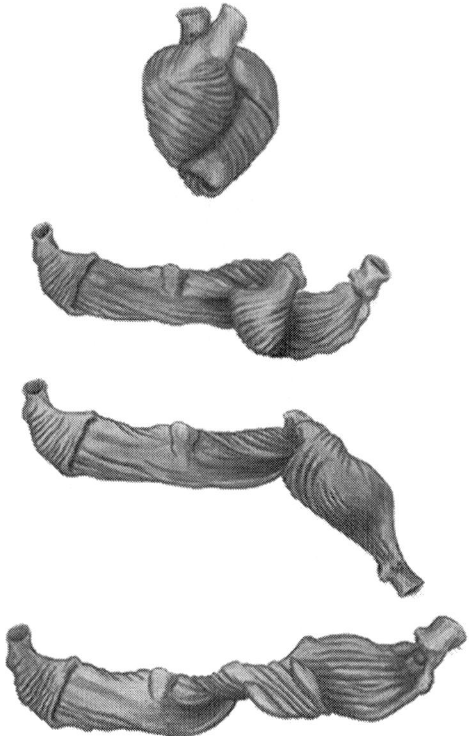

Figure 4: Helical Ventricular Myocardial Band of Torrent-Guasp showing (top image) the intact heart has a wrap and a helix that has a vortex at its tip. Beauty is simplicity, as the second image shows unwrapping, and how the inner and outer shells form the helix. The heart is made of a simple rope, as seen on the third and fourth images where the helix is unfolded.

In the same way, Stonehenge has the sun, which may be considered as its "conical tip," and which we can view each summer solstice by looking through Stonehenge's structural portals. (**Figure 9**) How extraordinary that the space between the outside of the inner arms of Bluestone Horseshoe — and inside the surrounding Sarsen Circle — reflects a buttress for Stonehenge's conical central area. I saw an architectural pattern in this gigantic megalithic structure that I needed to explore further. I wanted to see how it might mimic the cone and base of the heart (as you will see later in **Figure 9**).

Still, I wondered if this parallel configuration was merely a visual coincidence that I conceptualized to justify my desire to see a similarity. I did not yet know the answer.

Seeking the Balance

I needed to go deeper than focusing only upon the surface. So I began to question whether Stonehenge's construction had a *measurable composition* that matched the heart's configuration.

The key to this analysis must be simplicity. Such clarity conforms to how other scientists have linked mathematics to nature, like da Vinci and Einstein. Doczi explored this theme in *The Power of Limits,* offering a breathtaking demonstration of the interaction of basic mathematical components within Stonehenge's stark construction. The structural breakdown is amazing, as we find this unique megalithic structure contains the circle, a square, rectangles, Pythagorean triangles, as well as displays of the harmonic matching (or reciprocal) relationships between rectangles — all marvelously merged into a single structure. (**Figure 5 and 6**)

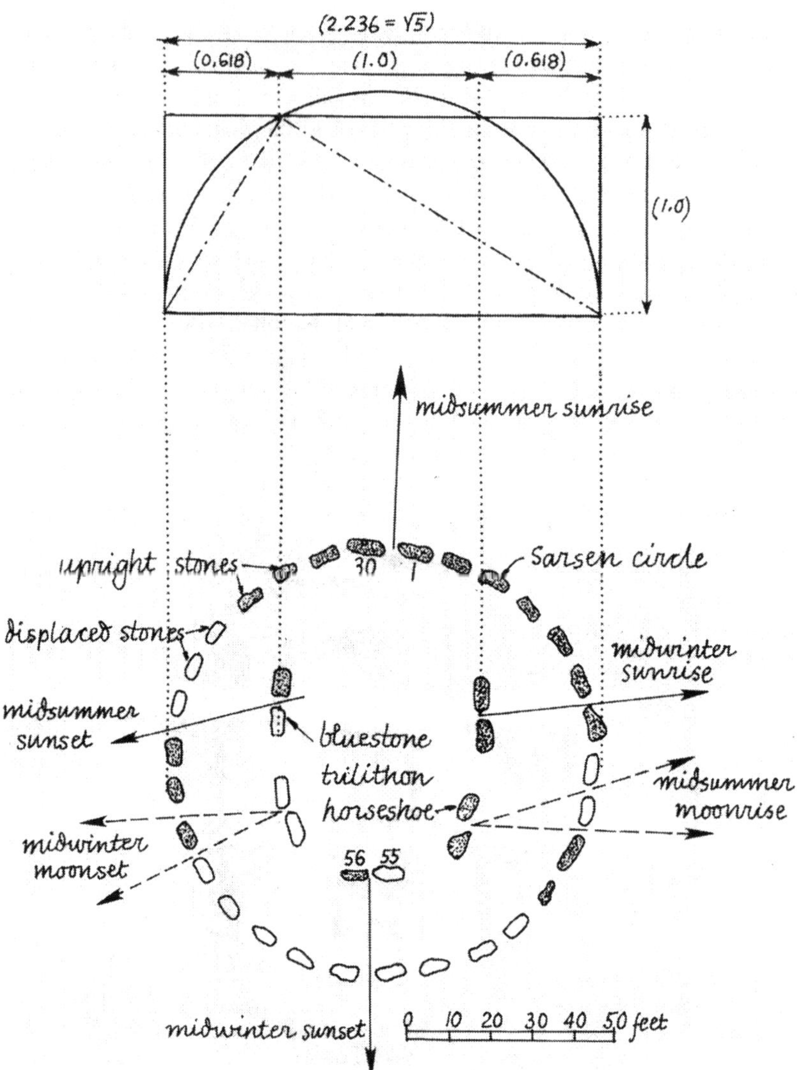

Figure 5: Mathematical representation of Stonehenge from Doczi that shows the Sarsen Circle, and how the inner Bluestone Trilithon Horseshoe interfaces to reflect a square and reciprocal rectangles, and conforms to the Golden Section (shown in upper box where measurements equal 0.618...), where the small is to the large, as the large is to the whole.

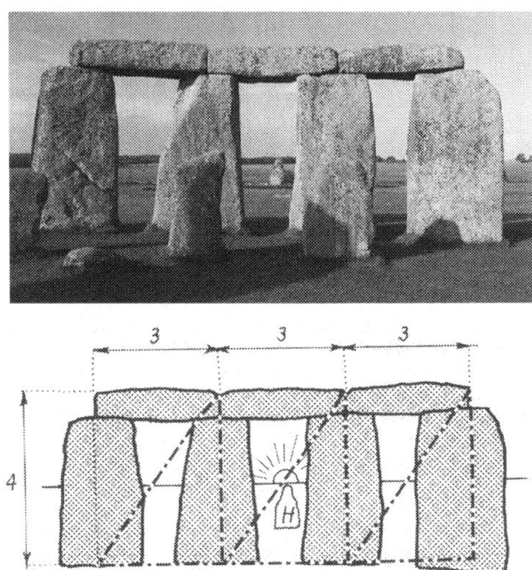

Figure 6: The beams and supporting stones that frame views of summer solstice beyond the Heel Stone contain triangles with Pythagorean dimensions.

A stunning concept, as these vital geometric shapes within Stonehenge incorporate the conceptual seeds behind many things we observe mathematically.

Astounding, yes. *But where is the heart?*

Broader View

This was only the first step into finding the similarity between Stonehenge's design and the heart's architectural form. The challenge was to cite what was known, and then broaden our view.

The Greeks originated this concept of "broadening our view" and it offered rich significance. They knew that many people would look at something, but go no further. They would add no new insights, nor undertake investigations. In response, the Greeks adopted the mantra of searching where nobody has searched before to expand their understanding. I've adopted this concept in my research and clinical career, and use this approach in this memoir. I hope that my *simply looking* — has evolved into *my having vision*.

My conceptual leap to compare Stonehenge and the heart was not a capricious undertaking. Sir Theodore Cook's 1914 book, *The Curves of Life,*[140] defines how nature reproduces its most efficient patterns and displays them in vastly different arenas. The essence of his teaching became clear to me during my Helix and the Heart presentation at the AATS. This allowed me to show that the heart's design includes a *macroscopic helical (spiral)* weave of muscles, and simultaneously show a similar interweavings of *microscopic* helical patterns — within the collagen that forms the ventricle's framework, in the proteins that make the heart muscle move (such as actin, myosin, and tropomyosin), within the chemical calcium ions that excite this motion, and finally throughout the helical electrical network of nerves that stimulate the muscles to perform their movement.[108, 141] This same spiral pattern abounds in nature.

Importantly, humans have leaned upon these natural governing patterns as they design their own constructions. Da Vinci observed the aortic whorls of blood flow in the heart — spirals that are linked mathematically to patterns created on architectural pillars adorning Greek temples, as well as to mazes atop Neolithic tombs in Ireland in 3000 BC — whose designs ultimately match the gigantic spiral galaxies.

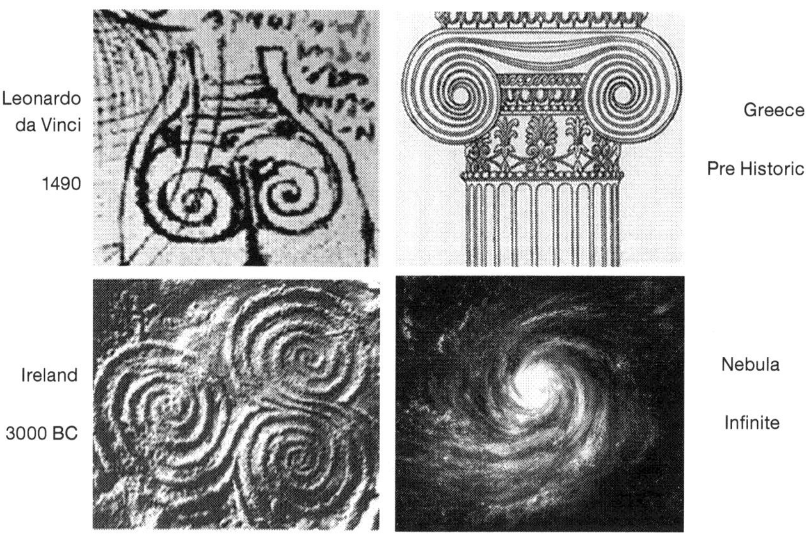

Figure 7: The harmony of natural spirals. The aorta by da Vinci, prehistoric Greek columns, spiral mazes in Ireland, and the cosmos.

But *broadening my view* toward Stonehenge and the heart required that I move beyond spirals. I had already explored Pythagoras' introducing the golden section to describe another mathematical principle that is a unifying feature recurring throughout nature's forms. **Figure 8** repeats a previous diagram because I believe this fundamental concept underlies the central focus of my search for uncovering similarities within nature's grand design.

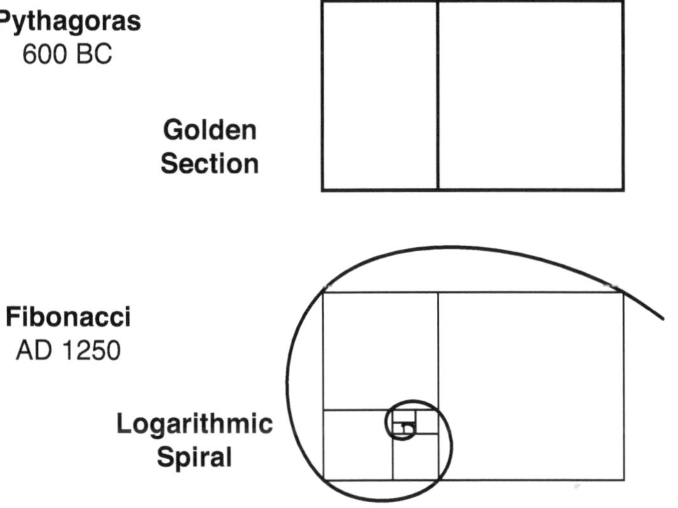

Figure 8: Upper is the golden section by Pythagoras in 600 BC, where small is to large, as large is to whole. Lower is interface of golden section to create logarithmic spiral by Fibonacci in AD 1250.

Finding Analogies

The emergence of this novel broader view enabled me to search for *other* mathematical similarities within Stonehenge's basic construction, some of which might parallel the heart's geometric form. To my delight, clear, straightforward, and sensational findings emerged.

To begin, the outer Sarsen Circle of Stonehenge (**Figures 5 and 9**) is a *circle* that contains within it:

a) a *square* in the center, whose width and length are defined by the arms of the inner Bluestone Trilithon Horseshoe

b) matching *rectangles* whose outer corner edges touch the outer walls of the Sarsen Circle. A startling harmonic relationship is revealed: if the square size is given a 1.0 value, these two components that touch the Sarsen Circle will each have a 0.618 proportion as they form rectangles. This is the golden section mathematical relationship. (**Figures 5, 8, and 9**)
c) 3 *Pythagorean triangles* appear within the 4 Sarsen outer wall pillars. (**Figure 6**) The summer solstice sunrise is seen as you look through them.

How wondrous that Stonehenge's creators integrated the core mathematical elements of circle, square, rectangle, Pythagorean triangles, *and* the golden section ratios *before* these forms were even known! They dramatically preceded Pythagoras (570–495 BC), who formulated his theorems a thousand years later!

The composite of these structural shapes is simply incredible. Was it happenstance that these prime mathematical relationships are an integral part of Stonehenge? This seems unlikely, as these elements are repeated in nature, and through their presence in Stonehenge, certify they instinctively exist within the mind of the human.

And finally, in the midst of recognizing all of these forms... I found the cardiac analogy.

Uncovering the Answer

My guideline of "elegance is simplicity and confusion is complexity" pointed me toward concentrating upon three specific endpoints: *an apex, a conical shape, and a surrounding wrap.*

I began with Stonehenge's view from the circle's centerpiece (Altar Stone) toward the perpetual summer solstice sunrise. The sun becomes an "*apical tip*" beyond the megalithic structure — one that is equivalent to the heart's *apex*, so vital to its function. (**Figure 9**)

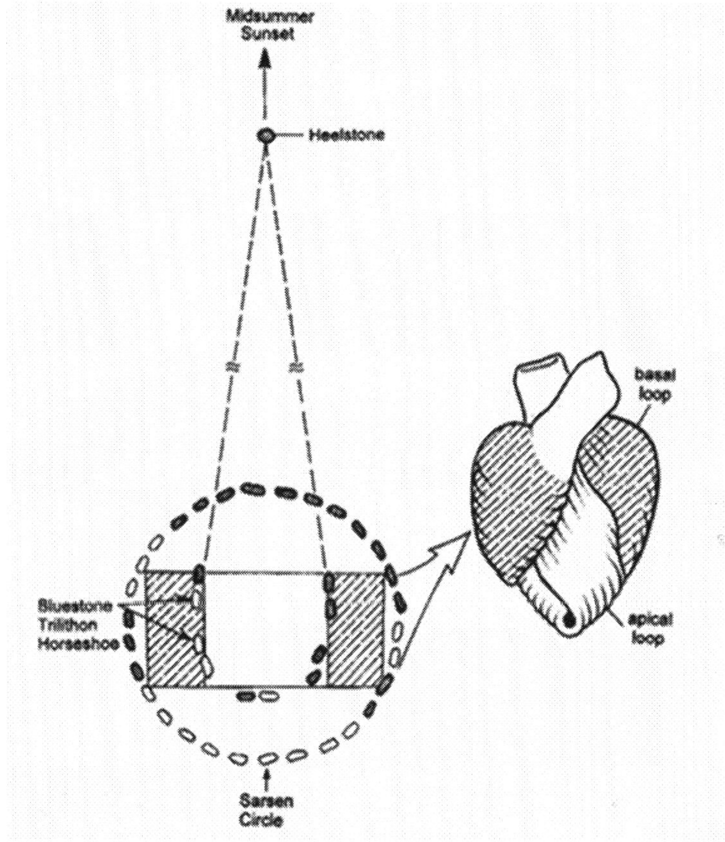

Figure 9: Relationship between Stonehenge and heart.
Each has a conical tip: Stonehenge has the Midsummer sunset
and the heart has its vortex. Stonehenge's "conical body" is surrounded
by "a circular wrap," whose shaded sections mirror the golden section.
Likewise, the heart's apical loop is circumferentially wrapped by the basal loop.

Stonehenge's *conical shape* then becomes apparent by creating a simple line drawing extending from each of the U-shaped arms of the Bluestone Trilithon Horseshoe toward this tip (**Figure 9**) — mimicking the conical shape of the normal heart's construction.

I was enthralled to discover that the side distances between the horseshoe arms and their surrounding Sarsen circle create an "*external buttress*" as seen in **Figure 9** (I clarified this concept by shading the two outer rectangle boundaries), which mirrors the heart's buttress-like wrap muscle. Remarkably, these "supporting structures" *become the small* (area within the shaded rectangles) *that relate to the large* (area in the larger rectangle that includes the central unshaded square) — within Stonehenge construction.

The Heart's Golden Proportion

I found it extraordinary that the heart's architecture parallels the construction of Stonehenge. How astounding that the proportionality between the arms of the Trilithon Horseshoe and Sarsen Circle has the same harmonic relationship that exists within the heart's inner and outer helical arms... a cardiac parallelism that **Figure 10** re-emphasizes.

This dramatic and matching construction between the megaliths and the heart leads to one conclusion: *unity wins.*

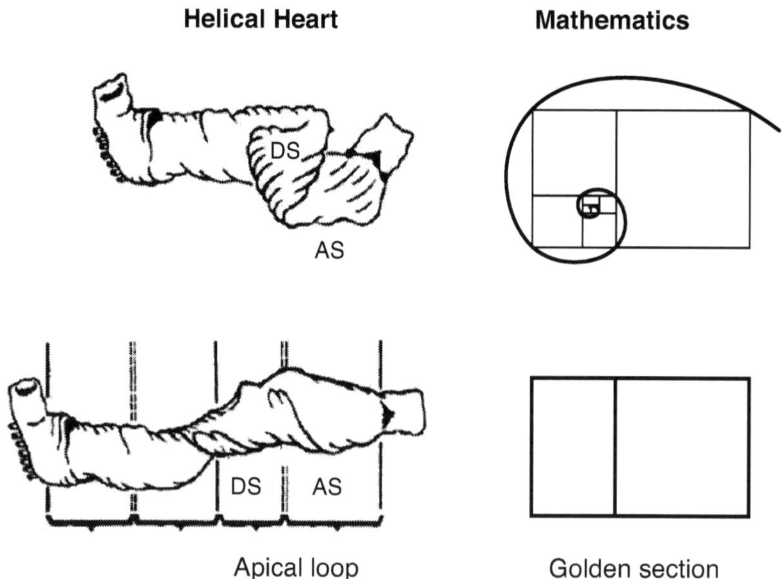

Figure 10: Relationship of helical heart to mathematics.
Above, the helical heart, whose spiral is partially unfolded...
adjacent to the spiral of mathematics formed by golden proportion.
Below, the helix is unwrapped, and the proportional size of the descending (DS) and ascending (AS) segments is in complete harmony with the golden section.

Strength of Opposites

In *The Power of Limits*, Doczi introduces the term "dinergy" to describe opposite energies creating internal support through complementary actions. Doczi's meaning is quite evident in the interactions of the helix and its surrounding wrap muscle in the heart. When the heart twists to pump, its stability is ensured because the circumferential wrap contains and prevents the twisting spiral helix from "exploding" as it develops powerful torsion to eject blood to the body. Similarly, the same wrap prevents the cardiac "implosion" that would occur as the helix uncoils to create an inward suctioning motion to rapidly fill the heart. In contrast, imagine the helical whorl of a hurricane where no wrap exists. The swirling expands over many miles to produce massive destruction since there is no complimentary force to contain it.

The equivalent to dinergy in Stonehenge's geometry is more representational. (**Figure 9**) Its presence is evident in the two shaded reciprocal rectangles that surround the conical shape aimed toward the Heel Stone. Though the effect of this speculative counterforce upon function within Stonehenge is unclear, dismissing its existence as just a coincidental observation may reflect a shortsighted view, since the golden section's reciprocal ratios conspicuously exist within this megalithic structure. We simply won't understand the reason until others uncover the rest of Stonehenge's mysterious history.

Relating to a Greater Whole

But Stonehenge and the heart are not isolated entities. Each connects to the world around them. Stonehenge is surrounded by the universe, and as far as we can tell, humans created this megalithic structure to allow them to focus upon the Earth's place within the ever-moving galaxy that surrounds it. The heart possesses a similar pattern, with its location allowing it to constantly circulate nourishing blood to the surrounding body.

In the truest sense, the heart's life-giving function has allowed humans to create Stonehenge's spectacular architectural form. These massive stone markers, in turn, permit us to peer at the patterns generated by the grandeur of nature that encompasses us.

Greater Purpose?

The precise objectives of Stonehenge are unknown, though theories range from a "temple to the sun" to an astronomical calculator (that may predict eclipses as well).

But perhaps the perpetual wonder of Stonehenge is linked in part to the enticing simplicity of *interdependence* in construction that includes the basic mathematical elements: circle, square, rectangle, and triangle. Together, they perennially guide the light of the summer solstice sunrise to its apex, as well as other functions still to be understood. The same wonder applies to the heart, where its inter-functioning parts will efficiently beat together forever.

Everlasting Elegance

A more abstract similarity also exists between the heart and Stonehenge. It relates to longevity. The configuration of our heart structure is eternal, persisting in generation after generation, and sustained the humans who constructed Stonehenge, which has its own longevity. Our pumping heart began beating over 400 million years ago in fish, and evolved about 100,000 years ago into the human form we have today. Stonehenge was constructed with a corresponding permanence, as those who built it created a megalith configuration that continued long past their own limited spans of time on Earth. The camaraderie between Stonehenge and the heart may further be that they share an *enduring elegant simplicity.*

What does seem absolutely clear to me is that nature provides us with guiding principles based on harmony and interrelatedness. We humans learn from nature and use this knowledge to introduce beauty and balance into our creations. Our intuitive recognition leads us to build structures with similar patterns and principles. Examples given earlier include the Gothic design of cathedrals

(**Figure 11**) that express the same complementary support (dinergy) that nature employed in icebergs formed many millennia ago. Humans obviously did not participate in their formation, yet our heart's shape and Stonehenge's design have the same predictable architectural imprint. How fascinating.

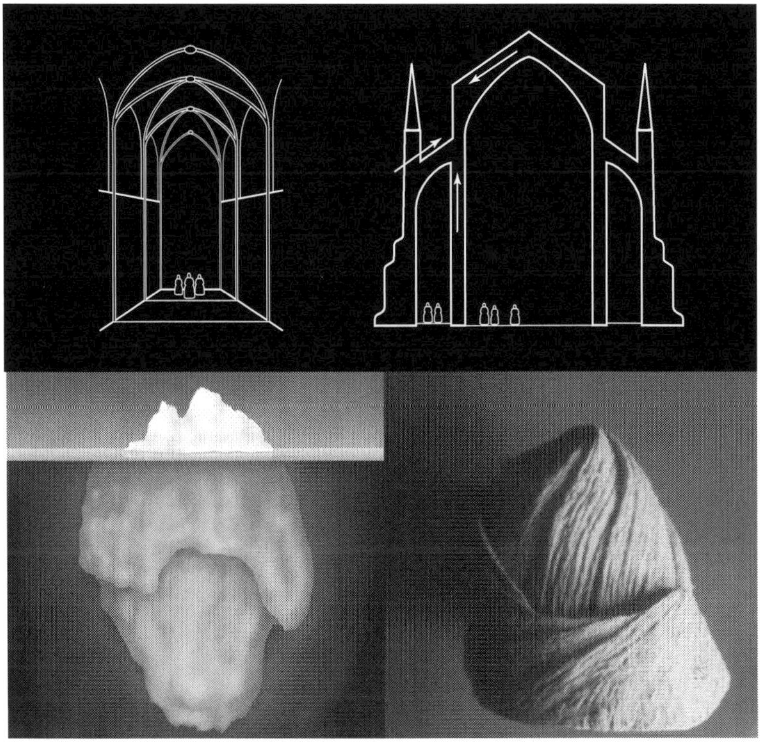

Figure 11: Architectural commonality:
On left, a gothic dome church with external buttress support and gothic contour of a church on right. Lower left shows iceberg, and lower right demonstrates how the heart's apical loop is surrounded by circumferential wrap

Examining Stonehenge in this manner has been the most "out of the box" exploration I have ever pursed, and has resulted in my discovering some marvellous commonalities. The beauty of our interaction with nature is reflected in the parallels that exist between the design of this magnificent megalithic structure, and within the hearts of those who built this landmark over 1,800 years ago.

Intriguingly, the heart that has existed for eternity is only now beginning to be truly understood.

Perhaps Stonehenge will soon follow!

I summarized the structural and functional connections between Stonehenge and the heart in an editorial entitled, "Stonehenge and the Heart: Similar Construction," in the *European Journal of Cardio-Thoracic Surgery*, and share this with the reader.

Link to Stonehenge and the Heart: Similar Construction:

https://academic.oup.com/ejcts/article/29/Supplement_1/S286/379460/Stonehenge-and-the-heart-similar-construction

CHAPTER 26

The Helix and Cardiac Disease: The Riddle of Pacemakers

Let's revisit the current world of understanding heart function, reflected by how a high school science teacher, a medical school physiology professor, or a cardiologist might mimic cardiac action as "clenching a fist to squeeze" for ejection, and "opening all fingers together" for filling. The hand takes on the role of the heart, but this pantomime fails to mirror reality, because the heart primarily *twists.*

I have cited this discrepancy numerous times in this book because its persistence explains why many cardiac treatments are not more successful. Since disease reflects a departure from normal, the objective of a successful treatment should be to restore normality. But when conventional medicine has a misconception of what is normal — how can they treat a disease?

This is the reason I became so passionate about sharing Paco's concept of the helical ventricular myocardial band with the medical world. Paco introduced an incredible discovery, but before I would write about and publish what he had uncovered, there were a number of primary questions I had to answer for myself (understanding the right ventricle, the septum, etc.). The last of these queries was *how the electrical currents that stimulate the heart can cause the helical muscles to function as they do.* (The events described in this chapter took place from 2002 to 2005, but are presented at this point to take advantage of your more complete understanding of the heart.)

I knew that the heart twisted and uncoiled. But why did this happen? I was a cardiac surgeon who possessed limited knowledge of the electrical system, a restriction that imposed a built-in obstacle to my quest. Yet as it would turn out, these absences in my understanding led me to uncover something that was entirely unexpected.

I would discover a vast gap in medical treatment — one that adversely affected millions of people worldwide.

Those who have pacemakers.

Measuring the Electricity

I began my exploration simply enough, by looking at the traditional starting place for calculating electrical impulses in the heart: the EKG.

In movies and in real life, in emergency and non-emergency situations, whenever there is a problem with someone's heart, a physician will order an electrocardiogram (EKG or ECG). This is the classic approach, since it is electricity that stimulates a heart's actions and the EKG measures those impulses. A patient lies down and electrodes are attached to the skin on their chest and each arm and leg. These are wired to a device that records the heart's electrical signals.

An entire field of physicians, called electro-physiologists, focus on detecting and treating diseases from abnormal cardiac electrical impulses. Because of that, EKGs are not something a cardiac surgeon like myself becomes deeply involved with. I needed to start by acquiring a better understanding of this test.

What I knew was that the electrocardiogram records the flow of electrical current within the heart as it travels from one place to another, and this information is displayed as a "tracing" on a continuous grid. (**Figure 1**)

The tracing shows high and low points (spikes and dips) that are called waves. The terms P wave, QRS wave, and T wave indicate electrical signals that are associated with the heart's different mechanical movements. The P wave has mild deviations and its impulses cause contraction of the atrium. In contrast, the QRS wave has very dramatic height changes. It appears to be where all the electrical action happens and I thought it represented the contractions of the ventricles. Finally, the medical texts I read indicated that the T wave reflects repolarization of ventricular muscle fibers... meaning they recover to resting levels.

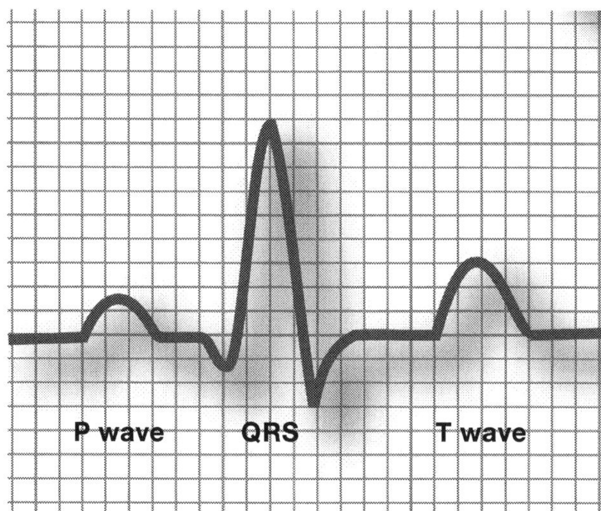

Figure 1: Electrocardiogram, with typical tracing showing the P wave (when atrium contracts), QRS wave (initiation of electrical activity in ventricle), and T wave (recovery of ventricular muscle fibers).

When an EKG reveals a slow heart rate or other irregular rhythms, the most common and well-known solution is to implant a pacemaker to restore a normal heart rhythm and function.

Everyone, including me, believed all would be well after this remedy. But as I would uncover, this was not necessarily true.

Right Terms, Wrong Meanings

While grateful for the knowledge I gained through my novel understanding of the heart structure described by Paco Torrent-Guasp, his unique contribution did not help in my search for explaining how electrical impulses caused the helical heart to function.

Electro-physiologists refer to what they study as "excitation-contraction coupling" — a term that describes the relationship (coupling) between how the observed EKG impulses "excite" a muscle, and how that causes it to contract to produce the heart's movements. But, as we have seen, the conventional description of the heart's motion during contraction is wrong. So there was a challenge ahead to uncover how impulses actually stimulate *the twisting heart*.

More Answers Lead to More Questions

I realized I needed help. Fortunately, I knew just the person to provide it.

This is when I brought Paco with me to visit Jim Cox (the visit that was cited in Chapter 19 about creating my AATS lecture). Jim is the previously mentioned master surgeon and renowned electro-physiologist, who was Chairman of Cardiac Surgery at Georgetown University, and just elected to be the President of the American Association of Thoracic Surgery.

I began by having Paco explain his concept of how the heart functioned. This was Jim Cox's first introduction to the helical heart and he thought it was nothing less than extraordinary.

The primary purpose of the visit was to discuss how the heart's electrical system explained its function. Apparently, some of my conclusions were wrong. Jim explained that while *it appears* that most of the heart's mechanical action takes place during the "explosion of electrical energy" displayed during the dramatic QRS wave — very little movement occurs then. Most of the muscular activity takes place during the much more modest-looking T wave interval, though no one entirely understands how.

In fact, while Jim Cox generously shared his knowledge about the interactive muscular relationships reflected by the QRS and T waves, he also highlighted his frustration at the scarcity of knowledge about what causes these heart motions.

I finally said, "Jim, I still don't understand the relationship of the EKG to the helical heart that Paco just explained to you."

Jim's honest reply was, "I don't either."

So here I was in the office of one of the most esteemed individuals in the field of heart electro-physiology, and I left with more questions than answers. Of course, that's not uncommon when interacting with people at the top of their field. The essence of research is that each new answer evokes a fresh question. That meeting was the catalyst for our undertaking the electrical impulse studies that this chapter will describe.

But all my enthusiasm hardly prepared me for the shocker I would encounter.

"All Together Now" (But Not Really)

In medicine, understanding the true harmony of nature is crucial, since disease reflects a divorce from nature, and its damage can be mended *only if* we know what is normal so we can restore it.

Life is motion. Such elegant beauty of movement is nowhere more prevalent than in the heart's twisting sequence during each heartbeat. Nature provides examples of sequential movement everywhere. Just imagine sitting atop a hill during a late summer evening, thrilled to observe the flickering lights of fireflies during their dazzling dance. If you watch long enough, you realize this twinkling progression is not arbitrary. Nobody knows for certain what the patterns mean, but the fireflies do not all glow at once. The light show of sequential displays repeats over and over within each group.

A comparable mechanism exists within the heart, determining its series of movements, as evidenced in the helical heart uncovered by Paco and explored further in my own studies.[104–106] Therefore, in order to develop a treatment that corrects a disruption of the heart's exquisite rhythmical pattern — we must take into account how electrical stimulations to the helix and wrap produce the heart's series of narrowing, shortening, lengthening, widening, twisting, and uncoiling motions.[105]

Unfortunately, it's difficult to research this due to the way physicians conventionally interpret EKG results, which reflects their belief that the EKG impulse tracings represent the heart squeezing all at once... like a fist.

This misunderstanding is further evidenced by the persistent use of terms like "synchrony" for normality — and "resynchronization" as a treatment to return synchrony when movement in different areas of the heart becomes out of balance. The cardiology world thinks these parts (both ventricles and septum) *beat at the same time synchronously*. But like the pantomime of the clenched fist, the idea of synchrony does not match reality.

As cited in a previous chapter, a source of this confusion was that two-dimensional echocardiogram tests made it appear that the left and right ventricle and septum (the muscular curtain between the right and left ventricles) all squeezed at once. But this portrayal became dramatically challenged following the development of three-dimensional echo studies that showed the heart twisting. The twisting's natural sequential motions (different parts of the heart contracting one after another) were confirmed during our initial ultrasonic crystal probe study to validate Paco's model of the heart's helix and wrap.[142]

Pacemaker Perils

Pacemakers are a remarkable invention. Starting with the first implantable version invented in 1958, these medical devices are now used by over 5 million people in the United States alone. If a patient's heart is not beating sufficiently fast, or if there is a block, a pacemaker delivers electrical impulses to stimulate and maintain a normal heart rate. It is a truly a miraculous, wonderful device. But as I would find out, it's not as miraculously wonderful as commonly believed.

Though pacemakers are nearly always put in now by cardiologists, I used to put them in all the time, and as far as I knew, they worked perfectly fine. As a cardiac surgeon, I did not perform the long-term follow-up of these patients. I just believed pacemakers improved lives and returned patients to normalcy.

That is why I was shocked during my research to learn that 30% of patients who get pacemakers do not obtain the expected improvement.[143]

Equally unsettling was that no one knew why.

How can this be? How could these marvelous devices that successfully delivered minute electrical currents to stimulate the heart's contractions... not deliver the promised results?

Suddenly, my looking into the relationship between the EKG and the helical heart would launch a whole new, compelling investigation.

Following the Leads

In designing treatments, devices are created to reproduce nature. But it is humans, not nature, that must determine the actions performed by these devices. How well they work will reveal if our belief about the true nature of the heart is correct.

As I looked deeper into the problem, my first clues revolved around where the leads (wires) are connected to the heart, as they carry the electrical impulses from pacemakers. Our choice of the stimulation site reveals an enlightening story... but only if we listen.

When a person has a slow heart rate because the atrium is slow to contract (the ventricles are fine), the atrium can be stimulated by a pacemaker (without placing any additional leads to stimulate a ventricle). This approach is very successful, as the natural sequence of ventricular twisting is maintained in these patients.

However, when the pacemaker lead is directly placed *in ventricular muscle to stimulate that ventricle* — then problems may occur.

I began to wonder if directly exciting the ventricles with an electric current might cause an irregularity in their contraction, so that twisting might disappear. If that were the case, would the heart then contract like a fist (as conventional medicine believes it *only* does)... or might it develop an irregular beat?

I knew that without twisting, the heart will not function as it normally should. Might *this* account for why the pacemaker does not satisfactorily correct their problem in almost a third of these patients?

Of course, this possibility would not be considered by physicians who do not accept that the heart twists in the first place. In fact, cardiac resynchronization therapy (CRT) began as a means to recreate what they *believed* to be normality — by simultaneously pacing (stimulating) the septum and left ventricle — to make them squeeze at the same time (synchronously). This approach was based upon recognizing that irregular ventricular contractions caused damage in patients... since mortality rises if different parts of their hearts beat at different times.[144] This delay in stimulation makes one part of the ventricle contract — while the other part stretches — a combination that makes the mitral valve leak and impairs the heart's efficiency.

It is true that CRT's simultaneous pacing can counteract this problem by making the septum and the left ventricle wall contract at the same time. All seems to look good as the septum bulging disappears and the mitral valve stops leaking. A serious condition appears avoided.

Unfortunately, 30 to 40% of patients receiving CRT have no improvement.[145] Why not? Stimulating the muscles to make them squeeze simultaneously is not the ideal objective. The correct goal is to make the helix twist as it squeezes — the link to restoring normality.

CRT's "biventricular pacing" highlights an "all at once stimulation" approach that *fails* to reproduce normal heart function. The natural twisting motion of the left ventricle, septum, and right ventricle requires a *sequential pattern of stimulation* to function normally.

At this point, I still had more questions than answers. Yet I could not imagine that I was the first person to make these connections.

Not surprisingly, I wasn't. Not even close.

Searching Forward by Looking Backward

I recognized the focus of my search would be to understand the heart's wiring conduction system, the heart's helical design, and the natural twisting motion that occurs during each heartbeat. Curiously, though much of this knowledge was not available in 1925, I found that Carl Wiggers, a famed physiologist, addressed the same questions back then.[146]

He described a cardiac muscle dysfunction that he called "asynergic beats" (meaning "not organized," since "synergy" means cooperative interaction). This occurred when an electrical stimulus, like that generated by a pacemaker, was placed at the right ventricular (RV) apex — instead of *through the heart's natural conduction system*. While we've had this knowledge of asynergic beats for over 90 years (since 1925), pacemaker leads are *still* being placed at the same RV apex spot that creates the uncoordinated beats. There has simply been little consideration given to Wiggers' work, and nothing has changed.

Natural Conduction System

I started looking closer into how the heart normally begins to ignite ventricular contractions. The answers are well-established.

Impulses are initiated within a clump of muscle tissue cells that reside on the top of the septum. Called the AV node (atrioventricular node), this clump functions like a generator. Jim Cox explained to me that from here, these generated electrical impulses travel over a collection of nerve fibers called the *bundle of His* (pronounced "Hiss"). This moves down the heart along the septum, where the bundle then separates into two branches — called, appropriately enough, *the left and right bundle branches.* (**Figure 2**)

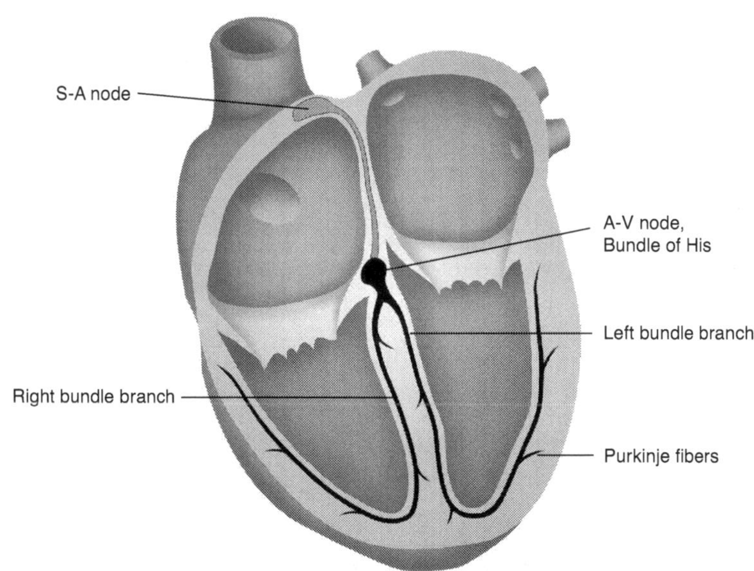

Figure 2: Electrical circuitry of heart, showing artio-ventricular (A-V) bundle on top of septum, branching into left and right bundle branches, and penetration into muscle by Purkinje fibers.

From there, many smaller "twigs," called "Purkinje fibers," divert off these two branches. These fibers are part of the Purkinje system (discovered by Czech anatomist and physiologist Jan Evangelista Purkinje in 1839). They conduct the electrical impulses to the left and right ventricles.

I wondered: could studying this natural conduction system provide a solution to the pacemaker issues?

Though this system was recognized in the medical community, it too had its own mystery. You can actually see this natural wiring (these nerves are visible to an anatomist), but just after the Purkinje fibers touch the surface of each ventricle — their visible nerve connections with muscle suddenly stop. They only go into 15% of the muscles. There is nothing perceptible that connects these nerves to allow them to stimulate the remaining 85% of the heart muscle! *With no evidence of any other internal wiring system,* we simply do not know how electrical impulses reach the muscles that must contract.

Once more, I was running into a brick wall. This was not my area of expertise, and I knew I needed help.

And again, I knew the right person.

Cecil Coghlan

Good fortune fell upon me, as Cecil Coghlan, a remarkable cardiologist, became another mentor as I explored the wondrous scheme of natural electrical design.

I first met Cecil after my presentation about Paco's helical heart at a Birmingham conference, and we became good friends. Yet this comradery started after he told me that our team had created the wrong ventricular shapes — after I showed him examples of hearts that retained a circular form instead of an ellipse — following our early ventricular restoration procedures. Our initial concentration was on exclusion of the scar, as we had not yet focused upon the importance of ventricular shape.

My learning credo is that *opposition requires responses, not reaction.* I asked Cecil to meet with us the next day to further explain his thoughts. His knowledge of the heart was extraordinary. He showed me my error — and my critic eventually became my mentor. So now, while investigating the relationship between electrical excitation and heart function, I visited him again at his home and at his University of Alabama office. I brought up my concerns about electricity and the helical heart... and the puzzle of why pacemakers were not satisfactorily helping patients in nearly a third of cases.

Cecil wasted no time in providing me a definitive answer. "It is simply not possible for the heart to maintain its twisting motion when a pacemaker stimulates the ventricles directly."

The conviction of his statement was somewhat startling, but as I would find, his reasoning was sound. And very revealing.

He continued, "You know the heart has its own electrical conductive system, starting with the bundle of His and continuing into the Purkinje system. If a pacemaker is only stimulating the atrium, the heart's own system is still utilized and twisting can be maintained and the heart can function well. But if the ventricles are *stimulated directly* — using a method that bypasses the heart's natural system — it then replaces normality with one not nearly as effective."

I interjected, "This is despite their successfully pacing the heart to beat at a higher rate?"

"Exactly," Cecil confirmed. "Here's the problem. When they directly stimulate the ventricles, the electrical impulses now travel much more slowly through the ventricle — muscle cell by muscle cell. This only happens *at one-tenth of the speed* that impulses normally travel by the heart's natural circuitry [actual numbers being 0.3 mm vs. 3.0 mm/millisecond]. That's not fast enough to preserve the heart's sequential motions [one part after the next] that create twisting and uncoiling."[147]

"So now the spiral motion is replaced by an irregular, uncoordinated contraction," I surmised, "which perhaps explains why 30% of patients report unsatisfactory improvement following use of a pacemaker."[143]

"It very well could," Cecil agreed. "But there's more, too."

Cecil continued. "This slower distribution of impulses can cause worse issues. If an electrical impulse to a region is delayed by 120 milliseconds — while an adjacent region is contracting — this non-stimulated region won't contract as it suddenly bulges like an aneurysm, and the ventricle's overall efficiency is impaired. This disharmony happens when pacemakers *fail* to stimulate a region of heart muscle via the natural conduction of the bundle of His and Purkinje pathways."

It was all finally making sense to me. I offered, "Then perhaps a solution would be to find a way to take advantage of the natural conduction system that's already in the ventricles."

Cecil nodded, thoughtfully. "That could be true... if anyone understood what that system was."

Cecil was referring to the fact that the Purkinje fibers only penetrated 15% of the ventricle muscles. How the electrical impulses then get to the other 85% to stimulate the ventricles' movement — was still not understood.

"But here's what we do know," countered Cecil. "There *has to be another system* that we cannot yet detect, over which the electrical impulses travel rapidly through the ventricles. How do we know this? Since the heart naturally twists, the impulses must somehow quickly get to all muscle areas."

Cecil's point was that if pacemaker electrical signals going to this other 85% of the ventricle muscles *only* traveled at the very slow one-tenth of normal speed (as exists when they only stimulate muscle cells)... the impulse would not get to the areas where it was needed in time to generate twisting. Thus, a dilemma might arise as contraction occurs when a pacemaker lead stimulates only one area... while *non-stimulated regions bulge or billow during each heartbeat.* Cecil was fascinated by the magic of the unique natural system that ignites the entire heart muscle to produce sequential twisting. His enthrallment was not hampered by our failure to understand this process.

Then Cecil added optimistically, "I have been working on a theory about what this could be... but I still don't know yet."

I smiled and told Cecil that what he had just revealed to me was remarkable. The key to healthy and vigorous heart function seemed to be its ability to *efficiently conduct* electric impulses through the ventricles.

"More than you might realize," Cecil said with a gleam in his eyes. "Let me tell you something that is every bit as remarkable as what I've already said."

I eagerly listened. He was right. What he revealed next was truly stunning.

Ontogeny and Phylogeny: Phenomenal Lessons from Nature

Cecil proceeded to explain this importance of electrical conduction through the ventricles by comparing how it functioned in the anatomy of different species — an intriguing theme that addressed both "ontogeny" and "phylogeny" relationships.

Ontogeny describes the origin of an organism and how it originally developed, while phylogeny describes how it evolved over time. The dramatic variations of the excitation-contraction relationship in different animals demonstrate why vigorous conduction in the ventricles is vital to every species. Cecil's idea was that the way in which the impulses travel through a ventricle muscle exerts a striking effect on the animal's ability to function in its world.

Paco had unfolded hearts across a broad spectrum of species, ranging from birds to mammals, and found that the helical ventricular band exists in each of them. In every case, the beginning of the bundle of His/Purkinje system is always positioned on top of the septum. While that was consistent, the hearts of different species had vastly different capabilities, and different rates at which they beat. Cecil now offered me the alluring theory about this connection: that these diverse capabilities in different species were due to how deeply the wiring system had *penetrated* into their ventricular muscles.

I knew that the human heart rate rarely exceeds 180 beats per minute, even during severe physical or emotional stress. As Cecil pointed out, that is dramatically different from hummingbirds, whose hearts beat nearly 1,500 times per minute in order to maintain their incredibly rapid wing motion during flight. A similarly high rate occurs in canaries, at around 1,000 beats per minute. Cecil learned that each of these species has a specialized type of Purkinje system penetration — one that *touches every heart muscle fiber* within their ventricles. Rather than the conduction system in humans that only penetrates 15% of the ventricle muscle... in hummingbirds, it touches 100%. This direct connection of the wiring system to the working muscle explains the never-ending speed of their wing motion. Nature avoided the 85% gap between the Purkinje system and muscle that exists in humans.

On the other hand, the wild boar has Purkinje fibers that almost reach the outer ventricular wall (extending through two-thirds of the ventricle). This explains why boars are able to escape from a lion or cheetah. The boars do not run out of gas, while the lion or cheetah will tire after an intense, but short chase.

In dogs, the Purkinje system fibers extend *halfway* through the ventricular muscular wall. While they have the same resting heart rate as humans of about 80 beats per minute, they can achieve higher heart rates than us, and have increased endurance. This may draw from the dog having descended from the hardy wolf, and account for the wolf's capacity to roam over great expanses of terrain in search of food.

The fact that the human heart's conductive nerves barely penetrate the inner muscle of the ventricles may explain why our heart rates never exceed about 180 beats / minute despite urgent needs from exercise or fright. This inherently limits both our speed and our stamina.

Cecil's understanding of electrical connections in different hearts fascinated me from a clinical point of view. While one might wonder if some day we could find a way for pacemakers to enhance our heart's abilities beyond normal human capacity, my interest was more immediate than that.

I wanted to find out how we can get the most out of what nature has already provided us.

Even though the medical community (including Cecil) did not understand how the wiring system functioned in the ventricles after impulses leave the Purkinje system... perhaps there was a way that pacemakers could *use the conduction system already in the ventricles* (rather than bypass it as they presently do by directly stimulating ventricles).

A new goal loomed on my horizon.

Heart Movement: The Natural Order of Things

The motion of the heart is like a cardiac symphony, with different areas contracting in sequence as they are activated, each playing their part precisely.

My focus now turned toward finding a way for pacemakers to preserve this complex series of motions. We knew that the QRS was simply an ignition key – the initiation of electrical activity that stimulated the efficient natural system that exists within the ventricles.

Recognizing this, I saw my true task: *find a way to stimulate the bundle of His directly* — and allow the heart's own conduction system to transmit those electrical impulses to the rest of the heart in its natural fashion.[148] In this way, we might preserve the heart's natural twisting function and help almost a third of the patients who do not get satisfactory improvement following conventional pacemaker treatment.

I knew the potential benefit to patients was vast, since over 5 million patients in the United States have pacemakers, and over 1 million patients worldwide receive new or replacement pacemakers (such as when the prior pacemaker's battery depletes) every year. These numbers reflect an astounding pool of people who could benefit by having their hearts' electrical support delivered into their natural conduction pathways.

Praise for Pacemakers

It should be noted again that despite the cited drawbacks to how nearly all of these medical devices are wired into the body, ventricular pacemakers as used now do have enormous lifesaving importance. Electrical firing from these units prevents sudden death in patients who have complete heart block (where electrical impulses do not travel from the atrium to the ventricle). It also bestows a more rapid heart rhythm to patients with slow heart rates (below 50 beats per minute).

Still, direct ventricular stimulation will only cause the heart to squeeze, but can never restore the natural sequential twisting motion. It may even cause heart function to worsen, and possibly instigate heart failure in patients with dilated hearts.[149] The frequency of these specific adverse effects is uncertain, but it is known that at least 30% of patients receiving pacemakers do not obtain clinical improvement.[143, 145] This could mean patients who had symptoms of easy fatigue will not improve. If they had shortness of breath, that will not change.

Willie Sutton: Go Where the Money Is

Admittedly, the pursuit of a medical approach to restore a heart's natural contraction rhythm is not a typical one for a cardiac surgeon. It is the cardiologists known as electro-physiologists that usually conduct this type of treatment. Surgeons rarely put in pacemakers today, except when we find the heart isn't working correctly (as when there's a heart block) at the conclusion of an operation. We then insert the leads and implant the pacemaker.

Given all this, why would I (a surgeon) be drawn to uncovering a way to directly stimulate the bundle of His? My answer would mirror the reply given by Willie Sutton, the famed bank thief, who when asked why he robbed banks, replied, "Because that's where the money is."

My curiosity led me to the bundle of His because "that's where the money is." From there, we may stimulate electrical nerve transmission along normal circuitry. Yet theory is only as good as it can be shown to reflect reality. This still needed to be tested: if the leads of a pacemaker were placed in this bundle of His... would it re-establish the *sequential* heartbeat that restores natural twisting action?

Testing the Theory

This is what I hoped to find out experimentally. But to do that, I had to find a way to access the bundle of His in order to place a pacemaker's leads. (**Figure 3**) I needed to discover some means to get to this internal site *from outside the heart.* We certainly did not want to perform open-heart surgery to place the leads of a pacemaker.

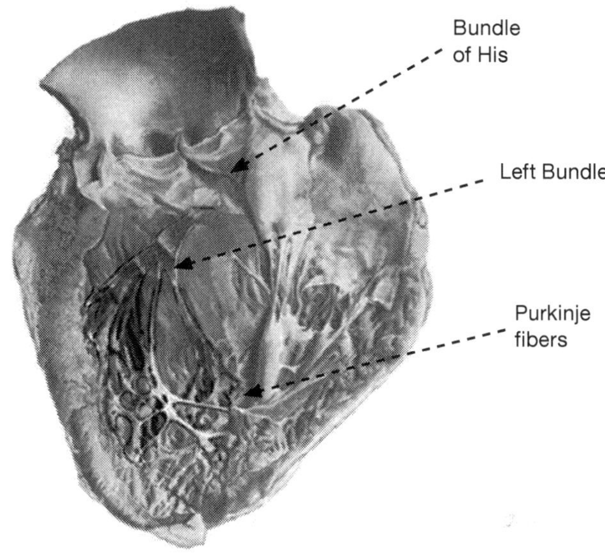

Figure 3: Anatomic display of electrical circuitry, showing bundle of His, left bundle and its fan-like splay of bundle branches, and how Purkinje fibers only touch the surface of ventricle muscle.

Trying to figure this out in my lab, I had the idea to unravel Paco's model of the helical ventricular myocardial band as my guide. Unfolding the heart replica, I first found where the bundle of His was exactly represented on the top of the septum. (**Figure 4**)

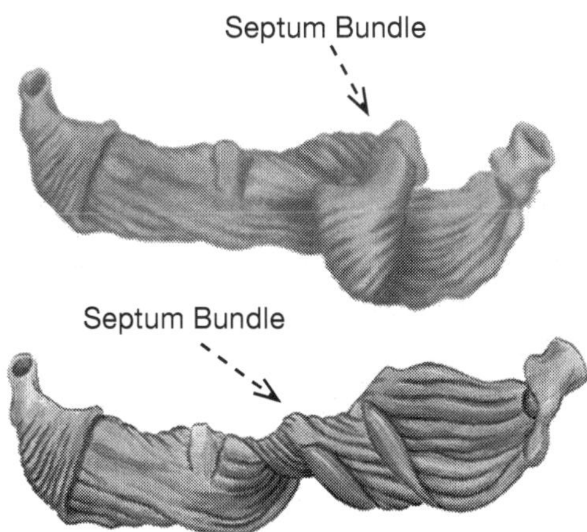

Figure 4: Identification of septum bundle of His by Torrent-Guasp model. It exists where the basal loop folds to start the helix. Clearly evident, this site is called "septum bundle" in these two images.

I then folded the heart model back together and determined that if we punctured the ventricle through a specific location... we could thread wire leads through it to reach the top of the septum that contains the bundle of His![150]

I clearly saw its location work on the model. But would it work in reality?

On an animal test subject, we selected the puncture site outside the top of the right ventricle and inserted a lead through a needle conduit into the location. (**Figure 5**)

With everything in place, it was time to simulate the stimulus of a pacemaker. It was, as we say, the moment of truth.

The result was immediately obvious, as *a normal twisting beat followed each electrical stimulation!* We had successfully reproduced the heart's ability to pace by the natural pathway! It was unbelievable! We were thrilled (though not entirely surprised, since we had simply followed nature).

We had paced the right atrium and stimulated the bundle of His — and restored the natural twisting action. The consistency of our success was confirmed by additional studies on more animals — we reached the bundle of

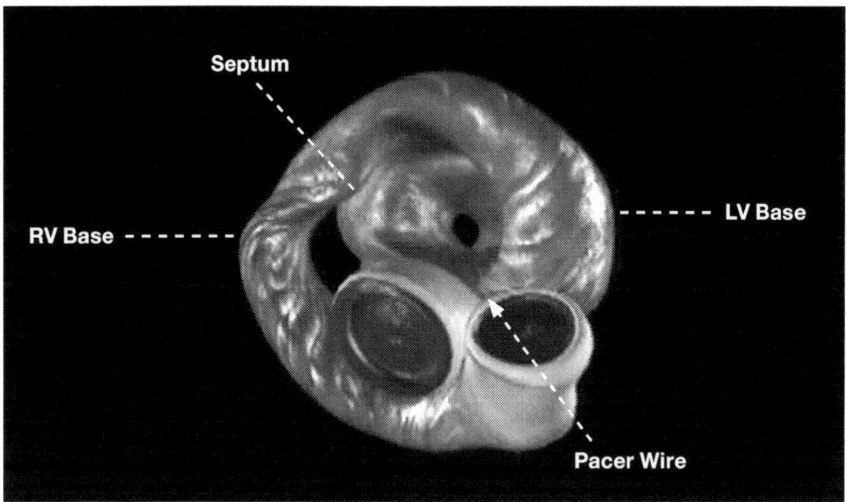

Figure 5: By using a top view of anatomic landmarks of the heart's surface, we insert a catheter (with a pacer wire, represented by arrow) into the upper septum. This is done by entering from the pulmonary artery, advancing it into the left ventricle, and implanting the wire on top of the septum. Another example of using this model to answer a riddle never before solved.

His every time. But truthfully, one look was worth a thousand words, as my two research fellows and I witnessed as the heart began twisting again. The success of our search to generate pacing via the natural conduction pathways meant that *Willie Sutton had found the bank.*

Ours was *Not* the Only Study. So Where are the Changes?

Interestingly, my further exploration of the medical literature revealed that we were not the only ones testing this approach. I uncovered groups of cardiologists who had done what we had. These experienced electro-physiologists reported superb findings after they used pacemaker leads to stimulate the bundle of His,[151–153] but their findings were not well publicized. Their results avoided the abnormal heart contractions that were typically produced by today's pacemakers that place the leads in a manner that Wiggers had warned us about 90 years ago. Clearly, we were long past due for a new pacemaker treatment approach that would restore a natural twisting motion to our patients' hearts.

We were excited by the enormous volume of candidates that could benefit from this new approach. This included patients with slow heart rates (called bradycardia), those with wide QRS intervals (their EKG showing different parts of their heart being stimulated in an abnormal pattern), those having left bundle branch block ("LBBB" — a blockage in the left branch of the bundle of His), and of course, those with uncoordinated heart contractions from traditional pacemakers stimulating the RV apex.

Despite all this, progress in making changes in the use of pacemakers has not occurred. Even though the limited number of reports so far has consistently documented excellent findings — interest in pursuing this new approach has spawned scant studies.

In 2010, only 59 patients were included, but this was the world's largest report of the great success that followed bundle of His pacing.[154] A more recent study on 75 patients receiving bundle of His pacemakers has reported an 80% success rate in ventricular performance at a follow-up 12 months after pacemaker placement.[153]

Perhaps more frustratingly, an eight-year combined South European and Southern Italy study reported on *just 570 patients* treated by pacemakers that stimulated the bundle of His or its adjacent fibers. While larger than the other studies, 570 is still a tiny number considering there are many millions of people who need pacemakers worldwide. Predictably, each of these 570 patients developed a normal electrocardiogram pattern, with functional ventricular contractions that matched those of athletes (the study compared their results to athletes, since athletes could be regarded as having the epitome of healthy heart function).[151]

They too published results proving the advantages of stimulating the heart's natural ignition point, but nobody wanted to listen. These dramatically improved outcomes have not altered conventional cardiac approaches. It seems that even with other available pacing options, many physicians continue wearing the same shoes, even though the toe is still being stubbed.

Persistence of Resistance

So why would there be opposition to change when the pool of those who could benefit is so vast? Well, this "sea change" *demands significantly different actions from pacemaker manufacturers and from cardiology electro-physiologists*, and that is the likely problem.

Manufacturers would have to redesign and produce new types of pacemakers and leads, but they already have a willing and eager marketplace for those they presently make. Cardiology electro-physiologists would have to learn new techniques, rather than perform the ones they have "successfully" used for years. They would need to give up the current simplicity and ease of quickly installing leads at the apex stimulation site. But this kind of thinking reflects a *physician-related* benefit — rather than a choice that may optimally serve the patient.

Nobody wants to change from a system that is already making a lot of money. It would require an investment of funds by manufacturers. Plus, it would involve an investment in education by the cardiologist. Acquiring proficiency in this new method is a little harder at first, but once learned, the procedure only requires about 20 more minutes. Yet such a learning curve must be undertaken before *any* new approach can be done smoothly and easily.

But the now-documented benefits of pacemakers utilizing the heart's normal circuitry should justly override those considerations, as it improves upon a treatment still producing the abnormalities first described in 1925.

Today, cardiologists and electro-physiologists still have not embraced the benefits of using natural circuitry when placing pacemakers. This attitude will hopefully change following their appreciation of ongoing reports that document how its use can restore the natural twisting pattern of contraction... a goal never achieved by traditional pacemaker treatment.

Where Goeth the Electricity? The Grand Mystery

I had more than accomplished my original mission of understanding the final missing piece before publishing about Paco's discovery. I now understood how the heart's electrical currents cause the helical muscles to function. They must sequentially reach each muscle fiber to allow the normal twisting action to occur. Yet my search went far beyond this, as we now also had a proven approach to stimulate the bundle of His — and confirmed that its use completely restored the heart's natural twisting and contraction movements — essential to returning normal heart function.

But there still remained a mystery.

It was an enigma unsolved by all fields of cardiology. Yet the truest tribute to learning is maintaining an openness to hear and welcome new ideas, even if they are as yet untested.

Join me on one further journey into uncharted territory.

This was our puzzle: we had identified the main "thoroughfares" over which electrical stimuli travel in the heart, including the bundle of His, the RV apex, and the Purkinje system. Yet as I have described, anatomists knew that the last part of this conduction system — the Purkinje fibers — only penetrates into 15% of the ventricular muscles in humans and then suddenly stops.

So once electricity passes over these known conduit channels — how does it get to its final destination — the muscle cells (called myocytes) that are essential to stimulating the normal twisting action that creates efficient cardiac contraction?

Nobody knew.

Yet once understood, this could open the door to innovative treatments for the heart. We simply do not know what might be possible.

My "traveling to learn" approach brought me again to Cecil Coghlan, the brilliant and distinguished cardiologist described earlier in this chapter, who shared my fascination with the helical ventricular myocardial band. It would prove to be an incredible trip.

In his office, I brought up the riddle of electrical impulses.

I knew Cecil had been searching for that answer as well. He had arrived at a theory, and revealed the "conceptual seeds" that might someday lead to a solution.[147]

"Heart architecture is more complex than just the two-dimensional world of electrical fibers and muscle cells," he began. "Instead of only looking at the muscles and nerves, we should look at *the framework*."

Cecil proposed that the heart was formed upon a "scaffold" of connective tissue (collagen) that served as the foundation of its natural ventricular shape. This "mesh framework" existed as a fine sheath-like layer of connective tissue that surrounded the electrical pathways (the His/Purkinje system) — *as well as each microscopic heart muscle cell.*

Cecil suggested, "There may be certain chemical substances in this matrix that cause the current to move so quickly. There is an intriguing tiny protein in anatomy called proteoglycans that in part bind water and cations (positively-charged ions, such as sodium and potassium) within the internal cellular structures."

Not familiar with them, I asked, "You believe they might be part of this matrix?"

"Yes, and they may in some way act like little generators to spread the electrical impulses quickly and smoothly along this entire framework and the ocean of muscle fibers."

My eyes were opened. I listened intently as Cecil explained that electrical impulses could move from cell to cell by what he called "proton hopping."

This process would transmit the impulses over the surface of each muscle cell. It could do this at *a velocity that is consistent* with those conduction speeds needed for the natural twisting movement, and for everything else required for the heart to function as it does.

As he finished, I finally said, "This is absolutely amazing."

Each of Cecil's ideas was new to me, particularly since my knowledge of electro-physiology was limited. But I believed they made sufficient sense, such that I said, "Jim Cox has invited me to create a book unveiling Paco's work, to publish through the American Association for Thoracic Surgery's journal as part of their Seminars on Thoracic and Cardiovascular Surgery. I would like you to write a chapter on electricity and the heart as part of the book."

Cecil was happy to do so. After he turned it in to me, I gave it to Jim Cox, who has spent his life learning about this. In the same manner that I have come to understand the heart, he understands electricity in ways nobody ever has before. Jim declared Cecil's chapter the most innovative paper he had ever read on this subject.

It was creative new thinking. Of course, I knew that does not necessarily make the concept right, but bright folks with open minds (like Jim Cox) welcome new ideas. Jim wanted to ask Cecil some questions about the chapter regarding his own research. They exchanged notes. I suggested Jim co-author the chapter with Cecil, who readily agreed.

The Future

Cecil Coghlan made a thoughtful postulation, but subsequent testing was needed to determine if he is correct. But how to test it?

As it turns out, nature may have given us a means to evaluate his concept.

We know that heart failure patients with an enlarged dilated ventricle develop ventricular rhythm problems causing abnormal beats, sometimes progressing to develop ventricular fibrillation that causes sudden death. Could these rhythm issues occur as the ventricle dilates and stretches... because this enlargement also stretches Cecil's proposed collagen network?

That got me thinking.

We understood that our surgical ventricular restoration returned a dilated spherical heart back to its normal elliptical shape. The result was that both natural ventricular twisting and contraction were recovered[155–156] — with only rare development of sudden death.

This supported Cecil's concept.

A return to nature, rather than use of electrical devices, had solved this otherwise lethal problem. Instead of using pacemakers to treat the rhythm problem, *the rebuilt ventricular form* solved the excitation-coupling issue — and proper rhythm was immediately restored. Now, we also presumed it returned the collagen network to its normal size and shape. Unknowingly, we corrected the very issue that Cecil's theory may have suggested as the cause of lethal ventricular rhythms.

If accurate, this means we may have a different way to counter abnormal rhythms and sudden death.

Unlike previous chapters, this one ends with a question rather than an answer. As Einstein said, "The important thing is to never stop questioning." Is Cecil's premise correct? Further exploration certainly seems warranted, and studies should be pursued to confirm the answers.

If proven true, who knows what other kinds of extraordinary treatments might evolve from this knowledge?

CHAPTER 27

Life: My Art and My Science

"My Art and My Science" is the final chapter of my memoir, and reveals how art has interwoven with my lifelong scientific pursuits. It identifies how such artistic connections have surprisingly guided me toward uncovering solutions to the unsolved medical conditions.

The fields of art and science have more in common than one might think. Both involve goal selection, drive, development of the pursuit, and perseverance... long-standing qualities that are similarly reflected in other areas, such as my preparing for and then completing marathons in running and swimming.

These strides toward innovation in art and science have a remarkable similarity. The first actions are conventional, as we must "walk where others walked before." The artist observes and copies the masterful works of others, with a mentor looking over their shoulder as they learn how others have done things. This bears close resemblance to the learning curve in medical school and in specialty training that is needed before self-starting your scientific future. The cardiac surgeon mimics the known work of others as he or she trains with a mentor surgeon that directs the placement of every stitch.

First Art, then Science

I began drawing when I was ten years old, but had no formal art training. A fun adventure unfolded for me as I began by copying pictures. My wall today still displays a portrait of my father, made at age thirteen. Looking back, I can see the mindset of the researcher surfacing early in myself, as my subsequent drive to investigate new medical areas may have been mirrored during my untrained childhood. For example, my desire to play in new artistic arenas led to me buying an oil color set so that I could explore ways to amplify a picture's depth.

Though the artistic seeds were planted early, my drive to become a doctor became my total focus and would overshadow my artistic interests. I did no drawings in college, medical school, or during the beginning of my residency training at Johns Hopkins Hospital. Leisure time finally came into my life for the first time when I transferred to UCLA. My initial medical chores did not require long hours. Instead, I worked a typical eight-hour day during my six-month rotation in pathology (to learn about disease patterns), and during six more months in the outpatient clinic.

I sought activities to fill this free time, and my stimulus would come from a dear friend and colleague, Don Paglia. We met during my rotation in the Department of Pathology, where he was an assistant professor. He was an established painter and sculptor whose work had appeared in numerous shows. Don took a three-month voyage to Japan, acting as a physician on a Coast Guard cutter. During this time, I had the opportunity to live in his home. It was an astounding experience to be surrounded by his artwork, whose excellence burst from the pictures that covered his walls. My fascination with his artistic activity made me think, "If he can make this part of his life, perhaps I can have art as an aspect of mine as well."

I had found a world that I wanted to play in again. But to follow this path, I needed to learn if my childhood love of drawing had endured.

Promising Start

My first drawing would be a surgeon's hand. It was an interesting first choice, especially since many artists steer away from drawing the hand due to the difficulty of accurately portraying its many angles, twists, and turns. But modeling was easy. I looked at my own hand, imagining it making an incision. I created a slew of paper sketches to improve and overcome these inherent challenges before beginning an oil color painting. The challenge of having no trained knowledge in oils did not deter me from vigorously chasing this artistic objective.

I was delighted. I had my first completed picture in almost 20 years. (**Figure 1**) Don Paglia returned home and complimented the work, with his

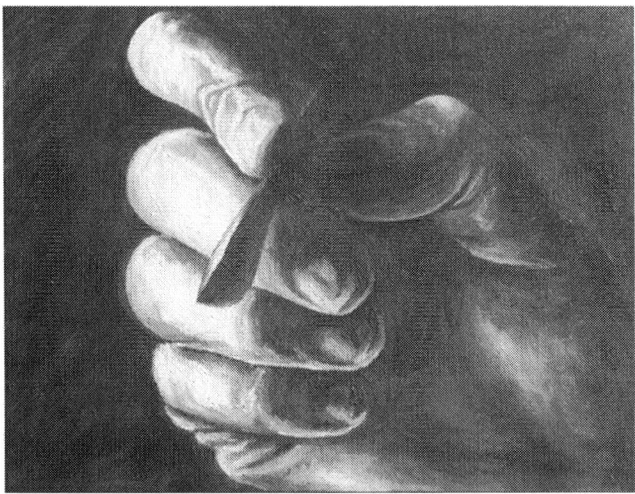

Figure 1: A surgeon's hand.

only critique relating to my rendering of anatomy. He was disturbed by my very flat thumb. It seemed abnormal and needed a more natural angulation. Solving this problem was easy, as I simply "exchanged" his thumb for mine in the painting, a maneuver that also reflected my deep gratitude to him for supplying the enticement to re-engage with art.

Don suggested I submit the painting to The Festival for Arts competition at The Los Angeles Physicians Art Society. I was flattered and took his advice, but was unable to attend the festival's award ceremony because I was in the operating room. So we came downtown the next day, but found the building closed. We asked a janitor, who happened to have a strong accent, if he knew who had won. He wasn't sure of the winner's name, but told us that a "bigga hand wit a bigga knife" had a gold ribbon around it. We all laughed, overjoyed at the unexpected reward for my first venture.

Back to the Back Burner

Despite this encouraging recognition, I had to abandon my artwork once more, due to the long hours required for patient care. But my residency was immediately followed by two years in the Air Force. I was stationed in Dayton,

Ohio, where I lived in an off-base cabin at the corner of a large state park. This allowed me to walk into a backyard surrounded by nature, and let me focus again upon art.

My fascination with the hands remained. I tried painting from the viewpoint of a patient on the operating table, encircled by the operating team. The patient is touched by the graceful hands of the caregivers, whose bodies appear smaller as they fade into the background. As the doctors and nurses perform a surgical procedure, their hands dominate the foreground while the team's masked faces focus upon the patient. Illumination comes from the central surgical light above the operating table. (**Figure 2**)

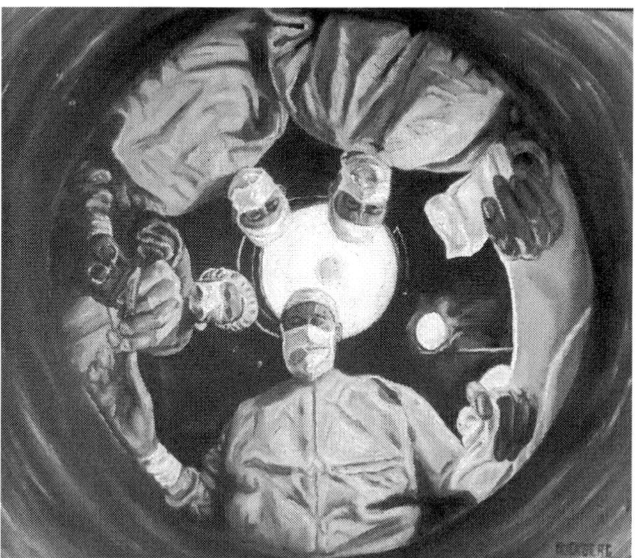

Figure 2: The patient's view.

The final challenge was framing the circular image that naturally arose from the patient's point of view. I used my clinical experience to help me capture this spherical view. I envisioned it as if peering through a sigmoido-scope to blend depth, perspective, and record the foreground and background to amplify the drama of a surgical scene. This imagery permitted the viewer to focus on the intensity of the operating room as the background's various details melted away to emphasize the surgical team's concentration upon patient care.

The selection of hands became an important ingredient within the many pictures I drew then and in those I continue to create. Hands have always appealed to me, as they seem to be a true reflection of the individual, unlike facial expression or body language, which are constantly being modulated. Further, they reflect the union of thinking and acting. Michelangelo said, "The eye and the mind create with the hands." His profound vision certainly describes how I have used my hands during my lifelong ventures into art and science.

Creation was the focus of Michelangelo's comment, and it remains the driving force in art — and science. Many descriptions for creation exist. Mine is that it "fills an empty room with new ideas, then tests them with ongoing change during learning." This process uses your spirit to contribute fresh input into the vacant space, all the while knowing it is just the first step of an innovative exploration. We must retain the freedom to learn new things during its pursuit. This is the hallmark of the artist, the physician, and anyone else that is inventive.

The Artistry of Discovery

Learning always brings challenges.

The only choice is to walk toward such new things, even though the road may appear to lead to a dead end. Ignoring a problem or turning around to go elsewhere is not an option. The goal must be to determine what that "dead end" means, and then to determine how to change it. Such curiosity creates leaders, rather than the passive acceptance that defines the traditionalists in both the world of art — and of science. This was demonstrated previously when we abandoned simply congratulating ourselves for a medical treatment that yielded a 80 to 90% survival rate... and moved toward the next phase, where we asked the fundamental question, *"Why are 10 to 20% still dying?"*

The early example of this in my own career occurred in 1975, when ventricular fibrillation was routinely used during operations to replace the aortic valve. This mechanical method kept the heart quiet so that cardiac surgeons could more easily operate. Yet patients who had thick heart walls did not fare well, and when they died, these losses were simply deemed to be part of that percentage in which the operation wasn't successful. But I wanted to know why, and our research revealed the answer (the left ventricle's inner shell becomes damaged when a thickened heart undergoes induced ventricular fibrillation). Such treatments on those types of patients were abandoned.

I remember presenting these scientific results at a major meeting in New Orleans. A surgeon from Chicago sought me out afterward. He told me how much he appreciated my talk, but did so in a unique way. He stated that while he watched my presentation, he thought of Renoir making another beautiful canvas. He enjoyed seeing the evolution of my thinking, and compared it to how Renoir kept working to make a painting more and more beautiful, each step a progression.

What a lovely comment that bridged my two worlds.

Momentous Mentors

An underappreciated aspect of art-making is the perseverance to complete a project. This requires an uninterrupted span of time. As I've described, the availability of such extended periods would fluctuate during my life, as my cardiac surgeon responsibilities did not let me fully focus upon another time-consuming endeavor. Yet my preoccupation with choosing only larger, demanding art projects was self-generated. Moreover, having had no artistic training or mentor, I thought you started directly with a painting and ended up with a canvas, correcting your numerous mistakes and revising your painting until its final form.

I hadn't learned that sketching was an integral part of the process in producing a painting and that making such simpler drawings can be fulfilling on their own — until I enrolled in a UCLA Extension Program. I did this with Don Paglia, as we started from scratch in a beginner's drawing class. Though already an accomplished artist, Don always wanted to learn new things. This capacity to never be afraid to learn further blends perfectly with my approach to science.

Through this class, Joe Blaustein and Jan Stussy became the two giant mentors of my artistic life, each teaching me lessons that also profoundly impacted my scientific career. Through them, I found how meticulous step-by-step sketches could play an essential role in the ultimate discovery of a completed painting.

Most importantly, for the first time... I learned *how to see* rather than simply how to look.

Joe had us look at the paintings of Rembrandt *to see* the grandeur of his talent. How easy it is to become enthralled by the beauty of each of Rembrandt's dashing images that exist within the larger painting. But if you stop there, you miss appreciating the majesty of his vision. These compelling, yet separate parts, do not tell the picture's deeper story. He taught us that they are vital accessories within the grand design, as Rembrandt takes us on the journey of foreground, mid-ground, and background space within the total canvas. Focusing only upon the small lovely images will deprive us of a greater vision that is the power of what Rembrandt had given to us. For therein lies the full depth and meaning of his work.

My eyes truly opened, as I could clearly see how this translated to my medical research. All too often, the medical field focuses on the individual "pieces" of an illness — its assortment of symptoms — and tries to correct those with medications or a procedure. But if we can *see* the whole picture — the whole disease — and correct *that,* many symptoms will fall away as we rectify the grander issue.

It is easy to list all the things wrong with someone, but you have to figure out *why they went wrong.* You have to bring it down to something simple, for that is elegance. Conversely, many will typically say it's too complicated. But that's because they don't understand it. "Complexity" conveys lack of understanding. This is the essence of my mantra that "elegance is simplicity, confusion is complexity."

This approach to appreciating *vision* is exemplified by my early work within the world of reperfusion damage. Rather than simply trying to note and counter each of the various symptoms, I explored the larger picture to develop an answer that would solve the core disease. This opened a broad new universe of learning not only about heart surgery, but also heart attacks, lung damage, blue babies, liver injury, leg injury, and brain damage. All of this flowed from seeing the hidden yet greater scheme that existed in a new world that contains previously unappreciated connections.

The same concept proved true with congestive heart failure. If you focus only on the symptoms, you miss the bigger answer of addressing the ventricle — its source. Conventional medicine still looks at smaller issues and uses drugs to treat dilated hearts. But that doesn't work. Why? The heart's geometry is the problem. The natural elliptical football shape has changed to a circular basketball contour. Hearts simply cannot get better while they stay circular. Correct the wrong anatomy, which returns the natural elliptical form, and the problem is solved.

Over 50 years of my life have been spent in education (as both teacher and learner), and how grateful I am to have had Jan Stussy as my artistic mentor. Jan's rare blend of support and challenge were his yin and yang. He spent many hours setting up the artistic environment (model and background) for each class, yet we were never allowed to come in and begin our artistic work. Instead, we had to take time to walk around the studio to see the model and his or her surroundings in order to select where we wanted to start to draw. We were encouraged to consider what our particular talents might be and the paints we could best employ. In other words, he forced us to become more than an artist that only arrived for a night of rendering, and expanded our thinking by making us integrate the complete process. It was like with Rembrandt's paintings — the whole is greater than the sum of its many parts. You were no longer simply an instrument, but would become the orchestra, focusing beyond the various parts of a medical illness to perceive the fuller picture. This innovative scheme enabled us to not just look, but to see... mirroring the scientific work described throughout this volume.

Gently and firmly, Jan evaluated the output of each student. He chastised those who did what they had done before. "You know this, why are you here? Do not show up if you need credit for work accomplished previously. Grow, expand, have fun." We used these newly uncovered talents to fill the *empty rooms of our canvas* — we continued to learn. The rigid approach of traditionalists would impair their capacity to grow from Jan's teaching.

Jan's mandate to his students — "Never remain comfortable with what you do; you've already done it, move on" — is really the story of life. Never be satisfied with only what you did yesterday. Choose something else for tomorrow.

Moving Beyond Self-Limiting Beliefs

A staggering spread of talent (with students possessing different levels of prior experience) existed within our classes, yet every one of us was astounded by how we grew artistically during each session. Jan taught us how to demand more from ourselves, and through this, we achieved more than we could imagine. This passion also translated directly into my research work, where I aimed beyond what the medical world presumed was possible. This drive formed a significant role in igniting the adventures that characterize my scientific career as chronicled here. I never knew where we would end up, but I always believed it would be in the right place.

Foreground, Mid-ground... *Background*

Working with Don Paglia and Elyse Wyman (another friend and colleague from the Stussy course), we developed inventive ways to place water in an oil pan, and add turpentine and oil colors to create a mixture of hues. Sliding a sheet of drawing paper through this mélange produced an array of tints and shapes on the paper's surface. Each of us looked at the whirling patterns, then glimpsed an idea for a picture. This imagery created a new vision, an intrinsic treasure that now existed but without the need to utilize a model placed into provocative surroundings. Instead, the painter's mind became the source of inspiration, as we took a breathtaking expedition into the unknown. (**Figure 3**)

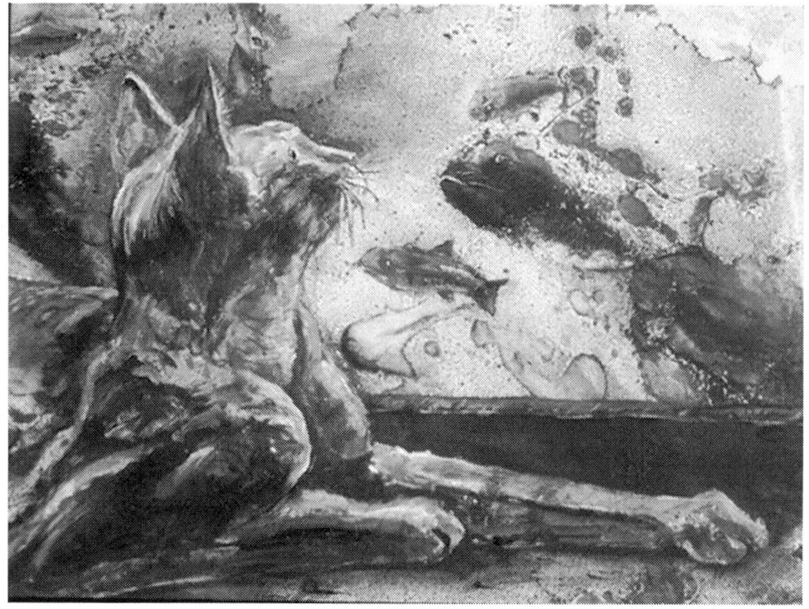

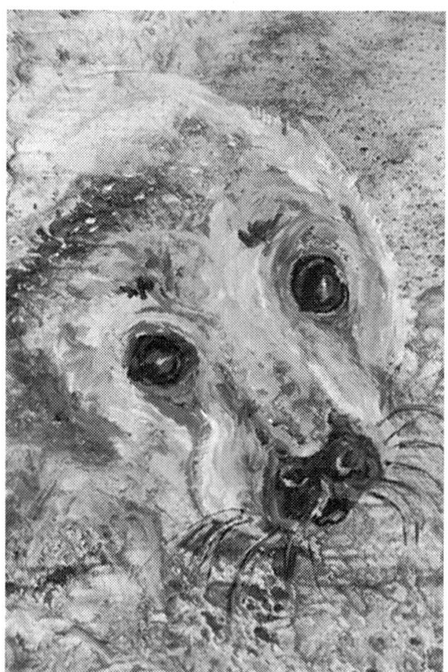

Figure 3: Cat and aquarium (top), Harp Seal (bottom)

Many unique pictures were made in this fashion, and I was as surprised as others to see the outcomes. Joy filled me during the rendering as I applied the new techniques I had learned with each painting, which then built toward my next endeavor.

For my sketching, my favorite subjects were Albert Einstein and Arturo Toscanini (acclaimed Italian conductor), as a spectacular grace and worldliness characterized their faces. (**Figure 4, 5**) Their wrinkles were the result of many years of curiosity and learning, and their resulting beauty reigned wonderfully over their gentle images.

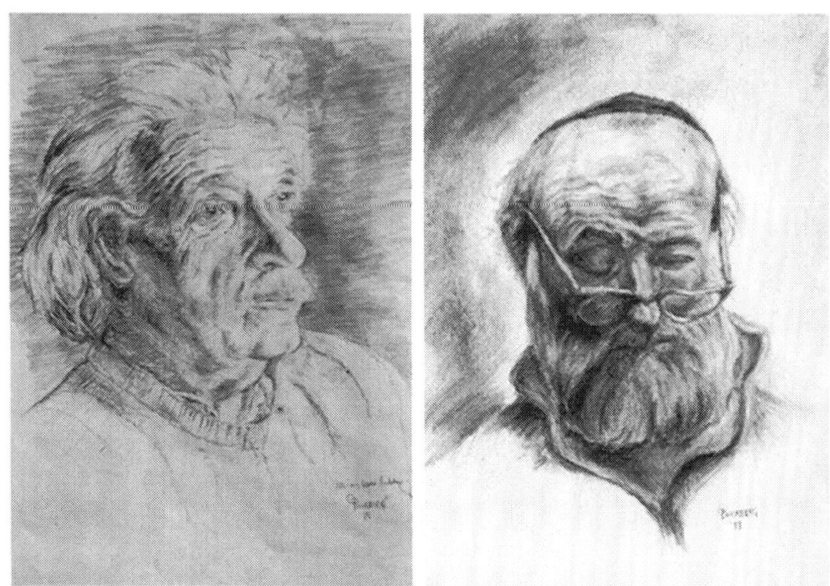

Figure 4: Einstein (left), Rabbi (right).

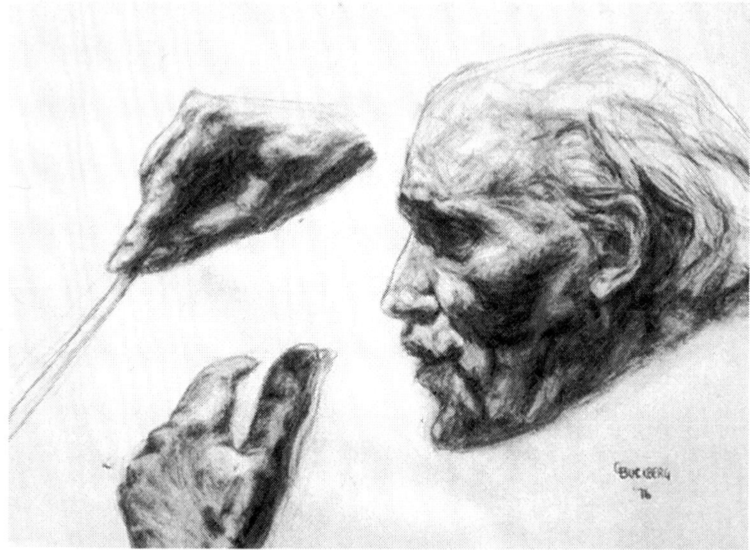

Figure 5: Toscanini

This led me to combine the faces of aging men with their hand motions. This composition had completeness, as these hands with their soft, pliable, purposeful, and elegant posture — paired together with these radiant faces — kindled a candid portal into their personality. A complete message arose from an image containing only hands and faces, as our brain now allowed us to understand and appreciate how they portrayed their human source.

Life in Reverse

From those colorful fertile backgrounds created by Don Paglia, Elyse Wyman, and myself, emerged spontaneous pictures containing depths that could not be intended, but were very powerful. The wonder of surprise creates the added thrill that arises when new directions are explored.

This experience occurred in dramatic fashion to me one evening while I was on Catalina Island with my children. After they had gone to bed, I had a beer and decided to draw. I wiped black charcoal across the paper surface to create a rough monochromatic background, then used an eraser to rub away portions of this dark backdrop to reveal the facial features of Toscanini. The process took less than five minutes, but the face was delightfully captured! Not only that, but the rubbed out areas unveiled two more heads, one on each side. (**Figure 6**)

This picture remains one of my favorites. It was unplanned, employed a method never used before by me (eraser), and captured a beauty within the background, resulting in an innovative creation.

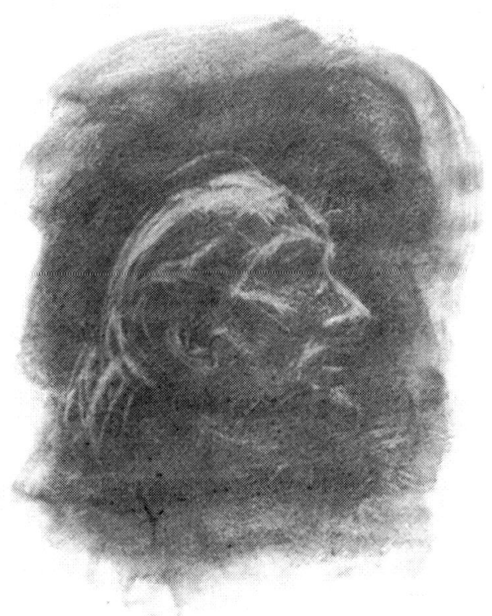

Figure 6: Toscanini

The Unforeseen Road

The hunt for scientific answers can take similar and often equally unanticipated pathways. We just have to be willing to go where the journey leads us.

Take, for example, my search to understand the helical heart. This new knowledge overcame prior voids in our understanding of previously unsolved cardiac problems. It led to development of innovative ways to remedy heart failure in the dilated heart, understand diastolic dysfunction, recognize right ventricle and septum issues, as well as improve pacemaker function. The vibrancy of knowledge gained from this new look at the heart will continue to open doorways... provided we traverse these new portals.

Discovery takes tenacity. Such doggedness to finish a process we believe is correct is really a lifestyle attitude. Training for my running and swimming marathons drew upon the same determination that guided me through the pictures just described, and propelled the scientific journeys detailed within this memoir.

That's not to say it is easy. I found that even with the immense satisfaction of finishing each race, sporting endurance events take their toll. I recall running my first of three Los Angeles Marathons, and realizing that big people like myself may be better suited for swimming, as my only focus after crossing the finish line was to relax. I placed my back against a large nearby tree and shimmied down to a prone position. My daughter Gia, then nearing twenty years old, found me splayed out, eyes closed, completely still. Her natural thought — "Oh my, Daddy's dead" — caused her to douse me with the contents of two water bottles. It was the perfect antidote, as I sprung to life to join my loving family to celebrate.

Similar amusing scenarios occurred when I did my ten-mile marathon swims on 11 different occasions. A person is always needed to paddle on a surfboard near each swimmer to guide them along the Pacific Coast ocean waters between Huntington Beach where we entered, and Seal Beach where we finished. The son of a colleague was my first paddler. As we approached the finish, he said, "Dr. B, do you want the good news or bad news? Well, the good news is we beat someone. The bad news is he only had one leg."

One year, I was delayed because my paddler that day could not finish (he developed gastrointestinal distress and went ashore). I had to follow a sailboat while swimming along my ocean route to finally arrive at Seal Beach. Gia, who has my sense of humor, said, "Daddy, I am so proud of you. The one-legged man finished only 12 minutes ago, then a blind man came to the end of his swim 7 minutes ago, and just before you emerged from the ocean, a 76-year-old man completed the ten-mile swim. We are so happy you finally got here!"

The Thirst to Grow

Humor aside, *persistence* is required with science projects for a reason that goes well beyond discovery: it must confront the barriers established by critics. Yet these roadblocks are false, and they must be overcome by the truth that prevails in science. Doing only what is expected is the true obstacle to progress. The need to overcome such rigid barriers also exists with art. Van Gogh's innovative ways departed from expectations, and for that reason he was rewarded with initial rejection. Yet our current culture is so much better off now because his truth eventually won.

As I complete this final chapter, which sets parallels between art and science, it becomes ever clearer to me that creativity in both disciplines has been my source of stimulation. They share the exciting allure of challenging goals, unbridled energy to evolve new ideas, joy in finding answers amid early futile attempts, and the thrills of giving to others (patient or art viewer). Ultimately, they bestow the most coveted gift of having accomplished: *meaningful work.*

For me, "My art is my science, and my science is my art."

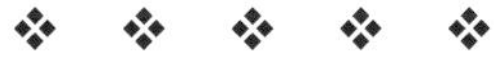

EPILOGUE

My Journey

Looking back at my life story makes me consider what may have been my guiding lights. Two come primarily to mind. The first is an attitude about life, and the second is the scientific springboard that launched and steered so many of my voyages.

I learned early from my family that the world is made by giving and not by taking. This principle has led to my greatest joys. The highest reward is to help someone — to see them happy, smiling, and comfortable. Givers are the truly rich people. I complete this memoir with the hope that I have accomplished *meaningful work,* for this prize of helping others remains my grandest goal.

For many, the bible is the main guide. Claude Bernard's *Introduction to the Study of Experimental Medicine* is my medical and scientific equivalent, and second guiding light. I buy numerous copies and liberally distribute them to other physicians. Simplicity is my mainstay, and his illumination of the movement between observer and experimenter and back to observer identifies how we must learn and grow. It is understanding nature, not affirming our preconceived beliefs, that is the centerpiece of our search, and curiosity is my driving force. Bernard's exasperations with rigidity — the never-ending barrier to growth — would continue today. I suspect that rigid people remain rigid... because their curiosity is absent.

I've learned that frustration and anger can never be the counterforce to such obstacles. Instead, I'm led by a steadfast commitment to make the truth even clearer. This memoir confirms that each scientific answer is correct, as each passed through the steps of making an observation of abnormality, testing it experimentally, reinforcing it by application in patients, and then making efforts to teach these new ideas to create a fundamental shift in how to care for these disastrous diseases.

Despite reporting solid evidence for these novel and successful treatments — for acute heart attack, sudden death (cardiac arrest), congestive heart failure, re-oxygenation injury in babies, lung and leg problems after blood flow restoration, damage to the heart's septum, utilizing pacemakers to restore normal cardiac twisting, and the potential for greatly improved treatments linked to a deep understanding of the structure / function relationship within the helical heart — *the promise of these breakthroughs remains unfulfilled*. Ongoing inflexibility prevents the blossoming of the seeds that underlie a *major revolution in thinking* about health care.

Tragically, progress remains hampered by medical community rigidity, just as it was for my hero Claude Bernard, and for Semmelweis, who in the 1800s told the titans of medicine to wash their hands to avoid childbed fever — but they refused.

Today's losers are the patients, whose diseases have not been cured.

Considering this further leads to a fascinating insight into the oftentimes adversarial views of cardiology and cardiac surgery. Let's look at the noninvasive methods that have evolved in the cardiologist's catheterization lab — ones that try to match what occurs during heart surgery operations. At first, intense resistance to the goals of innovative surgical treatments are expressed by the cardiology community. Yet as soon as those same treatment objectives become achievable by the development of catheter-based (cardiology) approaches that *they* can use — this rigidity suddenly turns into vigorous enthusiasm.

Evidence of this goes back to the introduction of coronary angioplasty — to replace surgical coronary artery bypass grafting. Then catheter-based mitral procedures became all the rage to replace using surgical procedures to repair or replace the mitral valve.

Today, cardiology's resistance to the concept of treating congestive heart failure by restoring the heart's normal form is finally turning into advocacy — as the cardiologists now are investigating how to insert a cone-shaped ventricular device in the cath lab — to reshape the spherical ventricle back into its natural elliptical form.

These winning changes will bring new blood flow beyond narrowed arteries, restore leaky valves, and rebuild natural form in stretched dilated failing hearts. *Yet the patients have borne the brunt of this dilemma*, for while their disease can now be treated by using either non-invasive (cardiology-based) or surgical methods... the ability for *them to receive this benefit* has been delayed by resistance. They had to wait until the cardiologists had their own new tool to deliver it. Providing life-saving treatments must be everyone's goal — regardless of who supplies it.

"Scientific truth wins, but only God knows the timing." Galileo taught us this lesson, after obstructionists let 500 years pass before his findings were finally accepted. In 2016, science "discovered" and acknowledged the truth about Einstein's 1916 theories on gravitational waves. My sincerest hope is that exploration and testing of the revelations described in my book will take only a fraction of this time.

I'm frequently asked, "What is your stimulus to never stop 'fighting the fight' of transmitting new ideas, when rejection has prevailed for so long?" My answer is that the excitement of uncovering nature's secrets and using these discoveries to help others, ignites a thrill and vigor that consistently rewards such useful contributions. Yet this prize can never overshadow the sheer joy that the cardiac surgeon experiences after someone is directly improved by his or her surgical skills. ...But there is more.

Many years ago, I visited a dear friend. I helped him do four operative procedures in one day, and he shared his gratefulness for being able to work in a medical center that had sufficient patients to support such a busy practice. I concurred, but advised him that I also want my surgical contribution to touch people in numbers that extends beyond my operating room. I recently received a book written by a legendary heart surgeon, whose fame and talent allowed him to individually operate on "100,000 hearts." I marveled at his astonishing accomplishment. Then I thought about blood cardioplegia, which has been used in 25 million patients, *and realized that part of my dream has already happened.*

My life's purpose has been, and remains, to powerfully overturn the stagnant barriers against new thinking. Patients will greatly benefit, as adopting these new approaches will offset the devastating symptoms and shortened lifetimes caused by these major diseases whose remedies are revealed in this memoir.

My discoveries happened because of the collaborative efforts of many research fellows, colleagues, and especially my mentors, upon whose shoulders I stood to see the next peak ahead. Now my memoir reaches out to those most affected by our current inability to counter major heart diseases — those of you reading these pages. My wish is that your passionate concern for your health and the health of your loved ones will motivate you to share the information contained in this book with those you turn to for your medical care.

The answers exist now. So please join me on this quest.

RESOURCES / OVERVIEW

Brief Summaries of the life-saving answers discovered during my lifelong journey are available in PDF format on a "Summaries of Discovery" page at **www.GeraldBuckberg.com.**

These may help the non-medical reader better understand each chapter's contents, so they may also more easily share them with others.

The summaries include:

Blood Cardioplegia: Protecting Hearts During Surgical Operations (Chs. 6 & 7)

Acute Heart Attacks: New Treatment to Avoid Lasting Injury (Chs. 8 & 9)

Re-oxygenation Injury: Protecting Vulnerable Babies (Ch. 10)

Sudden Death: Bringing the Dead Back to Life (Ch. 11)

Unwitnessed Arrest: Beating the Unbeatable Foe (Chs. 12 & 13)

Heart Failure: Solving the Unsolvable Challenge (Chs. 16 & 17)

Paco Torrent-Guasp's Amazing Discovery: Why the Heart Works (Ch. 18)

The Helical Heart: Solving Heart Failure's Unanswered Puzzles (Ch. 20)

Diastolic Dysfunction: Uncovering its Cause and Finding its Solution (Ch. 22)

The Septum: Preventing Unnecessary Damage during Cardiac Operations (Ch. 24)

Pacemakers: The Riddle Solved (Ch. 26)

REFERENCE LIST

1. Buckberg GD, Luck JC, Payne DB et al. Some sources of error in measuring regional blood flow with radioactive microspheres. *J Appl Physiol.* 1971;31:598–615.
2. Buckberg GD, Olinger GN, Mulder DG et al. Depressed postoperative cardiac performance. *J Thorac Cardiovasc Surg.* 1975;70:974–988.
3. Melrose DG, Dreyer B, Bentall HH. Elective cardiac arrest. *Lancet.* 1955;2:21.
4. Kirsch U, Rodewald G, Kalmar P. Induced ischemic arrest. Clinical experience with cardioplegia in open-heart surgery. *J Thorac Cardiovasc Surg.* 1972;63:121–130.
5. Tyers GFO, Todd GJ, Niebauer IM. The mechanism of myocardial damage following potassium citrate (Melrose) cardioplegia. *surg.* 1975;78:45.
6. Gay WA, Ebert PA. Functional, metabolic, and morphologic effects of potassium-induced cardioplegia. *surg.* 1973;74:284–293.
7. O'Blenes SB, Friesen CH, Ali A et al. Protecting the aged heart during cardiac surgery: the potential benefits of del Nido cardioplegia. *J Thorac Cardiovasc Surg.* 2011;141:762–770.
8. Domanski MJ, Mahaffey K, Hasselblad V et al. Association of myocardial enzyme elevation and survival following coronary artery bypass graft surgery. *JAMA.* 2011;305:585–591.
9. Khuri SF, Healey NA, Hossain M et al. Intraoperative regional myocardial acidosis and reduction in long-term survival after cardiac surgery. *J Thorac Cardiovasc Surg.* 2005;129:372–381.
10. Cooley DA, Reul GJ, Wukasch DC. Ischemic contracture of the heart: "stone heart.". *Am J Cardiol.* 1972;29:575–577.
11. Shumway NE, Lower RR. Hypothermia for extended periods of anoxic arrest. *Surg Forum.* 1959;10:563.
12. Piper HM, Garcia-Dorado D, Ovize M. Review: A fresh look at reperfusion injury. *Cardiovascular Research.* 1998;38:291–300.
13. Bernard C. An Introduction to the Study of Experimental Medicine. New York: Dover Publications, 1957.

14. Brazier J, Hottenrott C, Buckberg GD. Noncoronary collateral myocardial blood flow. *Ann Thorac Surg.* 1975;19:425–435.

15. Nelson RL, Fey KH, Follette DM et al. Intermittent infusion of cardioplegic solution during aortic cross-clamping. *Surg Forum.* 1976;27:241–243.

16. Follette DM, Steed DL, Foglia RP et al. Advantages of intermittent blood cardioplegia over intermittent ischemia during prolonged hypothermic aortic clamping. *Cardiovasc Surg.* 1978;58:1–200.

17. Follette DM, Mulder DG, Maloney JVJr et al. Advantages of blood cardioplegia over continuous coronary perfusion or intermittent ischemia. *J Thorac Cardiovasc Surg.* 1978;76:604–619.

18. Buckberg GD, Brazier JR, Nelson RL et al. Studies of the effects of hypothermia on regional myocardial blood flow and metabolism during cardiopulmonary bypass. I. The adequately perfused beating, fibrillating and arrested heart. *J Thorac Cardiovasc Surg.* 1977;78:87–94.

19. Rosenkranz ER, Okamoto F, Buckberg GD et al. Safety of prolonged aortic clamping with blood cardioplegia. III. Aspartate enrichment of glutamate-blood cardioplegia in energy-depleted hearts after ischemic and reperfusion injury. *J Thorac Cardiovasc Surg.* 1986;91:428–435.

20. Lazar HL, Buckberg GD, Manganaro AM et al. Myocardial energy replenishment and reversal of ischemic damage by substrate enhancement of secondary blood cardioplegia with amino acids during reperfusion. *J Thorac Cardiovasc Surg.* 1980;80:350–359.

21. Loop FD, Higgins TL, Panda R et al. Myocardial protection during cardiac operations. *J Thorac Cardiovasc Surg.* 1992;104:608–618.

22. Mahrholdt H, Wagner A, Parker M et al. Relationship of contractile function to transmural extent of infarction in patients with chronic coronary artery disease. *J Am Coll Cardiol.* 2003;42:505–512.

23. Gaudron P, Eilles C, Kugler I et al. Progressive left ventricular dysfunction and remodeling after myocardial infarction. Potential mechanisms and early predictors. *Circulation.* 1993;87:755–762.

24. Torabi A, Cleland JG, Rigby AS et al. Development and course of heart failure after a myocardial infarction in younger and older people. *J Geriatr Cardiol.* 2014;11:1–12.

25. Gerber Y, Weston SA, Enriquez-Sarano M et al. Atherosclerotic Burden and Heart Failure After Myocardial Infarction. *JAMA Cardiol.* 2016;1:156–162.

26. Bolognese L, Neskovic AN, Parodi G et al. Left ventricular remodeling after primary coronary angioplasty: patterns of left ventricular dilation and long-term prognostic implications. *Circulation*. 2002;106:2351–2357.

27. Allen BS, Rosenkranz ER, Buckberg GD et al. Studies on prolonged regional ischemia. VI. Myocardial infarction with LV power failure: A medical/surgical emergency requiring urgent revascularization with maximal protection of remote muscle. *J Thorac Cardiovasc Surg*. 1989;98:691–703.

28. Sjostrand F, Allen BS, Buckberg GD et al. Studies of controlled reperfusion after ischemia: IV. Electron microscopic studies: Importance of embedding techniques in quantitative evaluation of cardiac mitochondrial structure during regional ischemia and reperfusion. *J Thorac Cardiovasc Surg*. 1986;92/3:512–524.

29. Allen BS, Rosenkranz ER, Buckberg GD et al. Studies of controlled reperfusion after ischemia: VII. The high oxygen requirements of dyskinetic cardiac muscle. *J Thorac Cardiovasc Surg*. 1986;92:543–552.

30. Buckberg GD, et al. Studies of controlled reperfusion after ischemia. *Journal of Thoracic and Cardiovascular Surgery*. 1986;92:483–648.

31. Okamoto F, Allen BS, Buckberg GD et al. Studies of controlled reperfusion after ischemia: VIII. Regional blood cardioplegic reperfusion on total vented bypass without thoracotomy: A new concept. *J Thorac Cardiovasc Surg*. 1986;92/3:553–563.

32. Allen BS, Okamoto F, Buckberg GD et al. Studies of controlled reperfusion after ischemia. XV. Immediate functional recovery after six hours of regional ischemia by careful control of conditions of reperfusion and composition of reperfusate. *J Thorac Cardiovasc Surg*. 1986;92:621–635.

33. Vinten-Johansen J, Buckberg GD, Okamoto F et al. Studies of controlled reperfusion after ischemia: V. Superiority of surgical vs medical reperfusion after regional ischemia. *J Thorac Cardiovasc Surg*. 1986;92:525–534.

34. Reimer KA, Jennings RB. The "wavefront phenomenon" of myocardial ischemic cell death. *li*. 1979;40:633–644.

35. Allen BS, Buckberg GD, Schwaiger M et al. Studies of controlled reperfusion after ischemia: XVI. Early recovery of regional wall motion in patients following surgical revascularization after eight hours of acute coronary occlusion. *J Thorac Cardiovasc Surg*. 1986;92:636–648.

36. Allen BS, Buckberg GD, Fontan F et al. Superiority of controlled surgical reperfusion vs. PTCA in acute coronary occlusion. *J Thorac Cardiovasc Surg*. 1993;105:864–884.

37. Roger VL, Go AS, Lloyd-Jones DM et al. Executive summary: heart disease and stroke statistics — 2012 update: a report from the American Heart Association. *Circulation.* 2012;125:188–197.

38. Lehmann C. Economic Benefits of e-Technology in Managing Congestive Heart Failure. 2005. American Association of Homes and Services for the Aging.

39. Taussig HB, Blalock A. The tetralogy of Fallot; diagnosis and indications for operation; the surgical treatment of the tetralogy of Fallot. *surg.* 1947;21:145.

40. Miller BJ, Gibbon JH Jr., Greco VF et al. The production and repair of interatrial septal defects under direct vision with the assistance of an extracorporeal pump-oxygenator circuit. *J Thorac Surg.* 1953;26:598–616.

41. Patz A. Current status of role of oxygen in retrolental fibroplasia. *Invest Ophthalmol.* 1976;15:337–339.

42. Gauduel Y, Duvelleroy MA. Role of oxygen radicals in cardiac injury due to reoxygenation. *J Mol Cell Cardiol.* 1984;16:459–470.

43. Buckberg GD, et al. Studies of Hypoxemic/Reoxygenation Injury. *J Thorac Cardiovasc Surg.* 1995;110:1163–1286.

44. Halldorsson A, Kronon M, Allen BS et al. Controlled reperfusion after lung ischemia: implications for improved function after lung transplantation. *J Thorac Cardiovasc Surg.* 1998;115:415–424.

45. Allen BS, Barth MJ, Ilbawi MN. Pediatric myocardial protection: an overview. *Sem Thorac & Cardiovasc Surg.* 2001;13:56–72.

46. Allen BS. The reoxygenation injury: Is it clinically important? *J Thorac Cardiovasc Surg.* 2002;124:16–19.

47. Morita K. Invited commentary: surgical reoxygenation injury in myocardium of patients with cyanosis: how is it clinically important? *World J Pediatr Congenit Heart Surg.* 2012;3:317–320.

48. Jude JR, Kouwenhoven WB, Knickerbocker GG. Cardiac arrest. Report of application of external cardiac massage on 118 patients. *JAMA.* 1961;178:1063–1070.

49. Vayrynen T, Kuisma M, Maatta T et al. Medical futility in asystolic out-of-hospital cardiac arrest. *Acta Anaesthesiol Scand.* 2008;52:81–87.

50. Hamill RJ. Resuscitation: when is enough, enough? *Respir Care.* 1995;40:515–524.

51. Beyersdorf F, Acar C, Buckberg GD et al. Studies on prolonged regional ischemia. IV. Aggressive surgical treatment for intractable ventricular fibrillation after acute myocardial infarction. *J Thorac Cardiovasc Surg.* 1989;98:557–566.

52. Beyersdorf F, Kirsh MM, Buckberg GD et al. Warm glutamate/aspartate-enriched blood cardioplegic solution for perioperative sudden death. *J Thorac Cardiovasc Surg.* 1992;104:1141–1147.

53. Athanasuleas CL, Buckberg GD, Allen BS et al. Sudden cardiac death: Directing the scope of resuscitation towards the heart and brain. *Resuscitation.* 2006;70:44–51.

54. Clifton G, Miller E, Choi S et al. Lack of effect of induction of hypothermia after acute brain injury. *N Engl J Med.* 2001;344:556–563.

55. Follette DM, Fey K, Buckberg GD et al. Reducing postischemic damage by temporary modification of reperfusate calcium, potassium, pH, and osmolarity. *J Thorac Cardiovasc Surg.* 1981;82:221–238.

56. Nagao K, Hayashi N, Kanmatsuse K et al. Cardiopulmonary cerebral resuscitation using emergency cardiopulmonary bypass, coronary reperfusion therapy and mild hypothermia in patients with cardiac arrest outside the hospital. *J Am Coll Cardiol.* 2000;36:776–783.

57. Sung K, Lee YT, Park PW et al. Improved survival after cardiac arrest using emergent autopriming percutaneous cardiopulmonary support. *Ann Thorac Surg.* 2006;82:651–656.

58. Chen JS, Ko WJ, Yu HY et al. Analysis of the outcome for patients experiencing myocardial infarction and cardiopulmonary resuscitation refractory to conventional therapies necessitating extracorporeal life support rescue. *Crit Care Med.* 2006;34:950–957.

59. Allen BS, Buckberg GD. Myocardial protection management during adult cardiac operations. In: Baue AE, Geha AS, Hammond GL, Laks H, Naunheim KS, editors. Glenn's Thoracic and Cardiovascular Surgery. Norwalk: Appleton & Lange, 1995: 1653–1710.

60. Trummer G, Foerster K, Buckberg GD et al. Successful resuscitation after prolonged periods of cardiac arrest — a new field in cardiac surgery. *Journal of Thoracic and Cardiovascular Surgery.* 2009.

61. Allen BS, Ko Y, Buckberg GD et al. Studies of isolated global brain ischaemia: I. A new large animal model of global brain ischaemia and its baseline perfusion studies. *Eur J Cardiothorac Surg.* 2012;41:1138–1146.

62. Allen BS, Ko Y, Buckberg GD et al. Studies of isolated global brain ischaemia: II. Controlled reperfusion provides complete neurologic recovery following 30 min of warm ischaemia — the importance of perfusion pressure. *Eur J Cardiothorac Surg.* 2012;41:1147–1154.

63. Allen BS, Ko Y, Buckberg GD et al. Studies of isolated global brain ischaemia: III. Influence of pulsatile flow during cerebral perfusion and its link to consistent full neurological recovery with controlled reperfusion following 30 min of global brain ischaemia. *Eur J Cardiothorac Surg.* 2012;41:1155–1163.

64. Allen BS, Buckberg GD. Studies of isolated global brain ischaemia: I. Overview of irreversible brain injury and evolution of a new concept — redefining the time of brain death. *Eur J Cardiothorac Surg.* 2012;41:1132–1137.

65. Apostolakis EE, Baikoussis NG, Parissis H et al. Left ventricular diastolic dysfunction of the cardiac surgery patient; a point of view for the cardiac surgeon and cardio-anesthesiologist. *J Cardiothorac Surg.* 2009;4:67.

66. Schlensak C, Doenst T, Bitu-Moreno J et al. Controlled limb reperfusion with a simplified perfusion system. *Thorac Cardiovasc Surg.* 2000;48:274–278.

67. Beyersdorf F, Matheis G, Kruger S et al. Avoiding reperfusion injury after limb revascularization: experimental observations and recommendations for clinical application. *J Vasc Surg.* 1989;9:757–766.

68. Beyersdorf F, Mitrev Z, Ihnken K et al. Controlled limb reperfusion in patients having cardiac operations [see comments]. *J Thorac Cardiovasc Surg.* 1996;111:873–881.

69. Beyersdorf F, Schlensak C. Controlled reperfusion after acute and persistent limb ischemia. *Semin Vasc Surg.* 2009;22:52–57.

70. Allen BS, Hartz RS, Buckberg GD et al. Prevention of ischemic damage using controlled limb reperfusion. *J Card Surg.* 1998;13:224–227.

71. Halldorsson AO, Kronon M, Allen BS et al. Controlled reperfusion prevents pulmonary injury after 24 hours of lung preservation. *Ann Thorac Surg.* 1998;66:877–884.

72. Allen BS. Controlled pulmonary reperfusion: what is the optimal method of delivery? *Ann Thorac Surg.* 2000;70:1449–1450.

73. Lick SD, Brown PS, Jr., Kurusz M et al. Technique of controlled reperfusion of the transplanted lung in humans. *Ann Thorac Surg.* 2000;69:910–912.

74. Schnickel GT, Ross DJ, Beygui R et al. Modified reperfusion in clinical lung transplantation: the results of 100 consecutive cases. *J Thorac Cardiovasc Surg.* 2006;131:218–223.

75. Hong JC, Koroleff D, Xia V et al. Regulated hepatic reperfusion mitigates ischemia-reperfusion injury and improves survival after prolonged liver warm ischemia: a pilot study on a novel concept of organ resuscitation in a large animal model. *J Am Coll Surg.* 2012;214:505–515.

76. Harvey W. De Motu Cordis. 1628.

77. Klein MD, Herman MV, Gorlin R. A hemodynamic study of LV aneurysm. Circulation 35, 614–630. 1967.

78. Bonow RO, Maurer G, Lee KL et al. Myocardial viability and survival in ischemic left ventricular dysfunction. *N Engl J Med.* 2011;364:1617–1625.

79. Dor V, Sabatier M, Di Donato M et al. Efficacy of endoventricular patch plasty in large postinfarction akinetic scar and severe left ventricular dysfunction: comparison with a series of large dyskinetic scars. *J Thorac Cardiovasc Surg.* 1998;116:50–59.

80. Dor V, Sabatier M, Montiglio F et al. Endoventricular patch reconstruction of ischemic failing ventricle. a single center with 20 years experience. advantages of magnetic resonance imaging assessment. *Heart Fail Rev.* 2004;9:269–286.

81. Shah PJ, Hare DL, Raman JS et al. Survival after myocardial revascularization for ischemic cardiomyopathy: a prospective ten-year follow-up study. *J Thorac Cardiovasc Surg.* 2003;126:1320–1327.

82. Dahlberg PS, Orszulak TA, Mullany CJ et al. Late outcome of mitral valve surgery for patients with coronary artery disease. *Ann Thorac Surg.* 2003;76:1539–487.

83. Jatene AD. Left ventricular aneurysmectomy. Resection or reconstruction. *J Thorac Cardiovasc Surg.* 1985;89:321–331.

84. Roger VL, Go AS, Lloyd-Jones DM et al. Heart disease and stroke statistics — 2011 update: a report from the American Heart Association. *Circulation.* 2011;123:e18-e209.

85. Di Donato M, Toso A, Maioli M et al. Intermediate survival and predictors of death after surgical ventricular restoration. *Sem Thorac & Cardiovasc Surg.* 2002;13:468–475.

86. Migrino RQ, Young JB, ellis SG et al. End-systolic volume index at 90 to 180 minutes into reperfusion therapy for acute myocardial infarction is a strong predictor of early and late mortality. *Circulation.* 1997;96:116–121.

87. Buckberg GD. Editorial: Defining the Relationship Between Akinesia and Dyskinesia and the Cause of Left Ventricular Failure after Anterior Infarction and Reversal of Remodeling to Restoration. The Journal of Thoracic & Cardiovascular Surgery 116[1], 47–49. 1998.

88. Buckberg GD. Ventricular Structure and Surgical History. *Heart Failure Reviews.* 2004;9:255–268.

89. Athanasuleas CL, Buckberg GD, Stanley AW et al. Surgical ventricular restoration in the treatment of congestive heart failure due to post-infarction ventricular dilation. *J Am Coll Cardiol.* 2004;44:1439–1445.

90. Athanasuleas CL, Buckberg GD. Surgical ventricular restoration: where do we go from here? *Heart Failure Reviews.* 2015;20(1):89–93.

91. Babuty D, Lab MJ. Mechanoelectric contributions to sudden cardiac death. *Cardiovasc Res.* 2001 May;50(2):270–9.

92. Tomaselli GF, Zipes DP. What causes sudden death in heart failure? *Circ Res.* 2004;95:754–763.

93. Athanasuleas C, Stanley AW Jr, Buckberg GD et al. Surgical Anterior Ventricular Endocardial Restoration (SAVER) for Dilated Ischemic Cardiomyopathy. *J Thorac Cardiovasc Surg.* 2001;5:1199–1209.

94. Buckberg G, Athanasuleas C, Conte J. Surgical ventricular restoration for the treatment of heart failure. *Nat Rev Cardiol.* 2012;9:703–716.

95. Jones RH, Velazquez EJ, Michler RE et al. Coronary Bypass Surgery with or without Surgical Ventricular Reconstruction. *N Engl J Med.* 2009;360:1705–1717.

96. Oh JK, Pellikka PA, Panza JA et al. Core lab analysis of baseline echocardiographic studies in the STICH trial and recommendation for use of echocardiography in future clinical trials. *J Am Soc Echocardiogr.* 2012;25:327–336.

97. Michler RE, Rouleau JL, Al Khalidi HR et al. Insights from the STICH trial: change in left ventricular size after coronary artery bypass grafting with and without surgical ventricular reconstruction. *J Thorac Cardiovasc Surg.* 2013;146:1139–1145.

98. Athanasuleas CL, Buckberg GD, Conte JV et al. Surgical ventricular reconstruction. *N Engl J Med.* 2009;361:529–530.

99. Buckberg GD, Athanasuleas CL. The STICH trial: misguided conclusions. *J Thorac Cardiovasc Surg.* 2009;138:1060–1064.

100. Takaro T, Hultgren HN, Lipton MJ et al. The VA cooperative randomized study of surgery for coronary arterial occlusive disease II. Subgroup with significant left main lesions. *Circulation.* 1976;54:III107–III117.

101. Sheldon WC, Loop FD, Proudfit WL. A critique of the VA cooperative study. *Cleve Clin Q.* 1978;45:225–230.

102. Wijns W, Kolh P, Danchin N et al. Guidelines on myocardial revascularization: The Task Force on Myocardial Revascularization of the European Society of Cardiology (ESC) and the European Association for Cardio-Thoracic Surgery (EACTS). *Eur Heart J.* 2010.

103. Borelli GA. History of Cardiology. New York: Medical Life Press, 1927.

104. Buckberg G, Hoffman JI, Mahajan A et al. Cardiac mechanics revisited: the relationship of cardiac architecture to ventricular function. *Circulation.* 2008;118:2571–2587.

105. Buckberg G, Hoffman JI, Nanda NC et al. Ventricular torsion and untwisting: further insights into mechanics and timing interdependence: a viewpoint. *Echocardiography.* 2011;28:782–804.

106. Buckberg GD, Hoffman JI, Coghlan HC et al. Ventricular structure-function relations in health and disease: Part I. The normal heart. *Eur J Cardiothorac Surg.* 14 A.D.;47:587–601.

107. Robb JS, Robb RC. The Normal Heart: Anatomy and physiology of the structural units. *Am Heart J.* 1942;23:455–467.

108. Buckberg GD. Basic science review: the helix and the heart. *Journal of Thoracic and Cardiovascular Surgery.* 2002 Nov;124(5):863–83.

109. Sallin EA. Fiber orientation and ejection fraction in the human left ventricle. *Biophys J.* 1969 Jul;9(7):954–64.

110. Doczi G. The Power of Limits. Proportional Harmonies in Nature, Art, and Architecture. 1981. Shambhala Publications, Inc.

111. Suma H, Isomura T, Horii T et al. Role of site selection for left ventriculoplasty to treat idiopathic dilated cardiomyopathy. *Heart Failure Reviews.* 2005;9:329–336.

112. Suma H, Horii T, Isomura T et al. A new concept of ventricular restoration for nonischemic dilated cardiomyopathy. *Eur J Cardiothorac Surg.* 2006;29 Suppl 1:S207–S212.

113. Isomura T, Hoshino J, Fukada Y et al. Volume reduction rate by surgical ventricular restoration determines late outcome in ischaemic cardiomyopathy. *Eur J Heart Fail.* 2011;13:423–431.

114. Detaint D, Maalouf J, Tribouilloy C et al. Congestive heart failure complicating aortic regurgitation with medical and surgical management: a prospective study of traditional and quantitative echocardiographic markers. *J Thorac Cardiovasc Surg.* 2008;136:1549–1557.

115. Carabello BA. The changing unnatural history of valvular regurgitation. *Ann Thorac Surg.* 1992;53:191–199.

116. Sengupta PP, Korinek J, Belohlavek M et al. Left ventricular structure and function: basic science for cardiac imaging. *J Am Coll Cardiol.* 2006;48:1988–2001.

117. Sengupta PP, Krishnamorthy VK, Korinek J et al. Left ventricular form and function revisited: applied translational science to cardiovascular ultrasound imaging. *J Am Soc Echocardiogr.* 2007;20:539–551.

118. Krehl L. Kenntniss der fallung und entleerung des herzens. *Abhandl Math Phys.* 1891;29:341–362.

119. Bursi F, Weston SA, Redfield MM et al. Systolic and diastolic heart failure in the community. *JAMA.* 2006;296:2209–2216.

120. Nishimura RA, Tajik AJ. Evaluation of diastolic filling of left ventricle in health and disease: Doppler echocardiography is the clinician's Rosetta Stone. *J Am Coll Cardiol.* 1997;30:8–18.

121. Brecher GA. Experimental evidence of ventricular diastolic suction. *Circ Res.* 1956;IV:513–518.

122. Rademakers FE, Buchalter MB, Rogers WJ et al. Dissociation between left ventricular untwisting and filling. Accentuation by catecholamines. *Circulation.* 1992;85:1572–1581.

123. Tan YT, Wenzelburger FW, Sanderson JE et al. Exercise-induced torsional dyssynchrony relates to impaired functional capacity in patients with heart failure and normal ejection fraction. *Heart.* 2013;99:259–266.

124. Van Der TA, Barenbrug P, Snoep G et al. Transmural gradients of cardiac myofiber shortening in aortic valve stenosis patients using MRI tagging. *Am J Physiol Heart Circ Physiol.* 2002;283:H1609–H1615.

125. Stuber M, Scheidegger MB, Fischer SE et al. Alterations in the local myocardial motion pattern in patients sufering from pressure overload due to aortic stenosis. *Circulation.* 1999;100:361–368.

126. Castella M, Buckberg GD, Saleh S. Diastolic dysfunction in stunned myocardium: a state of abnormal excitation-contraction coupling that is limited by Na+-H+ exchange inhibition. *Eur J Cardiothorac Surg.* 2006;29 Suppl 1:S107–S114.

127. Chatterjee K, Massie B. Systolic and diastolic heart failure: Differences and similarities. *Journal of Cardiac Failure.* 2007;13:569–576.

128. Doyle A. The Sign of the Four. Lippincott's Monthly Magazine [6]. 1890. Lippincott's.

129. Starr I, Jeffers WA, Meade RH Jr. The absence of conspicuous increments of venous pressure after severe damage to the right ventricle of the dog, with a discussion of the relation between clinical congestive failure and heart disease. *Am Heart J.* 1943;26:291–301.

130. Sawatani S, Mandell C, Kusaba E. Ventricular performance following ablation and prosthetic replacement of right ventricular myocardium. *Trans Am Artif Intern Organs.* 1974;20B:629–636.

131. Cox JL, Bardy GH, Damiano RJ, Jr. et al. Right ventricular isolation procedures for nonischemic ventricular tachycardia. *J Thorac Cardiovasc Surg.* 1985;90:212–224.

132. Donald DE, Essex HE. Pressure studies after inactivation of the major portion of the canine right ventricle. *Am J Physiol.* 1954;176:155–161.

133. Brown SB, Raina A, Katz D et al. Longitudinal shortening accounts for the majority of right ventricular contraction and improves after pulmonary vasodilator therapy in normal subjects and patients with pulmonary arterial hypertension. *Chest.* 2011;140:27–33.

134. Reynolds HR, Tunick PA, Grossi EA et al. Paradoxical septal motion after cardiac surgery: a review of 3,292 cases. *Clin Cardiol.* 2007;30:621–623.

135. Isomura T, Horii T, Suma H et al. Septal anterior ventricular exclusion operation (Pacopexy) for ischemic dilated cardiomyopathy; treat form not disease. *Europ J Cardiothorac Surg.* 2006;29:S245–S250.

136. Buckberg G, Athanasuleas C, Saleh S. Septal myocardial protection during cardiac surgery for prevention of right ventricular dysfunction. *Anadolu Kardiyol Derg.* 2008;8 Suppl 2:108–116.

137. Bhaya M, Sudhakar S, Sadat K et al. Effects of antegrade versus integrated blood cardioplegia on left ventricular function evaluated by echocardiographic real-time three-dimensional speckle tracking. *Journal of Thoracic and Cardiovascular Surgery.* 2015;149:877–884.

138. Neragi-Miandoab S, Goldstein D, Bello R et al. Right ventricular dysfunction following continuous flow left ventricular assist device placement in 51 patients: predicators and outcomes. *J Cardiothorac Surg.* 2012;7:60.

139. Liakopoulos OJ, Ho JK, Yezbick AB et al. Right ventricular failure resulting from pressure overload: role of intra-aortic balloon counterpulsation and vasopressor therapy. *J Surg Res.* 2010;164:58–66.

140. Cook T. The Curves of Life. New York: Dover Publications, Inc., 1979.

141. Buckberg GD. Stonehenge and the heart: similar construction. *Eur J Cardiothorac Surg.* 2006;29 Suppl 1:S286–S290.

142. Castella M, Buckberg GD, Saleh S et al. Structure function interface with sequential shortening of basal and apical components of the myocardial band. *Eur J Cardiothorac Surg.* 2005;27:980–987.

143. van Eck JW, van Hemel NM, van den BA et al. Predictors of improved quality of life 1 year after pacemaker implantation. *Am Heart J.* 2008;156:491–497.

144. Kashani A, Barold SS. Significance of QRS complex duration in patients with heart failure. *J Am Coll Cardiol.* 2005;46:2183–2192.

145. Lustgarten DL, Calame S, Crespo EM et al. Electrical resynchronization induced by direct His-bundle pacing. *Heart Rhythm.* 2010;7:15–21.

146. Wiggers CJ. The muscular reactions of the mammalian ventricles to artificial surface stimuli. *Am J Physiol.* 1925;346–378.

147. Coghlan HC, Coghlan AR, Buckberg GD et al. 'The electrical spiral of the heart': its role in the helical continuum. The hypothesis of the anisotropic conducting matrix. *Eur J Cardiothorac Surg.* 2006;29 Suppl 1:S178–S187.

148. Brenyo A, Goldengerg I, Barsheshet A. The downside of right ventricular apical pacing. *Indian Pacing Electrophysiol J.* 2012;12:102–113.

149. Bank AJ, Gage RM, Burns KV. Right ventricular pacing, mechanical dyssynchrony, and heart failure. *J Cardiovasc Transl Res.* 2012;5:219–231.

150. Tomioka H, Liakopoulos O, Buckberg GD et al. The effect of ventricular sequential contraction on helical heart during pacing. *Europ J Cardiothorac Surg.* 2006.

151. Zanon F, Barold SS. Direct His bundle and paraHisian cardiac pacing. *Ann Noninvasive Electrocardiol.* 2012;17:70–78.

152. Kronborg MB, Mortensen PT, Gerdes JC et al. His and para-His pacing in AV block: feasibility and electrocardiographic findings. *J Interv Card Electrophysiol.* 2011;31:255–262.

153. Sharma PS, Dandamudi G, Naperkoswki A et al. Permanent His-bundle pacing is feasible, safe, and superior to right ventricular pacing in routine clinical practice. *Heart Rhythm.* 2015;12:305–312.

154. Barba-Pichardo R, Morina-Vazquez P, Fernandez-Gomez JM et al. Permanent His-bundle pacing: seeking physiological ventricular pacing. *Europace.* 2010;12:527–533.

155. Stanley AW, Jr., Athanasuleas CL, Buckberg GD. Heart failure following anterior myocardial infarction: an indication for ventricular restoration, a surgical method to reverse post-infarction remodeling. *Heart Fail Rev.* 2004;9:241–254.

156. Cirillo M, Campana M, Brunelli F et al. Time series analysis of physiologic left ventricular reconstruction in ischemic cardiomyopathy. *J Thorac Cardiovasc Surg.* 2016.

IMAGE CREDITS

p. 27, Figure 1. Photograph. From the author's collection. *Also:* p. 33, Figure 2. Photograph; p. 35, Figure 3. Photograph; p. 39, Figure 1. Photograph (right); p. 46, Figure 2. Graph; p. 49, Figure 1. Photograph (right); p. 57, Figure 2. Photographs; p. 58, Figure 3. Graph; p. 61, Figure 4. Graph; p. 62, Figure 5a. Photograph; p. 63, Figure 5b. Photograph; p. 99, Figure 1. Photograph; p. 116, Figure 1. Drawing (left); p. 144, Figure 1. Graph; p. 187, Figure 1. Chart; p. 258, Figure 1. Drawing (left); p. 263, Figure 2. Drawing; p. 268, Figure 4. Photograph; p. 269, Video; p. 273, Video 2; p. 284, Video 1; p. 299, Figure 1. Graph; p. 312, Video 1; p. 344, Figure 9a. Upper drawings; p. 350, Figure 12. Photograph (left); p. 360, Figure 1a. Drawing; p. 360, Figure 1b. Photographs; p. 402, Figure 1. Graph; p. 467, Figure 11. Upper drawings.

p. 36, Figure 4. By Frank Forney. Drawings used with permission. *Also:* p. 100, Figure 2; p. 271, Figure 5; p. 363, Figure 3; p. 427, Figure 1; p. 467, Figure 11, (lower left); p. 477, Figure 2.

p. 39, Figure 1. Photograph (left). Photograph Julius Comroe.

p. 49, Figure 1. Photograph (left). Used with permission of family.

p. 73, Figure 1. Painting. Used with permission of family.

p. 116, Figure 1. Photograph (right). *Heart Failure Reviews*, "Overview: Ventricular Restoration — A Surgical Approach to Reverse Ventricular Remodeling", Volume 9, 2005, pp. 233–9, Gerald D. Buckberg, with permission of Springer. *Also:* p. 258, Figure 1. Photograph (right); p. 263, Figure 2. Drawing.

p. 201, Video 1. Bradley S. Allen, Yoshihiro Ko, Gerald D. Buckberg, Zhong Tan, Studies of isolated global brain ischemia: III. Influence of pulsatile flow during cerebral perfusion and its link to consistent full neurological recovery with controlled reperfusion following 15 minutes of global brain ischemia, *European Journal of Cardio-Thoracic Surgery,* 2012, Volume 41, Issue 5, Pages 1155–1163, by permission of Oxford University Press. *Also:* p. 207, Video 1.

p. 265, Figure 3. *Heart Failure Reviews,* "Ventricular structure and surgical history", Volume 9, issue 4, 2005, pp. 255–268, Gerald D. Buckberg, with permission of Springer. *Also:* p. 349, Figure 11. Drawing.

p. 272, Figure 6. Drawing. By Gary Wind, MD. Used with permission of artist. *Also:* p. 361, Figure 2. Drawing.

p. 272, Figure 6. Drawing. Reprinted from *The Journal of Thoracic and Cardiovascular Surgery,* Volume 124, Issue 5, Gerald D. Buckberg, "Basic science review: The helix and the heart", pages 863–883, Copyright 2002, with permission from Elsevier. *Also:* p. 314, Figure 1. Photograph; p. 317, Figure 3. Photograph; p. 335, Figure 2. Drawing (left); p. 336, Figure 1. Screenshot from video; p. 340, Figure 6. Photograph (left); p. 343, Figure 8. Both upper drawings; p. 344, Figure 9b. Photograph; p. 346, Figure 10. All drawings; p. 391, Figure 3. Photograph (right); p. 467, Figure 11. Photograph (lower right).

p. 290, Video 2. From the studies of Vincent Dor 2003.

p. 315, Video 2. "The Helical Heart" video. Copyright Gerald Buckberg, 2005. *Also:* p. 319, Video 3; p. 342, Video 2; p. 486, Figure 5. Picture.

p. 316, Figure 2. Adapted from original by Peggy Firth. Used with permission of Firth Studios. *Also:* p. 367, Figure 4.

p. 317, Figure 3. Photograph. From Francisco Torrent-Guasp. *Also:* p. 344, Figure 9b. Photograph; p. 352, Figure 13. Photograph (left); p. 391, Figure 3. Photograph (right); p. 429, Figure 2. Photograph; p. 467, Figure 11. Photograph (lower right).

p. 320, Figure 4. Drawing. Reprinted from *The Journal of Thoracic and Cardiovascular Surgery,* Volume 13, Issue 4, WB Saunders, "Ventricular shape and function in health and disease", pages 324, Copyright 2007, with permission from Elsevier.

p. 327, Figure 5. By Peggy Firth. Drawings used with permission of Firth Studios. *Also:* p. 420, Figure 1; p. 456, Figure 4; p. 463, Figure 9; p. 485, Figure 4.

p. 327, Figure 5. Drawing. Reprinted from *Echocardiography,* Volume 28, Issue 7, Gerald Buckberg, Julien I.E. Hoffman, Navin C. Nanda, Cecil Coghlan, Saleh Saleh and Constantine Athanasuleas, "Ventricular Torsion and Untwisting: Further Insights into Mechanics and Timing Interdependence: A Viewpoint", pages 782–804, Copyright © 2011 John Wiley & Sons, Inc.

p. 333, Figure 1. Photograph. Reprinted from *The Journal of Thoracic and Cardiovascular Surgery,* Volume 134, Issue 5, Friedhelm Beyersdorf, Constantine Athanasuleas, "2007 American Association for Thoracic Surgery Scientific Achievement Award Recipient: Gerald D. Buckberg, MD, DSc", pages 1105–1108, Copyright 2007, with permission from Elsevier. *Also:* p. 495, Figure 1. Painting.

p. 335, Figure 2. Drawings. Cook, Theodore A., *The Curves of Life,* First Edition. London: Constable and Company, LTD, 1914. *Also:* p. 338, Figure 4. Drawing; p. 343, Figure 8. Drawing (upper right).

p. 336, Video 1. Thank you to Morteza Gharib and Scott E Fraser for their Zebra fish video.

p. 337, Figure 3. Daisy flower. Johan Larson / Shutterstock.com. Image used under license from Shutterstock.com.

p. 339, Figure 5. Drawing. *The Power of Limits,* by Gyorgy Doczi, © 1981 by Gyorgy Doczi. Reprinted by arrangement with The Permissions Company, Inc., on behalf of Shambhala Publications, Inc., Boston, MA. www.shambhala.com. *Also:* p. 343, Figure 8. Photograph (lower left); p. 346, Figure 10. Two drawings (on right); p. 458, Figure 5. Drawing; p. 459, Figure 6. Drawing (lower).

p. 339, Figure 5. Drawing. Buckberg, Gerald D, "Stonehenge and the heart: similar construction", *European Journal of Cardio-Thoracic Surgery,* 2006, Volume 29, Issue Supplement 1, pages S286–S290, by permission of Oxford University Press. *Also:* p. 343, Figure 8. Both upper drawings and photograph (lower left); p. 344, Figure 9a. Lower drawings; p. 344, Figure 9b. Photograph; p. 346, Figure 10. All drawings; p. 454, Figure 2; p. 456, Figure 4. Drawing; p. 458, Figure 5; p. 459, Figure 6. Drawing (lower); p. 463, Figure 9. Drawing; p. 467, Figure 11. Upper drawings and Photograph (lower right).

p. 340, Figure 6. Photograph (right). Vadim Sadovski / Shutterstock.com. Spiral Galaxy image used under license from Shutterstock.com. *Also:* p. 343, Figure 8. Photograph (lower right).

p. 341, Figure 7. Painting (upper left). Claude Monet, FineArt / Alamy Stock Photo. Haystacks (1890).

p. 341, Figure 7. Painting (upper right). Claude Monet / Shutterstock.com. Image used under license from Shutterstock.com. Wheatstacks, Snow Effect, Morning (© 1891), oil on canvas.

p. 341, Figure 7. Painting (lower left). Claude Monet. Artokoloro Quint Lox Limited / Alamy Stock Photo. Rouen Cathedral, West Facade (© 1894), oil on canvas.

p. 341, Figure 7. Painting (lower right). Claude Monet. Nigel Reed QEDimages / Alamy Stock Photo. Rouen Cathedral, oil on canvas.

p. 343, Figure 8. Drawing (upper left). Leonardo da Vinci, from Windsor Castle, Royal Library.

p. 346, Figure 10. Two drawings (on left). Reprinted from Torrent-Guasp F, Buckberg GD, Clemente C, Cox JL, Coghlan HC, Gharib M. the Structure and Function of the Helical Heart and its Buttress Wrapping. I. The Normal Macroscopic Structure of the Heart. *Semin Thorac Cardiovasc Surg.* 2001;13:301–19.

p. 350, Figure 12. Painting (right). Chagall, Marc (1887–1985) © ARS, NY. The Rabbi of Vitebsk. 1914. Oil on canvas. Photo Credit: Scala / Art Resource, NY.

p. 352, Figure 13. Photograph (right). Hurricane. Harvpino / Shutterstock.com. Image used under license from Shutterstock.com.

p. 355, Figure 14. Photograph. James Steidl © | Dreamstime.com.

p. 390, Figure 1. Photograph. Roman Coliseum. abadesign / Shutterstock.com. Image used under license from Shutterstock.com.

p. 390, Figure 2. Photograph (left). Dome of gothic cathedral. © Javarman |Dreamstime.com.

p. 390, Figure 2. Photograph (right). Flying Buttresses of Notre Dame Cathedral. Bill Perry / Shutterstock.com. Image used under license from Shutterstock.com.

p. 391, Figure 3. Photograph (left). Duomo Santa Maria Del Fiore and Bargello. kavalenkava / Shutterstock.com. Image used under license from Shutterstock.com.

p. 429, Figure 2. Photograph. Reprinted from *The Journal of Thoracic and Cardiovascular Surgery,* Volume 148, Issue 6, Gerald D. Buckberg, Julien I.E. Hoffman, "Right ventricular architecture responsible for mechanical performance: Unifying role of ventricular septum", pages 3166–71, Copyright 2014, with permission from Elsevier. *Also:* p. 438, Figure 3. Photograph.

p. 448, Figure 4. Photograph. Buckberg, Gerald D, "Right ventricular failure after surgical ventricular restoration: operation or myocardial protection problem?", *European Journal of Cardio-Thoracic Surgery,* 2017, Volume 52, Issue 6, pages 1018–1021, by permission of Oxford University Press.

p. 452, Figure 1. Photograph. Skyscan Photolibrary / Alamy Stock Photo. Photograph. Stonehenge. *Also:* p. 455, Figure 3. Photograph (upper).

p. 455, Figure 3. Photograph (lower). Stonehenge pillars. Copyright © 2007 Les Still. Used with permission of the copyright owner. http://mysticrealms.org.uk/

p. 459, Figure 6. Photograph (upper). Copyright © 2002 Kenny Ames. Used with permission of the copyright owner. www.Dragonknightphoto.com.

p. 471, Figure 1. Drawing. © Pjmorley | Dreamstime.com.

p. 485, Figure 3. Drawing. *Atrioventricular Bundle Dissected in the Left Ventrice.* Sobotta Atlas of Human Anatomy © Elsevier GmbH, Urban& Fischer, Munich. Anatomy: A Regional Atlas of the Human Body. Carmine Clemente. Fourth Edition.

p. 495, Figure 1. Painting. By the author. *Also*: p. 496, Figure 2. Painting; p. 502, Figure 3. Paintings (upper and lower); p. 503, Figure 4. Drawings (left and right); p. 504, Figure 5. Drawing; p. 505, Figure 6. Drawing.

INDEX

T

ABOUT THE AUTHOR

Gerald D. Buckberg is a Distinguished Professor of Cardiac Surgery at UCLA's David Geffen School of Medicine. He is the recipient of the 2007 American Association for Thoracic Surgery Scientific Achievement Award, the highest honor the Association bestows, and his groundbreaking achievements have been lauded with international recognition. His early research led to the landmark discovery of blood cardioplegia (a method that safely stops the heart during surgery), which has dramatically increased the safety of open heart operations. The procedure is currently used by over 85% of surgeons in the United States and 75% of surgeons worldwide. Over 25 million patients have benefitted from the technique.

Dr. Buckberg did residency training at Johns Hopkins Hospital and UCLA, received Cardiothoracic training at UCLA Medical Center, and did research training at the Cardiovascular Institute at the University of California, San Francisco. A member of multiple surgical societies, including the American Association of Thoracic Surgery, American Surgical Association, and the Society of Thoracic Surgeons, his teams have developed new treatments for acute myocardial infarction (heart attacks) that save and restore healthy function and avoid the development of congestive heart failure that often follows heart attacks.

He later formed a team of leading surgeons and cardiologists from the U.S., Europe, Asia, and South America to treat congestive heart failure in dilated hearts. Initial success in 1198 patients was followed by an additional 5,000 highly successful procedures worldwide.

Further innovative studies have led to breakthroughs that have helped treat sudden death syndrome (cardiac arrest), avoid heart muscle damage in blue babies, remedy disorders relating to the septum, and improve pacemaker effectiveness. His research has also led to a new structural understanding of why the heart beats normally, and yet fails during disease.

A marathon ocean swimmer as well as a marathon runner, Dr. Buckberg continues daily morning swims in UCLA's Masters Swim Club.

Further information is available on Dr. Buckberg's website, which includes videos and summaries of the treatments described in this book.

www.GeraldBuckberg.com

Made in the USA
Middletown, DE
19 June 2019